T0314261

Personality
Disorders

Personality
Disorders

Toward Theoretical and Empirical
Integration in Diagnosis and Assessment

Edited by **Steven K. Huprich**

American Psychological Association • *Washington, DC*

Published by
American Psychological Association
750 First Street, NE
Washington, DC 20002
www.apa.org

To order
APA Order Department
P.O. Box 92984
Washington, DC 20090-2984
Tel: (800) 374-2721; Direct: (202) 336-5510
Fax: (202) 336-5502; TDD/TTY: (202) 336-6123
Online: www.apa.org/pubs/books
E-mail: order@apa.org

In the U.K., Europe, Africa, and the Middle East, copies may be ordered from
American Psychological Association
3 Henrietta Street
Covent Garden, London
WC2E 8LU England

Typeset in Goudy by Circle Graphics, Inc., Columbia, MD

Printer: Maple Press, York, PA
Cover Designer: Naylor Design, Washington, D.C.

The opinions and statements published are the responsibility of the authors, and such opinions and statements do not necessarily represent the policies of the American Psychological Association.

Library of Congress Cataloging-in-Publication Data

Personality disorders (Huprich)
  Personality disorders : toward theoretical and empirical integration in diagnosis and assessment / edited by Steven K. Huprich. — First edition.
     p. ; cm.
  Includes bibliographical references.
  ISBN 978-1-4338-1845-5 — ISBN 1-4338-1845-0
  I. Huprich, Steven Ken, 1966- , editor. II. American Psychological Association, issuing body. III. Title.
  [DNLM: 1. Personality Disorders—diagnosis. 2. Personality Assessment. WM 190]
  RC473.P56
  616.85'81075—dc23
                           2014024909

British Library Cataloguing-in-Publication Data
A CIP record is available from the British Library.

Printed in the United States of America
First Edition

http://dx.doi.org/10.1037/14549-000

In Memoriam
After the submission of their chapters, two legendary contributors to the study of personality and psychopathology passed away. Dr. Theodore Millon died on January 29, 2014, and Dr. Sidney Blatt died on May 11, 2014. I will be forever grateful to have their final contributions to the field in this book. Both were extremely generous and enthusiastic when working on their chapters. I benefitted from their support and wisdom and am sorry that they are not here to see the final product.

I also present this book in memory of James H. Hansell, PhD, who died on April 20, 2013. Dr. Hansell's influence on my professional development is immeasurable.

In Appreciation
In loving appreciation, I dedicate this book to Donna, Christie, and Katie Huprich. Their loving support fills my life with considerable riches every day. I love you all.

CONTENTS

CONTRIBUTORS

Emily B. Ansell, PhD, Yale University, New Haven, CT

Sidney J. Blatt, PhD, Yale University, New Haven, CT

Robert F. Bornstein, PhD, Adelphi University, Garden City, NY

Nicole M. Cain, PhD, Long Island University–Brooklyn, NY

John F. Clarkin, PhD, Weill Medical College of Cornell University, White Plains, NY

Tracy L. Clouthier, BA, Pennsylvania State University, University Park

Sarah A. Griffin, BA, Purdue University, West Lafayette, IN

Steven K. Huprich, PhD, Wichita State University, Wichita, KS

Katherine G. Jonas, BS, University of Iowa, Iowa City

Alex S. Keuroghlian, MD, MSc, McLean Hospital and Harvard University Medical School, Boston, MA

Kenneth N. Levy, PhD, Pennsylvania State University, University Park

W. John Livesley, MD, PhD, University of British Columbia, Vancouver, Canada

Patrick Luyten, PhD, University of Leuven, Leuven, Belgium; University College London, London, England

Kristian E. Markon, PhD, University of Iowa, Iowa City

Kevin B. Meehan, PhD, Long Island University–Brooklyn, NY

Theodore Millon, PhD, DSc, Institute for Advanced Studies in Personology and Psychopathology, Port Jervis, NY

Sharon M. Nelson, BS, Eastern Michigan University, Ypsilanti

Jonathan H. Porcerelli, PhD, ABPP, Wayne State University School of Medicine, Detroit, MI

Douglas B. Samuel, PhD, Purdue University, West Lafayette, IN

J. Wesley Scala, BS, Pennsylvania State University, University Park

Jonathan Shedler, PhD, University of Colorado School of Medicine, Denver

Caleb Siefert, PhD, University of Michigan–Dearborn

Kenneth R. Silk, MD, University of Michigan School of Medicine, Ann Arbor

Susan C. South, PhD, Purdue University, West Lafayette, IN

Stephen Strack, PhD, Veterans Affairs Medical Center, Los Angeles, CA

Christina M. Temes, MS, Pennsylvania State University, University Park

Irving B. Weiner, PhD, University of South Florida, Tampa

Aidan G. C. Wright, PhD, University of Pittsburgh, Pittsburgh, PA

Mary C. Zanarini, EdD, McLean Hospital and Harvard University School of Medicine, Lexington, MA

Johannes Zimmermann, PhD, University of Kassel, Kassel, Germany

Personality
Disorders

INTRODUCTION: PERSONALITY DISORDERS INTO THE 21st CENTURY

STEVEN K. HUPRICH

For those dedicated to studying the personality disorders (PDs), there is, perhaps, no period filled with greater irony in the history of modern clinical psychology and psychiatry than between 2005 and 2014. Indeed, some might find it amusing that those most interested in studying personality disorders experienced some of the most contentious debates in the move toward the fifth edition of the *Diagnostic and Statistical Manual of Mental Disorders* (*DSM–5*; American Psychiatric Association, 2013), only for the Board of Trustees of the American Psychiatric Association to retain the *Diagnostic and Statistical Manual of Mental Disorders* (4th ed., text rev. [*DSM–IV–TR*]; American Psychiatric Association, 2000) classification system for personality disorders that almost all agreed was dysfunctional, not empirically supported, and clinically not useful. If one were to invoke a musical metaphor to describe these series of events, one might consider 21st-century personality

http://dx.doi.org/10.1037/14549-001
Personality Disorders: Toward Theoretical and Empirical Integration in Diagnosis and Assessment,
S. K. Huprich (Editor)

disorder research nonmelodic, polyphonic, and, at times, atonal to the point of sounding rather cacophonous. However, with any serious piece of music, there are ways in which the composer takes the various themes and melodies and seeks to integrate them into something melodious and satisfying. In this case, the composer is the collective wisdom of scientific and scholarly activity. And, as editor of this volume, I could be described as a conductor of this highly talented orchestra of researchers and clinicians, who seek to take many themes and craft them together in a melodic fashion.

This is what this book is intended to do—to tell the story about the "cacophony" of attempts to label and define personality disorders over the past several years and to describe ways in which the future can be more harmonious. Stated within the scope of professional psychology, this book seeks to provide a framework for the diagnosis, assessment, and research on personality disorders that is theoretically and empirically sound, clinically robust, and of assistance to future generations of psychologists and mental health professionals.

Below, I provide a peek into this text by telling the story of how the cacophony swelled and how the themes are modulating. I first review the recent history and current directions for the study of PDs found in the Personality and Personality Disorders Work Group (PPDWG) proposals for *DSM–5*, the actual *DSM–5* personality disorder system, the *International Classification of Diseases* (10th and 11th eds.), and the *Psychodynamic Diagnostic Manual* (PDM Task Force, 2006) and its upcoming revision. Then, I provide an overview of how this book is organized. I first describe those opening chapters that focus upon issues involving the use of categories and dimensions to assess and diagnose personality disorders. This is followed by a discussion of those chapters dedicated to enhancing the research and assessment strategies surrounding the personality disorders. I then briefly describe those final chapters that seek to integrate different "melodies" (i.e., theoretical perspectives) into a more harmonious model of personality disorders. For clinicians and researchers alike, the intention of this text is to help readers expand their thinking about the personality disorders, consider ways in which the field has and should evolve over time, and offer new ways to think about the patients we treat and the system we use by which to assess and diagnose them.

THE *DSM–IV* TO *DSM–5* TRANSITION

In 2005, a white paper was published by Tom Widiger and Erik Simonsen in the *Journal of Personality Disorders*. It was the product of a group of personality disorder researchers who came together to offer important ideas about how the field should evolve in preparation for *DSM–5*. Shortly thereafter, the PPDWG for *DSM–5* was formed, chaired by Andrew Skodol, MD.[1] In August 2009, the PPDWG presented some of its initial ideas about necessary changes for the diagnosis and assessment of personality disorders at the biannual Congress of the International Society for the Study of Personality Disorders (held at the Mt. Sinai School of Medicine). Included in this presentation was a discussion of the need to consider both categorical and dimensional systems of assessing personality disorders, including the use of personality traits in lieu of the extant formal categories. In March 2010, these ideas were formally posted on the *DSM–5* website. Paranoid, Schizoid, Histrionic, Narcissistic, and Dependent PDs were proposed for elimination. The remaining personality disorders were described not as categories with a polythetic composition of symptoms but as prototypes. In this case, clinicians were asked to determine to what extent a patient matched the newly formulated prototype. In this system, a 37-trait, facet system for assessing personality was suggested as an additional model for diagnostic assessment. The Levels of Functioning Scale was proposed as well, in which individuals' self- and other-representations were to be evaluated for their level of adaptation toward social functioning (Skodol et al., 2011).

Reaction to this was substantial, and little was positive. Three journals (*Personality Disorders: Theory, Research, and Treatment*; *Journal of Personality Disorders*; and *Journal of Personality Assessment*) took up these issues in a series of fairly critical papers. Shedler et al. (2010) published an editorial in the *American Journal of Psychiatry* denouncing the deletion of PD categories. Widiger (2011), a longtime supporter of trait assessment for the personality disorders, criticized the PPDWG for its dismissal of the five-factor model of personality as a viable system upon which to build the *DSM–5* diagnostic system. And Bornstein (2011a) and Ronningstam (2011) offered strong criticisms of the idea of deleting Dependent and Narcissistic PDs, respectively. A year later, Huprich (2012) offered a critical commentary about the PPDWG's failure to follow its own rules when deciding to eliminate Depressive PD from the diagnostic manual.

In response to some of these criticisms, the PPDWG proposed retaining Narcissistic PD. In further evaluation of the pathological personality trait structure, the PPDWG also concluded that five broad trait domains with 25 corresponding facets would best assess personality structure in its pathological expression. It thus published the Personality Inventory for *DSM–5*

---

[1]Other members included Renato Alarcon, Carl Bell, Donna Bender, Lee Anna Clark, Robert Krueger, John Livesley, Les Morey, John Oldham, Larry Siever, and Roel Verhuel. For an interesting discussion of the membership of this work group, see Blashfield and Reynolds (2012).

(PID–5) in both a patient self-report version and a clinician-assessed version. It also decided against the use of a prototype system and opted for the retention of six personality disorder categories. In doing so, the PPDWG noted that each category also could be described by a constellation of some number of the 25 pathological traits. Furthermore, it reiterated that personality disorders eliminated from the *DSM* could be subsumed within the trait structure, as could any patient with a pathological manifestation of personality who did not adequately fit the *DSM* criteria for the six remaining PDs. Despite these changes, controversy remained. In my preparation for a roundtable discussion on the topic of *DSM–5* PDs at the 2011 annual meeting of the Society for Personality Assessment, I contacted Dr. Steven Hyman, chair of the *DSM–5* Diagnostic Spectra Committee, about some of the changes then being discussed. He wrote (personal communication, February 8, 2011),

> I am well aware of the controversy surrounding the proposed PD chapter in *DSM–5*. . . . I do not think that there was ever a serious notion of doing without a PD chapter in *DSM–5*, although there was a serious discussion of both distributing some PDs to other chapters and a serious discussion of cross-listing some disorders. There was a strong argument from diverse scientific sources to place schizotypal PD in a schizophrenia spectrum based on family, twin, cognitive, and imaging studies, and in accord with *ICD–10* practice. . . . The second serious debate was about placing antisocial PD in a chapter with a group of externalizing disorders including CD [conduct disorder] based on comorbidity, family, and twin data. The metastructure discussion concluded with two alternatives, either moving ASPD [antisocial personality disorder] to externalizing (favored) or cross-listing in externalizing and PDs. I do not know how that will ultimately be resolved.

In May 2012, a series of critical talks about the *DSM–5* Personality and Personality Disorders Work Group proposal were offered by myself and Drs. Robert Bornstein, Joel Paris, Mark Zimmerman, and John Livesley in a symposium at the American Psychiatric Association annual meeting. Dr. Andrew Skodol, chair of the work group, responded graciously to these concerns, reiterating the value of categorical and dimensional assessment, not to mention the utility of the Levels of Functioning Scale. However, on December 1, 2012, the Board of Trustees of the American Psychiatric Association opted not to adopt the PPDWG's proposal. Instead, it retained the current *DSM–IV–TR* (American Psychiatric Association, 2000) model (though the multiaxial approach of assigning personality disorders on Axis II was eliminated). The work group's proposal for a hybrid category and trait system was published in Section III of *DSM–5* (American Psychiatric Association, 2013). And so, after nearly five years of work and preparation for a change in the *DSM–5*, nothing fundamental had changed, leaving many disappointed by this series of events.

THE TRANSITION FROM *ICD–10* TO *ICD–11*

Planning for the next edition of the *International Classification of Diseases* is under way as this text is being published. Tyrer et al. (2011) described changes being proposed for the diagnosis and assessment of personality disorders in the *ICD–11*. These include classifying personality disorders mainly on the basis of the level of severity, providing a classification system that is based on five broad trait domains, and providing a rating procedure that allows a diagnosis to be made more easily than does the existing procedure. Like the PPDWG, the *ICD–11* work group has argued that the current labels for personality disorders are unsatisfactory, given the paucity of empirical support for some and their extensive overlap. It also has noted that wide varieties of disturbance in personality pathology and an artificial dichotomy between normality and abnormality are present in the current system. Finally, it has noted that the stigma associated with a personality disorder diagnosis often precludes use of the diagnosis in many clinical settings, which necessitates a change in the way personality disorders are assessed and diagnosed.

By way of describing their ideas more completely, Tyrer et al. (2011) proposed five levels of severity for personality disorders in the *ICD–11*: (a) None; (b) Personality difficulty—some problems in certain situations; (c) Personality disorder—well-demarcated problems in a range of situations; (d) Complex personality disorder—definite personality problems usually across several domains and across all situations; and (e) Severe personality disorder—complex disorders that lead to risk to self or others. Additionally, Tyrer et al. described five trait domains that reflect qualities seen from the time of Hippocrates (450 BC) to the present. They described these domains as Asocial/Schizoid, Dyssocial/Antisocial, Obsessional/Anakastic, Anxious/Dependent, and Emotionally Unstable.

As was the case for the *DSM–5*, reaction to the *ICD–11* proposal was mixed. For instance, Bateman (2011) questioned whether a radical change should be employed without any evidence that it will do better than the extant system. He also questioned what would happen to clinically useful categories, such as Borderline PD, if a trait system defined by severity were adopted. Davidson (2011) questioned the exclusion of assessing self and relational functioning, as well as the idea that the new system would decrease stigmatization. Finally, Silk (2011) noted that clinician subjectivity still is the ultimate criterion by which diagnosis is assigned. This has been a criticism across past editions of the diagnostic manuals and will not be solved with the current proposal.

THE DEVELOPMENT AND EVOLUTION OF
THE *PSYCHODYNAMIC DIAGNOSTIC MANUAL*

Though not as widely known as the *DSM* or *ICD*, the *Psychodynamic Diagnostic Manual* (PDM) was published in 2006 by the Alliance of Psychoanalytic Organizations. This group was composed of members from five different psychoanalytic and psychodynamic groups and was chaired by Nancy McWilliams and the late Stanley Greenspan.[2] It was the intent of these authors to create a manual informed by psychoanalytic and psychodynamic perspectives; more important, the *PDM* was meant to be clinician friendly and to describe the inner, subjective experience of patients—something that clinicians hear constantly and that most work with as part of their treatment for patients with personality disorder. The *PDM* was not intended to replace the *DSM* or *ICD* but to supplement them in a way that made it more clinically useful. As in the *DSM* system, several axes were described. The P Axis lists 15 types of personality disorders, seven of which have subtypes.[3] These categories were based on the extant psychodynamic literature and informed by a vast body of research, which included 300 text pages of empirical summaries listed in the last part of the *PDM*. Reviews of the *PDM* have been favorable (e.g., Clemens, 2007; Weiner, 2006), including one by Widiger (2006), who has been a strong advocate of the trait system. At present, the *PDM–2* revision is under way, being chaired by Vittorio Lingiardi and Nancy McWilliams (Huprich et al., in press).

The P Axis will be reformulated in in several ways in the *PDM–2*. First, a psychotic level of personality organization or "psychotic ways of functioning" may be added in the "Low Level of Borderline Personality Organization" subtype. Second, the types of personality disorders listed on the P Axis will be integrated and revised. Classification of these disorders will be guided by recent developments in the assessment research literature and could incorporate the findings of measures such as the Shedler–Westen Assessment Procedure (SWAP-200) and its new versions and applications (SWAP-II: Westen, Shedler, Bradley, & DeFife, 2012; SWAP-200-Adolescents: Westen, Shedler, Durrett, Glass, & Martens, 2003), the Psychodynamic Diagnostic Prototypes (Gazzillo, Lingiardi,

---

[2]The American Psychoanalytic Association, the International Psychoanalytical Association, Division 39 (Psychoanalysis) of the American Psychological Association, the American Academy of Psychoanalysis and Dynamic Psychiatry, and the National Membership Committee on Psychoanalysis in Clinical Social Work (subsequently renamed the American Association for Psychoanalysis in Clinical Social Work).

[3]The personality disorders listed in the *PDM* include schizoid, paranoid, psychopathic/antisocial (passive and aggressive subtypes), narcissistic (arrogant and depressed subtypes), sadistic and sadomasochistic, masochistic/self-defeating (moral and relational subtypes), depressive (introjective, anaclitic, and mixed subtypes), somatizing, dependent (passive-aggressive and counterdependent subtypes), phobic/avoidant, anxious, obsessive-compulsive (obsessive and compulsive subtypes), hysterical/histrionic (inhibited and demonstrative subtypes), dissociative identity, and mixed.

& Del Corno, 2012), the Inventory of Personality Organization (Kernberg & Clarkin, 1995), the Structured Interview of Personality Organization (Clarkin, Caligor, Stern, & Kernberg, 2004), and the Karolinska Psychodynamic Profile (Weinryb, Rössel, & Åsberg, 1991a, 1991b). Moreover, an Emotionally Dysregulated Personality Disorder, which roughly corresponds to the *DSM* description of Borderline Personality Disorder, may be added.[4] Given that the *PDM* does not have such a construct, such an addition may be empirically and clinically warranted.

Third, Blatt's (2008) conceptualization of two key configurations of psychopathology, anaclitic and introjective, is examined in greater depth in terms of the relationship of these concepts to the personality disorders. Introjective issues, centered on problems about the definition of one's identity, seem to predominate within Schizoid, Schizotypal, Paranoid, Narcissistic, Antisocial (Psychopathic), and Obsessive–Compulsive PDs. Anaclitic issues, related to the need to develop more stable and mutual object relations, seem more predominant in Borderline, Histrionic, and Dependent PDs.

Summary

As noted above, the creators of the *DSM*, *ICD*, and *PDM* frameworks all want to change the classification and diagnosis of personality disorders. *DSM* and *ICD* advocates have clear interests in incorporating a dimensional model by which to classify and describe personality pathology, and *PDM* advocates have more interests in retaining a typological system that is based upon the degree of fit between a patient and a particular prototype. In that sense, all three frameworks are moving toward recognizing a dimensional nature to the personality disorders. Likewise, the creators of all three manuals are interested in assessing an individual's level of functioning, though in slightly different formats—such as severity level (*ICD*), quality of relationships and interpersonal functioning (*DSM*), and level of personality organization, which de facto translates into an overall level of functioning across multiple domains.

Given what I have described above regarding the recent and upcoming changes in the diagnostic manuals, it should be clear that the field is set for a paradigm shift. How this shift should occur, however, has been the focus of much debate and, at times, sharp criticism. Nevertheless, there is a line of convergence among theories and research findings that can and should be

---

[4]Axis P does not consider some traditional *DSM* personality disorders, such as Schizotypal and Borderline. This arose out of early work with the SWAP in which many patients diagnosed with Schizotypal PD actually were best classified on the Schizoid prototype, and those diagnosed with Borderline PD were on the Histrionic, Emotionally Dysregulated, Dependent, and Masochistic factors.

integrated so that the field of personality disorders can move forward into the 21st century with greater clarity and unity of perspective. This is the intention of creating this book at this time.

In the paragraphs to follow, I provide a brief overview of what the contributors have offered in their discussion of assessment, research, and diagnosis of personality pathology. It is my intention that readers will find these chapters helpful not only as an overview but also as a way to think about how to integrate theory, practice, and research in ways that provide patients the best of what our science and practice have to offer.

PART I: CURRENT ISSUES IN THE DIAGNOSIS AND ASSESSMENT OF PERSONALITY DISORDERS

As noted, there has been considerable debate about the utility and validity of the current *DSM–IV–TR/DSM–5* personality disorder categories (e.g., Clark, 2007; Clarkin & Huprich, 2011; Huprich & Bornstein, 2007; Krueger, Skodol, Livesley, Shrout, & Huang, 2007; Widiger & Samuel, 2005). Research on clinicians' preferences for diagnosing personality pathology indicates that clinicians prefer a type-based system and can more accurately assign a diagnosis when assessing the degree of match between a given type and their patient (Rhadigan & Huprich, 2012; Rottman, Ahn, Sanislow, & Kim, 2009; Spitzer, First, Shedler, Westen, & Skodol, 2008; Westen, 1997). As Kenneth Silk (Chapter 1) discusses, diagnosis is an essential component of providing health care in that it recognizes that some set of problems or symptoms that have a unifying set of causes exists and that these problems or symptoms can be understood and treated. Diagnostic categories or types also allow for a more consistent way in which clinicians can talk with each other (Clarkin & Huprich, 2011). These points are elaborated upon by Kevin Meehan and John Clarkin in Chapter 4. They raise important questions about how the identification of personality traits (pathological or not) can inform what it is that is done in the clinical setting. (And, as chapters in Part III demonstrate, most contemporary models of personality disorders focus upon issues of how the individual thinks about and relates to him/herself and others and less upon traits.)

Yet, the problems with the current categorical systems—and clinicians' reliance upon their internalized representations of such categories and types—are well documented. These include (a) a failure to "carve nature at its joints," (b) lack of a meaningful or well-validated boundary between normal and disordered personality, (c) excessive heterogeneity within diagnostic categories, (d) excessive diagnostic co-occurrence across categories, (e) inadequate coverage of the full range of personality difficulties seen in clinical practice,

(f) questionable temporal stability of the diagnoses, (g) dissatisfaction among the clinicians with the current types, (h) questionable psychometric properties, and (i) problems in relying upon extant inner models and a failure to attend to all the data in front of the clinician. These issues are taken up directly by Douglas Samuel and Sarah Griffin (Chapter 2) and Kristian Markon and Katherine Jonas (Chapter 3). The authors of both chapters discuss the psychometric superiority and universality of dimensional models of personality and personality pathology. Markon and Jonas in particular describe benefits of a system of measurement that is based on unidimensional scales and traits and explain how the explanatory power of such measurement may exceed that of more heterogeneous, current diagnostic constructs.

Fortunately for the reader, the authors of these first four chapters offer ideas about how to integrate the disparate findings from their own points of view. They all recognize the necessity or implicit utility of categories and dimensions and view each framework as having strengths and weaknesses. Such ideas are not new;[5] however, it would seem the time has come for newer diagnostic systems to incorporate the strengths of both categories and dimensions.

PART II: RESEARCH AND ASSESSMENT STRATEGIES

How personality disorders are assessed and studied has a big influence on what can be learned about the individual being assessed, because each method of assessment has its own strengths and shortcomings (Huprich & Bornstein, 2007). Given this context, Part II of the book offers important information about recent developments in assessment and research methodologies and how they have and can inform our understanding of personality pathology. It begins with Aidan Wright and Johannes Zimmermann's (Chapter 5) comprehensive summary of a plethora of data analytic techniques that have been developed and refined over the past two decades, which will be interesting to both researchers and clinicians. In their discussion of these techniques—which includes a primer on the methods themselves—Wright and Zimmerman offer ideas about why current personality disorder assessment methods contribute to the problems of comorbidity and fail to provide adequate differentiation of patients in meaningful ways. They also discuss how more recent developments in statistical modeling (e.g., factor mixture models, latent class analysis) allow for the identification of both categories and dimensions, something that is sure to be more frequently utilized in years to come.

---

[5]See Widiger, Trull, Clarkin, Sanderson, and Costa (2005); Strack and Millon (2007); and Shedler and Westen (2004).

Chapter 6 is provided by Alex Keuroghlian and Mary Zanarini, who discuss the lessons learned from recent longitudinal studies of personality disorders. Two important longitudinal studies are the focus of their attention: the McLean Study of Adult Development and the Collaborative Longitudinal Study of Personality Disorders. The authors highlight how traits and symptoms tend to remain stable over time (some more than others) but that DSM-based PD diagnoses often remit, contrary to the idea that personality disorders are stable and untreatable.

The development of brain imaging techniques and genetic markers or substrates associated with personality traits has been an exciting area of research in the past decade or so. In Chapter 7, Susan South presents a comprehensive overview of the biological assessment of personality disorders. Like Wright and Zimmerman, South provides a primer of current methodologies used to study genetic influences on personality. She describes how twin and family studies can be statistically modeled to assess the unique effects of genes and environment on self-reported personality traits and how newer methodologies can account for the interaction of genetics and environment. Many believe that the latter area is most important for understanding how certain traits come to be expressed in those who go on to develop a PD or personality pathology (South & DeYoung, 2013). For those not particularly inclined toward biological models of personality and its pathology, South's chapter will be a pleasant surprise for its readability and how it sheds light on processes and qualities once believed too difficult to assess.

Shifting gears, the next chapter discusses something many clinicians know well—the problems patients with personality disorder have in regard to interpersonal relatedness and the defenses these individuals use to help manage their often difficult lives. In Chapter 8, Caleb Siefert and John Porcerelli provide a valuable overview of the theoretical and empirical literature on assessing interpersonal relatedness and defenses, showing that a key component of just about all personality pathology is the problematic ways in which the self and others are experienced and how individuals use specific patterns of defense to manage these concerns. Given the PPDWG's interest in assessing self- and other-representations in order to quantify an individual's level of functioning (Bender, Morey, & Skodol, 2011), this chapter highlights the need to address these issues more carefully in the descriptive nosology of personality disorders. Issues related to the self and other are almost always a pervasive topic in the consultation room. Even more interesting, Siefert and Porcerelli suggest that many of the personality disorder symptoms can be viewed as a constellation of defenses. They highlight the value of psychodynamically informed assessment of many personality disorders within this framework.

Following up on these ideas is Chapter 9 by Jonathan Shedler, who reviews the work he and Drew Westen have done for over 15 years on the utility of assessing clinicians and developing a diagnostic assessment procedure based upon their expertise. While discussing the value of clinician expertise in the development of an assessment and diagnostic system, Shedler describes the Shedler–Westen Assessment Procedure, which is a clinician-informed, empirically derived system of diagnostic personality prototypes that are seen in daily practice by clinicians. Unlike a number of researchers, Shedler suggests that prototypes offer considerable advantages over dimensionalized trait systems, the most significant of which is their clinical utility.

In Chapter 10, Irving Weiner provides a basic review of the differences in explicit and implicit assessment strategies. He reminds the reader that self-report methods have their place, while also highlighting some significant limitations that are often not given due attention when considering how to assess personality pathology. This section ends with Chapter 11 by Robert Bornstein. In his chapter, Bornstein highlights an experimental methodology known as process-focused assessment (Bornstein, 2011b) and explains how it can be used to understand the implicit and dynamic elements of personality and personality pathology. He provides a description of the principles of process-focused assessment, followed by representative exemplars of studies that have utilized such methodologies. In doing so, he highlights how intrapersonal and interpersonal processes can be detected in individuals with known personality styles or types that are often not well detected in self-reports.

PART III: MOVING TOWARD INTEGRATED AND UNIFIED MODELS OF PERSONALITY DISORDERS AND PATHOLOGY

The final section of this book advances the process of integrating the most common theories of personality disorders that have been utilized for assessment and treatment. For each chapter, the authors were asked not only to consider the major premises behind their respective theories but also to integrate more contemporary empirical findings (reviewed in this text) into the model. Though this latter request might have appeared difficult to accomplish, the authors of these chapters have done a thorough job of tying together ideas prominent in theories besides the ones for which they wrote. What is perhaps most interesting is that all chapters recognize the need to assess self- and other-representations, interpersonal relatedness, the ways in which individuals characteristically manage their psychological problems, the dynamic elements of all personality disorders, and the historical context in which such problems arise. The chapters explore psychodynamic

(Chapter 12 by Patrick Luyten and Sidney Blatt), attachment (Chapter 13 by Kenneth Levy, Wesley Scala, Christina Temes, and Tracy Clouthier), interpersonal (Chapter 14 by Nicole Cain and Emily Ansell), evolutionary (Chapter 15 by Theodore Millon and Stephen Strack), and cognitive/cognitive-affective processing (Chapter 16 by Steven Huprich and Sharon Nelson) models.

Chapter 17, by John Clarkin, Nicole Cain, and John Livesley, describes ways in which multiple theories of personality converge on particular ideas related to treatment. The authors suggest that while theoretical integration is not yet possible, an integrated treatment model for personality disorders—something they describe as integrated modular treatment—can and does exist. Although this text is not about treatment per se, I invited the authors to include this chapter because it is guided by the empirical literature on the assessment and diagnosis of personality pathology.

The curious reader may wonder why a five-factor model of personality disorder is not included in this section. This was intentional, mainly because a five-factor model and various trait models of PDs have been described for their capacity to assess and organize personality pathology, but there is very little in the literature that discusses how trait models can be used to inform and affect treatment. This remains a curious aspect of the personality disorder literature, in that there have been no formalized treatments described from a five-factor model. Although some have described five-factor profiles of patients and noted how the assessment can describe the qualities of the person being treated (Stone, 2005; Widiger & Lowe, 2007), the applicability of the model within the consulting room is notably absent. To be fair, however, theoretical paradigm shifts sometimes precede clinical applications; thus, it is possible that a five-factor or dimensionalized model of personality disorder treatment will be articulated more fully in the years to come. Fortunately, most of the authors in this section make some reference to trait theories, and Huprich and Nelson, in particular, describe how trait theory may be integrated into the cognitive-affective processing model.

CLOSING THOUGHTS

It is my intention that this book be of use to researchers and clinicians alike. I have organized this text around the recent and ongoing debates about how to assess and diagnose personality disorders. What I hope has been created is a text that paves the way for a new era of personality disorder conceptualization and research. Many past theories and ideas had the unintended effect of polarizing the field, which today seems inappropriate. Rather, today's task seems to be to discover how to integrate these various levels (e.g., molecular/genetic, trait, intra- and interpersonal, overt behavioral) and systems (e.g., self-report, behaviorally observed, clinician-guided, biologically organized) of analysis into a diagnostic system that makes the most sense clinically and is also well supported empirically.

As one example of how this integration might occur, consider as an analogy the treatment of bone fractures by orthopedists. Fractures are classified by those that are observed through physical or radiographic examination and their disruption on the mobility and motility processes. They are treated at a rather manifest level via open or closed reduction followed by immobilization and rehabilitation, supplemented by pain management and, for some, antibiotic medications. Yet, the pathophysiology of fractures is relatively well understood, and the biological mechanisms behind bone healing continue to be empirically investigated. Virtually no orthopedists would argue that classification of fractures should be organized around a cellular or molecular framework, nor would they suggest that the only course of treatment for most fractures would be pharmacological. However, research into the pathophysiology of fracture healing will continue, as it elucidates those mechanisms that differentiate who may benefit from enhancements to treatment (e.g., some form of pharmacotherapy; additional or reduced time immobilized; additional attention to other systems that might be adversely affected, such as vascular functioning in the injured limb). Orthopedists recognize that classification and treatment are managed through a particular framework, while understanding and equally valuing that the cellular dynamics of healing offers a different, though important, orientation to the fracture healing process. Knowing both domains is likely to make one a highly competent physician.

Thus, by way of comparison and example, just as the biological and trait researcher should value the subjective, psychodynamic, and interpersonal frameworks, so should dynamic and relational therapists recognize that genetic and neurobiological mechanisms underlie some of the "hard to operationalize" aspects of personality dynamics. For instance, it may be that more observable features of personality (e.g., self- and other-representations, adaptive and maladaptive mechanisms of managing distress) may make the most sense for a classification system, though having a system that is well described for its trait architecture and underlying biogenetic mechanisms will only serve to enhance ways in which the system is better understood for its strengths and limits. Of course, this may turn out not be the best way to organize the classification and diagnostic system. Nevertheless, attending to all the various frameworks by which personality disorders are studied will allow the cacophony to modulate into a new and richer melody.

REFERENCES

American Psychiatric Association. (2000). *Diagnostic and statistical manual of mental disorders* (4th ed., text rev.). Washington, DC: Author.

American Psychiatric Association. (2013). *Diagnostic and statistical manual of mental disorders* (5th ed.). Arlington, VA: Author.

Bateman, A. W. (2011). Commentary: Throwing the baby out with the bathwater. *Personality and Mental Health, 5,* 274–280. doi:10.1002/pmh.184

Bender, D. S., Morey, L. C., & Skodol, A. E. (2011). Toward a model for assessing level of personality functioning in *DSM–5*, Part I: A review of theory and methods. *Journal of Personality Assessment, 93,* 332–346. doi:10.1080/0022389 1.2011.583808

Blashfield, R. K., & Reynolds, S. M. (2012). An invisible college view of the *DSM–5* personality disorder classification. *Journal of Personality Disorders, 26,* 821–829. doi:10.1521/pedi.2012.26.6.821

Blatt, S. J. (2008). *Polarities of experience: Relatedness and self-definition in personality development, psychopathology, and the therapeutic process.* Washington, DC: American Psychological Association.

Bornstein, R. F. (2011a). Reconceptualizing personality pathology in *DSM–5*: Limitations of evidence in eliminating dependent personality disorder and other *DSM–IV* syndromes. *Journal of Personality Disorders, 25,* 235–247. doi:10.1521/ pedi.2011.25.2.235

Bornstein, R. F. (2011b). Toward a process-focused model of test score validity: Improving psychological assessment in science and practice. *Psychological Assessment, 23,* 532–544. doi:10.1037/a0022402

Clark, L. A. (2007). Assessment and diagnosis of personality disorder: Perennial issues and an emerging reconceptualization. *Annual Review of Psychology, 58,* 227–257. doi:10.1146/annurev.psych.57.102904.190200

Clarkin, J., Caligor, E., Stern, B. L., & Kernberg, O. F. (2004). *The Structured Interview of Personality Organization (STIPO).* Unpublished manuscript, Personality Disorders Institute/Weill Medical College of Cornell University, New York, NY.

Clarkin, J. F., & Huprich, S. K. (2011). Do the *DSM–5* proposals for personality disorders meet the criteria for clinical utility? *Journal of Personality Disorders, 25,* 192–205. doi:10.1521/pedi.2011.25.2.192

Clemens, N. A. (2007). The *Psychodynamic Diagnostic Manual:* A review. *Journal of Psychiatric Practice, 13,* 258–260. doi:10.1097/01.pra.0000281487.42441.f9

Davidson, K. (2011). Editorial: Changing the classification of personality disorders— An *ICD–11* proposal that goes too far? *Personality and Mental Health, 5,* 243–245. doi:10.1002/pmh.180

Gazzillo, F., Lingiardi, V., & Del Corno, F. (2012). Towards the validation of three assessment instruments derived from the *PDM* P Axis: The Psychodynamic Diagnostic Prototypes, the Core Preoccupation Questionnaire, and the Pathogenic Beliefs Questionnaire. *Bollettino di Psicologia Applicata*, *265*, 31–45.

Huprich, S. K. (2012). Considering the evidence and making the most empirically informed decision about depressive personality in *DSM–5*. *Personality Disorders: Theory, Research, and Treatment, 3*, 470–482. doi:10.1037/a0027765

Huprich, S. K., & Bornstein, R. F. (2007). Categorical and dimensional assessment of personality disorders: A consideration of the issues. *Journal of Personality Assessment, 89*, 3–15. doi:10.1080/00223890701356904

Huprich, S. K., Bornstein, R. F., Gazzillo, F., Gordon, R. M., Lingiardi, V., & McWilliams, N. (in press). The *Psychodynamic Diagnostic Manual* and the *PDM–2*: Opportunities to significantly affect the profession. *Psychoanalytic Inquiry.*

Kernberg, O. F., & Clarkin, J. F. (1995). *The Inventory of Personality Organization.* White Plains, NY: New York Presbyterian Hospital/Weill Medical Center of Cornell University.

Krueger, R. F., Skodol, A. E., Livesley, W. J., Shrout, P. E., & Huang, Y. Q. (2007). Synthesizing dimensional and categorical approaches to personality disorders: Refining the research agenda for *DSM–V* Axis II. *International Journal of Methods in Psychiatric Research, 16*(Suppl. 1), S65–S73. doi:10.1002/mpr.212

PDM Task Force. (2006). *Psychodynamic diagnostic manual.* Silver Spring, MD: Alliance of Psychoanalytic Organizations.

Rhadigan, C., & Huprich, S. K. (2012). The utility of the cognitive-affective processing system in diagnosing personality disorders: Some preliminary evidence. *Journal of Personality Disorders, 26*, 162–178. doi:10.1521/pedi.2012.26.2.162

Ronningstam, E. (2011). Narcissistic personality disorder in *DSM–5*: In support of retaining a significant diagnosis. *Journal of Personality Disorders, 25*, 248–259. doi:10.1521/pedi.2011.25.2.248

Rottman, B. M., Ahn, W., Sanislow, C. A., & Kim, N. S. (2009). Can clinicians recognize *DSM–IV* personality disorders from five-factor model descriptions of patient cases? *The American Journal of Psychiatry, 166*, 427–433. doi:10.1176/appi.ajp.2008.08070972

Shedler, J., Beck, A. T., Fonagy, P., Gabbard, G. O., Gunderson, J., Kernberg, O., . . . Westen, D. (2010). Editorial: Personality disorders in *DSM–5*. *The American Journal of Psychiatry, 167*, 1026–1028. doi:10.1176/appi.ajp.2010.10050746

Shedler, J., & Westen, D. (2004). Dimensions of personality pathology: An alternative to the five-factor model. *The American Journal of Psychiatry, 161*, 1743–1754. doi:10.1176/appi.ajp.161.10.1743

Silk, K. R. (2011). Commentary: The risks may be too high. *Personality and Mental Health, 5*, 296–300. doi:10.1002/pmh.187

Skodol, A. E., Clark, L. A., Bender, D. S., Krueger, R. F., Livesley, W. J., Morey, L. C., . . . Oldham, J. M. (2011). Proposed changes in personality and personality disorder assessment and diagnosis for *DSM–5* Part I: Description and rationale. *Personality Disorders: Theory, Research, and Treatment, 2*, 4–22. doi:10.1037/a0021891

South, S. C., & DeYoung, N. J. (2013). Behavior genetics of personality disorders: Informing classification and conceptualization on *DSM–5*. *Personality Disorders: Theory, Research, and Treatment, 4*, 270–283. doi:10.1037/a0026255

Spitzer, R. L., First, M. B., Shedler, J., Westen, D., & Skodol, A. E. (2008). Clinical utility of five dimensional systems for personality diagnosis: A "consumer preference" study. *Journal of Nervous and Mental Disease, 196*, 356–374. doi:10.1097/NMD.0b013e3181710950

Stone, M. H. (2005). Treatment of personality disorders from the perspective of the five-factor model. In P. T. Costa Jr. & T. A. Widiger (Eds.), *Personality disorders and the five-factor model of personality* (2nd ed., pp. 405–430). Washington, DC: American Psychological Association.

Strack, S., & Millon, T. (2007). Contributions to the dimensional assessment of personality disorders using Millon's model and the Millon Clinical Multiaxial Inventory (MCMI–III). *Journal of Personality Assessment, 89*, 56–69. doi:10.1080/00223890701357217

Tyrer, P., Crawford, M., Mulder, R., Blashfield, R., Farnam, A., Fossati, A., . . . Reed, G. M. (2011). The rationale for the reclassification of personality disorder in the 11th revision of the *International Classification of Diseases (ICD–11)*. *Personality and Mental Health, 5*, 246–259. doi:10.1002/pmh.190

Weiner, I. B. (2006). Enrichment of diagnostic classification [Review of the book *Psychodynamic Diagnostic Manual*, by the PDM Task Force]. *PsycCRITIQUES, 51*(50). doi:10.1037/a0006084

Weinryb, R. M., Rössel, R. J., & Åsberg, M. (1991a). The Karolinska Psychodynamic Profile: I. Validity and dimensionality. *Acta Psychiatrica Scandinavica, 83*, 64–72. doi:10.1111/j.1600-0447.1991.tb05513.x

Weinryb, R. M., Rössel, R. J., & Åsberg, M. (1991b). The Karolinska Psychodynamic Profile: II. Interdisciplinary and cross-cultural reliability. *Acta Psychiatrica Scandinavica, 83*, 73–76. doi:10.1111/j.1600-0447.1991.tb05514.x

Westen, D. (1997). Divergences between clinical and research methods for assessing personality disorders: Implications for research and the evolution of Axis II. *The American Journal of Psychiatry, 154*, 895–903.

Westen, D., Shedler, J., Bradley, B., & DeFife, J. A. (2012). An empirically derived taxonomy for personality diagnosis: Bridging science and practice in conceptualizing personality. *The American Journal of Psychiatry, 169*, 273–284. doi:10.1176/appi.ajp.2011.11020274

Westen, D., Shedler, J., Durrett, C., Glass, S., & Martens, A. (2003). Personality diagnoses in adolescence: *DSM–IV* Axis II diagnoses and an empirically derived alternative. *The American Journal of Psychiatry, 160*, 952–966. doi:10.1176/appi.ajp.160.5.952

Widiger, T. A. (2006). A diagnostic tour de force [Review of the *Psychodynamic Diagnostic Manual*, by the PDM Task Force]. *PsycCRITIQUES, 51*(50). doi:10.1037/a0006005

Widiger, T. A. (2011). The *DSM–5* dimensional model of personality disorder: Rationale and empirical support. *Journal of Personality Disorders, 25,* 222–234. doi:10.1521/pedi.2011.25.2.222

Widiger, T. A., & Lowe, J. R. (2007). Five-factor model assessment of personality disorder. *Journal of Personality Assessment, 89,* 16–29. doi:10.1080/00223890701356953

Widiger, T. A., & Samuel, D. B. (2005). Diagnostic categories or dimensions? A question for the *Diagnostic and Statistical Manual of Mental Disorders—Fifth Edition. Journal of Abnormal Psychology, 114,* 494–504. doi:10.1037/0021-843X.114.4.494

Widiger, T. A., & Simonsen, E. S. (2005). Alternative dimensional models of personality disorders: Finding common ground. *Journal of Personality Disorders, 19,* 110–130. doi:10.1521/pedi.19.2.110.62628

Widiger, T. A., Trull, T. J., Clarkin, J. F., Sanderson, C., & Costa, P. T., Jr. (2005). A description of the *DSM–IV* personality disorders with the five-factor model of personality. In P. T. Costa Jr. & T. A. Widiger (Eds.), *Personality disorders and the five-factor model of personality* (2nd ed., pp. 89–102). Washington, DC: American Psychological Association.

I

CURRENT ISSUES IN THE DIAGNOSIS AND ASSESSMENT OF PERSONALITY DISORDERS

1

THE VALUE OF RETAINING PERSONALITY DISORDER DIAGNOSES

KENNETH R. SILK

Merriam-Webster's Collegiate Dictionary (2003) defines *diagnosis* as both "the art or act of identifying a disease from its signs and symptoms" and "a concise technical description of a taxon" (p. 344), whereas *Dorland's Illustrated Medical Dictionary* (1965) states that diagnosis is "the art of distinguishing one disease from another" as well as "the determination of the nature of a case of disease" (p. 411). *Dorland's* definition further differentiates diagnosis into *clinical diagnosis*, which is what clinical psychology and psychiatry often simply refer to as "diagnosis based on the symptoms shown during life, irrespective of the morbid changes producing them" (p. 412). In other words, it is the act or art of identifying a disease. The process or steps that are gone through in identifying a *taxon* (the name given to a group within a formal system or nomenclature) are also seen as part of diagnosis. Thus, although diagnosis is often thought of as the specific taxon that is ultimately arrived at, diagnosis, by the definitions above, also includes the manner in which the diagnosis is

http://dx.doi.org/10.1037/14549-002
Personality Disorders: Toward Theoretical and Empirical Integration in Diagnosis and Assessment,
S. K. Huprich (Editor)

determined and the rules that are followed in order to proceed through the distinguishing process. The process is one of separation, or how to proceed in the sorting out of one group from another group and then bestowing the final label or name for that group.

This is an interesting point to keep in mind, given that ultimately the *DSM–5* Personality and Personality Disorders Work Group (PPDWG) not only proposed a change in the "criteria" leading up to identifying a taxon but also proposed new "rules" as to how to go about the identification process. The process would proceed from the general criteria proposed for personality disorder (PD) through the levels of personality functioning and then finally to the specific PDs or types. It would be driven more by the presence or absence of specific pathological personality traits than by specific criteria or behaviors, as outlined in the *Diagnostic and Statistical Manual of Mental Disorders* (4th ed., text rev. [DSM–IV–TR]; American Psychiatric Association, 2000, 2013).

In the development of the fifth edition of the *Diagnostic and Statistical Manual of Mental Disorders* (*DSM–5*; American Psychiatric Association, 2013), a number of changes were considered in the PD classification section with regard to what the final labels, or taxons, for these disorders (or *types* of personality pathology) would be. The question of how to arrive at a diagnosis of a PD type as well as what types (i.e., prior categories) were to be included or excluded became controversial, and a major split developed among PD researchers as to how to approach the diagnosis of these disorders (Clarkin & Huprich, 2011; Gunderson, 2010a, 2010b; Krueger et al., 2011, Livesley, 2011; Skodol, Clark, et al., 2011; Zimmerman, 2011).

The official section of *DSM–5* about the diagnosis of a PD is a replication of the diagnoses and categories as used in *DSM–IV–TR* (American Psychiatric Association, 2000). The final PPDWG proposal was rejected for the main diagnostic section of *DSM–5* (which is called Section 2), but it was retained as "Alternate *DSM–5* Model for Personality Disorders" and placed in Section 3, "Emerging Measures and Models." However, one thing that the PPDWG and all the other committees, commissions, and review groups of the American Psychiatric Association agreed upon was that Personality Disorders would not remain on Axis II. Axis II was eliminated, and Personality Disorders joined the other "mental disorders" in Section 2, which included those Axis I disorders from *DSM–IV–TR* as well as some diagnoses that have been added into *DSM–5*.

This chapter briefly reviews how two competing approaches to personality pathology diagnosis were derived. It concludes that tensions between these competing approaches may be less important than the need to consider and label the person who presents with psychiatric or psychological pathology. Considering the individual's personality style (i.e., how the person thinks of herself as a particular kind of person, recognizable to herself and to others) may be more important than how the label was obtained. After all, what diagnosis should primarily do is improve treatment and allow helpful and efficient communication among professionals.

WHY DIAGNOSES?

There exists the notion, though probably not a very realistic one, that if the process of diagnosis is done correctly, it can somehow approach biological "reality." In other words, some believe that there exists only one proper way of diagnosing mental disorders that can determine with minimal error whether a particular symptom is a member of a particular, well-defined group and not a member of any other group. Such a diagnosis is thought to reflect how nature is organized. This is often expressed by the concept that if diagnosis is to be truly a reflection of the natural biological order of the psychological universe, we will be able to "carve nature at its joints" (Campbell, O'Rourke, & Slater, 2011; Skodol et al., 2002). If this possibility exists, the process of diagnosis will approach some absolute, and that absolute has a basis in genetics and neurocircuitry (Jang, McCrae, Angleitner, Reimann, & Livesley, 1998; Paris, 2011; South & DeYoung, 2013). But that notion fails to take into account that experience, upbringing, and other environmental situations dramatically affect gene expression without in any way changing actual strands of DNA (Kandel, 1998).

Most discussions about diagnoses appear to reflect not the ideal but rather what different theoretical camps consider to be more or less "correct." This posture is true whether one approaches patients from a biological, psychodynamic, or even a behavioral perspective. Adherents of each perspective have their own thoughts about what would constitute the appropriate foundation upon which to base a diagnostic or classification system. Therefore, most of these arguments come down to positions of theoretical certainty rather than actual certainty. There will always be advantages and disadvantages in any approach, and these will be affected and modified by the political and theoretical considerations of the time in which diagnoses are being revised or rethought. Until research can arrive at sufficient empirical data, most probably in the fields of genetics and neuroscience, that reflect what we see in actual clinical practice, these arguments and disagreements about diagnosis will be more about theories, perspective, and influence on the future of the field.

It makes sense, at least since the third edition of the *Diagnostic and Statistical Manual of Mental Disorders* (*DSM–III*; American Psychiatric Association, 1980), that a diagnosis is more often based on collaborative compromise than on scientific fact or empirical data. After all, any empirical study of a diagnostic system set can be broken down and teased apart to reveal its limitations and then finally exposed as being no more empirically valid than the diagnostic approach it is vying to replace. But because the final product is more often than not a result of collaborative compromise does not mean that it is useless or that it lacks validity. It may be, in truth, the best product that weak, inconsistent, and inconclusive data can provide. And it certainly develops and defines labels or groups that are important in clinical work and research on all levels. Further, the final product may have involved compromising the validity supporting one theoretical perspective in order to increase the utility and acceptability of the system by as many practitioners as possible. After all, it may be necessary to apply a label to an uncertain entity so that it can be studied. And more practically speaking, not labeling a particular diagnosis runs the risk of the particular clinical phenomenon "disappearing," or at least of its being given a much lower level of importance or recognition in the eyes of funding agencies and insurance companies.

For example, Borderline Personality Disorder (BPD) was officially introduced into the *DSM* in 1980, and between 1981 and the current time, the number of manuscripts in Medline that listed BPD as a subject heading or a key word was 95 times greater than the number in the previous 32 years up to and including 1980. However, the number of manuscripts listing schizophrenia as a keyword or in a subject heading was only 3.7 times greater in the last 32 years than in the 32 years prior to *DSM–III*. And in these last 32 years, the amount of information gleaned about the psychology, psychobiology, genetics, symptoms, course, outcome, and treatments of BPD has been enormous (Gunderson, 2011; Leichsenring, Leibing, Kruse, New, & Leweke, 2011; Lieb, Zanarini, Schmahl, Linehan, & Bohus, 2004; New, Triebwasser, & Charney, 2008), even though some argued against the diagnosis then (Akiskal et al., 1985) and some have argued against the diagnosis more recently (Silk, 2010; Zimmerman et al., 2010).

If this is the best we can do, then why bother with diagnoses? As stated above, diagnostic labels are ways of trying to distinguish one category or taxon from another. Even after we decide on a primary "method" for deciding on diagnoses, we are left with the problem of asking what we call or how we label people who are known to have behaviors and affects deemed not in the normal range, but for whom there are no or very weak empirical data to support what it is that they display. Do we simply eliminate them from the diagnostic process? Do we just not count or categorize them? If that is the decision, there is the risk of ignoring specific data or information about a patient who is very similar but not exactly similar to other patients.

DSM–IV–TR did have the diagnosis or label attached to the categories of depression, anxiety, personality, and so on, of Not Otherwise Specified (NOS) for those patients who do not fit any more specific diagnostic category well enough. However, NOS simply conveys that there are people who clinically appear to be within the larger category (depression, PD) but do not meet enough criteria in any of the specific diagnoses to fit that diagnosis. But NOS does not convey why they do or do not meet a more specific diagnosis. In an attempt to be more specific as to why the patient fails to meet anything other than what was previously labeled as an NOS modification, the *DSM–5* has eliminated the NOS label and divided it into Other Specified and Unspecified modifiers. Other Specified allows for a statement as to why the patient failed to fit into any of the diagnoses in that grouping, and "Unspecified" does not provide a reason. But this division of NOS probably will not eliminate the common complaint, "We know he has a personality problem but I really do not know which one he would best fit into."

Another benefit of diagnoses is that labels imply certain assumptions or pictures about people. The diagnostic system allows us to use a word or a few words to describe an often complex set of behaviors, emotions, and clinical presentation. Thus, Major Depressive Disorder or Borderline Personality Disorder each conjures up a complex and lengthy set of descriptors. Many of these descriptors or pictures have been in existence for years, and when *DSM* committees modify these diagnoses, they are, to some degree, dissociating the labels from these clinical pictures or modifying the clinical picture attached to these labels through many iterations of the *DSM*. Some argue that there should be a substantial need and evidence for supporting a change, because any change, even the best of change, is accompanied by unintended consequences (Silk, 2012).

PERSONALITY DISORDER DIAGNOSES AND THE *DSM*s

PDs, at least historically in psychiatry, were thought to be the disorders that occupied the area between the neuroses and the psychoses (Deutsch, 1942; Grinker, Werble, & Drye, 1968; Hoch & Polatin, 1949). In classical psychoanalytic parlance, those with PDs were not people whose id regularly overran their ego, and they did not spend as much time in primary process thinking as did those people with true psychosis. Yet, they were also unlike people with neurosis, who seem to have a reasonably consistent and strong and intact ego, whose defenses in almost all instances are strong enough that there would not be a breakthrough of primary process thinking (Frosch, 1964). Rather, individuals with PD were thought to possess an ego that was less intact than that of people classified as neurotic (Kernberg, 1967). They could, at times, distort reality and behave and think in ways that demonstrated flawed thinking and compromised judgment and reality testing, but these periods were often transient, and these individuals never lost the ability to judge what reality was (Frosch, 1964). Kernberg in 1969 proposed a psychoanalytic classification of character disorder by describing pathology in the areas of ego and superego structure, internalized object relationships, and the expression and sublimation of aggressive and libidinal drives (Kernberg, 1970).

Although PDs were addressed in both the first edition of the *Diagnostic and Statistical Manual of Mental Disorders* (*DSM–I*; American Psychiatric Association, 1952) and the second edition, *DSM–II* (American Psychiatric Association, 1968), these diagnostic manuals were essentially ignored by the mental health community. PDs as delineated in these early manuals did not appear to promote further studies in the classification of PDs. For example, they were not really diagnoses as these have come to be understood. Rather, these two early *DSMs* were more of a collection of "Definitions of Terms of Mental Disorders" rather than a collection of criteria sets leading to specific diagnoses as they appeared in *DSM–III* and beyond. Under the definition of terms for PDs in *DSM–I* was the following:

> characterized by developmental defects or pathological trends in the personality structure, with minimal subjective anxiety, and little or no sense of distress. In most instances, the disorder is manifested by a lifelong pattern of action or behavior, rather than by mental or emotional symptoms. (p. 34)

In *DSM–II* one finds "deeply ingrained maladaptive patterns of behavior that are perceptibly different in quality from psychotic and neurotic symptoms. Generally, these are life-long patterns, often recognizable by the time of adolescence or earlier" (American Psychiatric Association, 1968, pp. 41–42). The PDs in *DSM–I* were divided into two subgroupings: (a) personality pattern disturbance that included Inadequate, Schizoid, Cyclothymic, and Paranoid types and (b) personality trait disturbance that included Emotionally Unstable, Passive-Aggressive, Compulsive, and Personality Trait Disturbance—Other. There was also a classification called Sociopathic personality disturbance, which included antisocial reaction, dissocial reaction, sexual deviation, and addiction. In *DSM–II* there were no longer these divisions within PDs. Inadequate, Paranoid, Cyclothymic, Schizoid, Obsessive-Compulsive (called Compulsive in *DSM–I*), and Passive-Aggressive types remained. Explosive (epileptoid), Hysterical (histrionic), Asthenic, and Antisocial types were added. There were also diagnoses for Other Personality Disorders of Specified Types and Unspecified Personality Disorder.

This all changed in *DSM–III* for a number of reasons. The *DSM–III* became a prominent manual through which diagnoses were expected to be made. There were a number of important differences in *DSM–III* from the *DSMs* that preceded it. First, the specific diagnoses (disorders) all consisted of lists of specific criteria in a polythetic form; second, it was claimed that *DSM–III* was supported by scientific evidence, though the amount of evidence and the rigor of the studies considered were not consistent from disorder to disorder; and finally, not only were PDs more specifically defined, but they also were put on their own axis.

By the placement of PDs on Axis II of a five-axis model, a number of goals were desired, though none were explicitly stated. By developing a model that contained five axes, it was hoped that clinicians would attempt to code or complete a comprehensive assessment of each patient by considering each of the five axes. The idea was that PDs (or at least the patient's personality) would not be ignored, at least in the initial evaluation. Even if the patient did not meet the full criteria for a PD, there was hope, and perhaps even the expectation, that the evaluating clinician might at least make some statement about the patient's personality or the patient's primary defensive style(s) on Axis II. Unfortunately, this never found its way into routine clinical practice, and why this never happened remains unclear. But, in initial and subsequent evaluations, clinicians more often than not filled in the Axis II category with terms such as *deferred* or *personality disorder NOS*. The high incidence of the use of the deferred and NOS categories was one of the arguments for adopting a more dimensional approach to diagnosing PDs in *DSM–5* (Bornstein & Huprich, 2011; Verheul, Bartak, & Widiger, 2007; Westen & Shedler, 1999).

Perhaps this ready dismissal or avoidance of dealing with the Axis II classification was also a product of the time when it was initiated. Psychiatry was moving away from the psychodynamic underpinning that, up until the early to mid-1970s, was essentially the default position for the theoretical basis of psychiatry. In the latter part of the 1970s, leading up to the publication of *DSM–III* in 1980, the theoretical approach in academic centers was becoming more biological, along with an acknowledgment that biological processes lay beneath not only all psychiatric disorders but also all of the ways that individuals think and feel and motivate themselves. The creators of *DSM–III* suggested that the manual was "atheoretical," being neither too biological nor too psychodynamic. However, many argued differently (Frances & Cooper, 1981; Klerman, Vaillant, Spitzer, & Michels, 1984). At the same time, there was a belief that the disorders of Axis II were not biological or that we had little evidence as yet for biological substrates underlying them. In fact, the treatments for Axis II disorders were thought to lie primarily in the psychotherapeutic camp, still being considered as disorders of nurture rather than nature (Gunderson & Pollack, 1985). Auchincloss and Michels (1983) suggested that the one group of disorders listed in *DSM–III* where psychodynamic psychotherapy was still paramount were the PDs.[1]

---

[1]Unfounded rumors claim that the creators of *DSM–III* "gave" Axis II to the psychotherapists to get support from the many American Psychiatric Association members who were primarily psychodynamic psychotherapists. These members were initially not in support of the *DSM–III* because it was too biological and was shifting patients away from psychotherapeutic to more biological interventions.

Psychiatry itself was changing. Clinicians were expected to make diagnoses at the initial appointment. It was (and still is) difficult to make a diagnosis of PD in a 60- to 90-minute initial interview (i.e., in a brief cross-sectional context). After all, these were disorders that were thought to be a collection of personality traits ("enduring patterns of perceiving, relating to, and thinking about the environment and oneself" that are "inflexible and maladaptive and cause either significant impairment in social or occupational functioning or subjective distress"; American Psychiatric Association, 1980, p. 305). How could one solidly determine and establish the presence of these patterns in a brief cross-sectional interview? And, on a somewhat different note, insurance companies often were unwilling to reimburse for the treatment of PDs. The consensus (at least that of the insurance companies) was that PDs were chronic and untreatable and were a waste of the therapist's time and the insurance company's money. For clinicians there was too little time allocated to actually feel confident that the interpersonal pattern they were witnessing was chronic and maladaptive. And more practically, clinicians may have asked themselves why they should engage in this kind of assessment at all, because arriving at a PD diagnosis often weakened the case for reimbursement from third-party payers (Plakun, 1996).

DETERMINING THE NEED FOR LABELS AND WHICH LABELS TO CHOOSE

While this was occurring in psychiatry, academic psychology was becoming more interested in the study of personality per se, though not necessarily PDs. Although it was evident that everyone had a personality, academic psychology was studying and describing personality traits in normal individuals while also exploring when and how those traits became pathological (Costa & McCrae, 1980; Watson, Clark, & Chmielewski, 2008). Everyone had traits, but in some people those traits existed in persistent and disruptive ways that if taken to the extreme could result in what was referred to as a PD (Costa & Widiger, 2002; Krueger & Eaton, 2010; Trull, 2005).

Thus, the belief developed that there was a continuum from the normal to the abnormal personality. Yet psychiatrists, who are physicians by training and approach, did not necessarily agree with this approach. For them, medicine deals with the pathological. In some instances medicine can appreciate the concept of degrees (a dimension) from normal to pathological (i.e., illness), such as in blood pressure or obesity or diabetes, but there are other disorders—for example, infectious diseases and cancer—that do not immediately reveal themselves on a dimensional continuum. There is a normal state and there is a pathological state, and although one might be able to define the two states in the particular organ or physiological system, the continuity (i.e., the dimensionality) from normal to abnormal is not readily evident. One might argue that, in these instances, there is a category for illness and a category for health, but the patient in the clinical setting with a particular illness does not necessarily move in dimensional increments from health to illness. Perhaps on a molecular or on a subclinically recognizable level the change does occur incrementally, but in the actual clinical presentation this is often hard to detect.[2]

Whether one ascribes to a categorical or a dimensional model, there is a need to retain labels for the various abnormal personalities or for the display of the various abnormal traits that people manifest. In medicine and psychiatry at the moment those labels are based, at least overtly, on categorical models. In discussions in the *DSM–5* PPDWG, there were attempts to decide which categories (now called *types*, to incorporate the possible dimensional aspects of the traits that make up the domains that come together to form the types) should be retained and which ones discarded. The decision to keep some and eliminate other labels initially created a storm of protest among clinicians studying and treating PDs (Bornstein, 2011; Clarkin & Huprich, 2011; Gunderson 2010a, 2010b; Ronningstam, 2011; Shedler et al., 2010), though it should be noted that in each prior iteration of the *DSM*, from *DSM–I* through *DSM–IV*, specific PDs were both added and eliminated with respect to the immediate prior edition. So, although what was labeled and what labels were given may have changed from edition to edition, there was always the need for some set of labels to define patients with personalities abnormal enough to reach PD status. In the PPDWG, the overall approach seemed rational in that it was intended to retain those types where there were sufficient data to support their continued existence as a valid diagnostic grouping (Skodol, Bender, et al., 2011).

But there may have been some unintentional work group biases impacting these decisions. The types or categories that were to be retained in *DSM–5* were those that had been studied in the Collaborative Longitudinal

---

[2]Many diseases in medicine can be seen in both categorical and dimensional terms. For example, if a patient is infected with a particular organism, the statement might be made that the patient has a specific pneumonia. That does not mean that within that episode of pneumonia there cannot be dimensional measures of severity (in this instance perhaps by measures of temperature or total white blood cell count, which are dimensional in that they are continuous). The same can be said about diabetes and high blood pressure. Although there are specific cutoffs in those dimensional measures that might then suggest that, above that cutoff, treatment should be initiated, those cutoffs are not rigid. Factors such as age, gender, and coexisting medical illness may influence the point at which treatment is recommended to begin and the type of treatment (e.g., behavioral modification of habits to improve cholesterol versus institution of pharmacotherapy with statins) to be instituted. Nonetheless, although cancers can be graded along some severity continuum and extent of spread within the body, the diagnosis of a specific cancer is categorical. The same might be said about an aneurysm, an ulcer, a fracture, or myriad other medical diseases.

Personality Disorders Study (CLPS; Skodol et al., 2005). The chair and vice chair of the PPDWG, as well as two other committee members, were involved in some aspects of the CLPS (Blashfield & Reynolds, 2012). Furthermore, the work group also had four members who had spent much of their academic careers developing assessment instruments of trait ratings of personality along dimensional models. The *Journal of Personality Disorders* article describing the CLPS (Skodol et al., 2005) related the following as to why the specific diagnoses were chosen for inclusion in that study:

> The four personality disorders selected for study represent each of the *DSM* personality clusters: schizotypal personality disorder (STPD) for Cluster A, borderline personality disorder (BPD) for Cluster B, avoidant personality disorder (AVPD) for Cluster C, and obsessive–compulsive personality disorder (OCPD) because factor-analytic studies have shown that it was separable from the three *DSM* clusters, despite its nominal assignment to Cluster C. . . .The four personality disorders chosen also correspond to the four psychobiological dimensions of psychopathology proposed by Siever and Davis (1991), are the most prevalent from their respective clusters, and derive from different theoretical frameworks. By focusing on these four divergent personality types, we estimated that we excluded only about 15% of treatment-seeking patients who meet criteria for any Axis II disorder. (Skodol et al., 2005, pp. 488–489)

Gunderson et al. (2000) provided a slightly different rationale for the decision to study these particular four personality disorders:

> The plan to study four PDs [Schizotypal, Borderline, Avoidant, and Obsessive-Compulsive], as opposed to all PDs, was based on a variety of conceptual and logistical issues. To attempt to study all PDs would have required a prohibitively large sample to allow us to evaluate the stability of the specific disorders; there would have been very uneven sample sizes, precluding meaningful comparisons for rarer disorders. The four personality disorders to be studied were selected on the basis of their phenomenological distinctions and their divergent clinical, conceptual and empirical bases. (pp. 303–304)

In addition to these four PDs, Antisocial PD was included by the *DSM–5* Work Group, and, late into its work, Narcissistic PD was retained after initially being proposed for elimination (Alarcon & Sarabia, 2012; Pincus, 2011; Ronningstam, 2013). Nonetheless, the CLPS seems to have had had a significant influence on the *DSM–5* PPDWG (Blashfield & Reynolds, 2012). But if the final selection of the types was related to the CLPS, there was a conceptual problem here. The CLPS was designed to study PDs in general and was not designed to decide what to keep or not keep as categories or types or labels in a future revision of a diagnostic manual. What became lost in the arguments was that diagnoses, whether types based on dimensions or categories based on criteria, are no more and no less than ways to label. The labels then become shorthand ways to reflect certain characteristics of individuals that are immediately and concisely conveyed when the label or type is mentioned. Although the information conveyed hopefully would be accurate, it is also in the specific PD labels that significant stigmas and transferential assumptions are made by clinicians and can become problematic.

Transferential issues and stigma were attached early to the diagnosis of AIDS, and, although diminished, they are still there to some extent. Stigma and transference/countertransference issues continue to attach themselves to substance misuse, sexually transmitted disease, obesity, and many other medical conditions. Nonetheless, this should not deter us from continuing to strive toward defining more precisely who such individuals are, why they are similar, and how they are different. Whether the labels describe types or categories is for future generations of diagnosticians to determine. At times, these disagreements seem to be "angels dancing on the head of a pin," for what is considered evidence today may no longer be so clear tomorrow. Consider the recent revelations about estrogen replacement therapy (Marjoribanks, Farquhar, Roberts, & Lethaby, 2012) or the discussion that the prostate specific antigen test is problematic because its uncertain specificity may lead to more morbidity and mortality than not having the test at all (Qaseem et al., 2013).

Whatever method for labeling is ultimately chosen, we should choose it by what it is we wish to convey by the label. Do we wish to convey clinically descriptive information about people, or do we wish to convey something about genes and physiological systems that are similar, even if they manifest themselves in widely different ways in clinical presentation? Are the labels that we design in a diagnostic system related to PDs meant to convey something about how people behave and interact with one another and society, about their feelings and the expression of those feelings, or are they meant simply to define groups of people who share genetic and physiologic similarities even if they appear differently from each other in the clinical setting? The former would appear to be very valuable to clinicians and the latter to researchers. We may never arrive at a place where the similarities that we know exist genetically and physiologically will be the same commonalities that we see in the office. Yet, is it not through the personality that we notice the differences in how similar people present? And it appears that if we ignore the personality, we hinder our own treatments and treatment approach.

It is well known that the comorbidity of an Axis II disorder impacts the presentation and perhaps clinical response to an Axis I disorder (Levenson, Wallace, Fournier, Rucci, & Frank, 2012; Oleski, Cox, Robinson, & Grant, 2012; Pinto, Liebowitz, Foa, & Simpson, 2011). And the comorbid presence of an Axis II disorder may impact the type of therapy that is found to be effective in an Axis I (Rakowska, 2011). Would defining a single trait or even a series of traits that come together to define a type lead to the same conclusion?

CONCLUDING REMARKS

What value would knowing about PDs be to medical students who have no plans to enter psychiatry or to clinical psychology students who do not see their work requiring a working knowledge of personality pathology? How might one present the concept of personality and PDs to them so they might find it relevant regardless of which branch or specialty of clinical practice they eventually choose? Thinking about the personality of each and every patient whom they see tells them something about the person who has the disease they are treating, and it may help them uncover better ways to approach and make a connection with the patient. It may also help them to better appreciate the reaction of the patient to the illness or problems, to disappointment, to tolerance of side effects, and to why certain medical patients may not have any visitors. There could be differences in terms of compliance, complaints, and interpersonal connections. Support systems and willingness for those systems to become involved with the patient might differ between a diabetic without strong specific personality traits and one with histrionic or obsessive–compulsive or even antisocial traits, types, or disorders Those traits or interpersonal styles, whatever they may be, eventually impact the outcome of the treatment of a medical disorder (Bornstein, 1995, 1998), and they may also for some reason make the patient more vulnerable to medical illnesses (Frankenburg & Zanarini, 2004). Then, personality issues—issues that need some form of label that could identify what or who it is that we may be encountering—may inform these future physicians and psychologists as to the most clinically and interpersonally useful ways of approaching the patient, as well as suggest how to convey information and present expectations with respect to compliance with treatment and treatment recommendations. And, if Frankenburg and Zanarini's (2004) work is accurate, there are many people with PDs who are seeking care for their medical illness(es).

Psychiatry and psychology are constantly searching for the "real" person we are treating. At times, that person (i.e., that personality of the patient) impacts the psychiatric disorder with which the person is presenting. And, at other times, it dominates the other disorder to the point that the other disorder is not the problem; the style and interaction of the person are what is paramount.

We need to retain labels or types so that we can convey, through those labels, something about the real person within the patient to whom we are administering care (Strack & Millon, 2007; Westen & Shedler, 2000).

Ideally, we should be able to combine dimensional measures so that no data are lost with categorical measures, so that what we are conveying can be succinctly expressed in clear definitive terms. A categorical-dimensional hybrid, which in truth is what the final *DSM–5* PPDWG proposal was, appears to be have been suggested over a number of years by many different personality researchers (Gunderson, Links, & Reich, 1991; Krueger, Skodol, Livesley, Shrout, & Huang, 2007; Oldham & Skodol, 2000). Prototypic matching approaches, which can also be thought of as a categorical-dimensional blend, may also be seen as useful and appropriate ways to label patients (Westen, DeFife, Bradley, & Hilsenroth, 2010; Westen & Shedler, 1999, 2000; see also Shedler, Chapter 9, this volume), and it appears that substantial groups of clinicians are attracted to prototypic matching (Rottman, Ahn, Sanislow, & Kim, 2009). There are of course the more purely dimensional models, which are discussed in this volume by Markon and Jonas (Chapter 3). Also, Samuel and Griffin (Chapter 2) discuss comparing the naming of disorders in categories versus types versus dimensions.

What to name these patients and how to go about choosing the name is not merely an academic argument. The labels given can impact dramatically the lives of our patients and how we and the world view them. Each ultimately arrives at the use of a label to describe a patient, but each of those labels conveys a somewhat different picture. None of those labels are "correct," because none describes the picture of a patient as the patient actually presents clinically. But before the field decides which particular labels to change or retain, and before it delineates what an old or new label might imply in a new method of classification, we need to be sure that the new label does not radically change what the old label depicted, conveyed, or implied. Whatever the new label or the implications of the new label, we need to assure not only clinical utility but also continuity with the concepts embedded in the old label. This effort is needed so that prior knowledge and research will not be lost but can be extended toward current research into and understanding of these patients who struggle so profoundly with their affects and interpersonal relationships (First et al., 2004; Morey, Krueger, & Skodol, 2013; Morey & Skodol, 2013).

REFERENCES

Akiskal, H. S., Chen, S. E., Davis, G. C., Puzantian, V. R., Kashgarian, M., & Bolinger, J. M. (1985). Borderline: An adjective in search of a noun. *Journal of Clinical Psychiatry*, 46, 41–48.

Alarcon, R. D., & Sarabia, S. (2012). Debates on the narcissism conundrum: Trait, domain, dimension, type, or disorder? *Journal of Nervous and Mental Disease*, 200, 16–25. doi:10.1097/NMD.0b013e31823e6795

American Psychiatric Association. (1952). *Diagnostic and statistical manual of mental disorders.* Washington, DC: Author.

American Psychiatric Association. (1968). *Diagnostic and statistical manual of mental disorders* (2nd ed.). Washington, DC: Author.

American Psychiatric Association. (1980). *Diagnostic and statistical manual of mental disorders* (3rd ed.). Washington, DC: Author.

American Psychiatric Association. (2000). *Diagnostic and statistical manual of mental disorders* (4th ed., text rev.). Washington, DC: Author.

American Psychiatric Association. (2013). *Diagnostic and statistical manual of mental disorders* (5th ed.). Arlington, VA: Author.

Auchincloss, E. L., & Michels, R. (1983). Psychoanalytic theory of character. In J. Frosch (Ed.), *Current perspectives on personality disorders* (pp. 2–19). Washington, DC: American Psychiatric Press.

Blashfield, R. K., & Reynolds, S. M. (2012). An invisible college view of the *DSM–5* personality disorder classification. *Journal of Personality Disorders, 26,* 821–829. doi:10.1521/pedi.2012.26.6.821

Bornstein, R. F. (1995). Interpersonal dependency and physical illness: The mediating roles of stress and social support. *Journal of Social and Clinical Psychology, 14,* 225–243. doi:10.1521/jscp.1995.14.3.225

Bornstein, R. F. (1998). Interpersonal dependency and physical illness: A meta-analytic review of retrospective and prospective studies. *Journal of Research in Personality, 32,* 480–497. doi:10.1006/jrpe.1998.2230

Bornstein, R. F. (2011). Reconceptualizing personality pathology in *DSM–5*: Limitations of evidence in eliminating dependent personality disorder and others *DSM–IV* syndromes. *Journal of Personality Disorders, 25,* 235–247. doi:10.1521/pedi.2011.25.2.235

Bornstein, R. F., & Huprich, S. K. (2011). Beyond dysfunction and threshold-based classification: A multidimensional model of personality disorder diagnosis. *Journal of Personality Disorders, 25,* 331–337. doi:10.1521/pedi.2011.25.3.331

Campbell, J. K., O'Rourke, M., & Slater, M. H. (Eds.). (2011). *Carving nature at its joints: Natural kinds in metaphysics and science.* Cambridge, MA: MIT Press.

Clarkin, J. F., & Huprich, S. K. (2011). Do the *DSM–5* personality disorder proposals meet the criteria for clinical utility? *Journal of Personality Disorders, 25,* 192–205. doi:10.1521/pedi.2011.25.2.192

Costa, P. T., Jr., & McCrae, R. R. (1980). Influence of extraversion and neuroticism on subjective well-being: Happy and unhappy people. *Journal of Personality and Social Psychology, 38,* 668–678. doi:10.1037/0022-3514.38.4.668

Costa, P. T., Jr., & Widiger, T. A. (Eds.). (2002). *Personality disorders and the five-factor model of personality* (2nd ed.). Washington, DC: American Psychological Association.

Deutsch, H. (1942). Some forms of emotional disturbance and their relationship to schizophrenia. *Psychoanalytic Quarterly, 11,* 301–321.

Dorland's illustrated medical dictionary (24th ed.). (1965). Philadelphia, PA: Saunders.

First, M. B., Pincus, H. A., Levine, J. B., Williams, J. B. W., Ustun, B., & Peele, R. (2004). Clinical utility as a criterion for revising psychiatric diagnoses. *The American Journal of Psychiatry, 161,* 946–954. doi:10.1176/appi.ajp.161.6.946

Frances, A., & Cooper, A. (1981). Descriptive and dynamic psychiatry: A perspective on *DSM–III. The American Journal of Psychiatry, 138,* 1198–1202.

Frankenburg, F. R., & Zanarini, M. C. (2004). The association between borderline personality disorder and chronic medical illnesses, poor health-related lifestyle choices, and costly forms of health care utilization. *Journal of Clinical Psychiatry, 65,* 1660–1665. doi:10.4088/JCP.v65n1211

Frosch, J. (1964). The psychotic character: Clinical psychiatric considerations. *Psychiatric Quarterly, 38,* 81–96. doi:10.1007/BF01573368

Grinker, R. R., Werble, G., & Drye, R. C. (1968). *The borderline syndrome: A behavioral study of ego functions.* New York, NY: Basic Books.

Gunderson, J. G. (2010a). Commentary on "Personality Traits and the Classification of Mental Disorders: Toward a More Complete Integration in *DSM–5* and an Empirical Model of Psychopathology." *Personality Disorders: Theory, Research, and Treatment, 1,* 119–122. doi:10.1037/a0019974

Gunderson, J. G. (2010b). Revising the borderline diagnosis for *DSM–V:* An alternative proposal. *Journal of Personality Disorders, 24,* 694–708. doi:10.1521/pedi.2010.24.6.694

Gunderson, J. G. (2011). Borderline personality disorder. *The New England Journal of Medicine, 364,* 2037–2042. doi:10.1056/NEJMcp1007358

Gunderson, J. G., Links, P. S., & Reich, J. H. (1991). Competing models of personality disorders. *Journal of Personality Disorders, 5,* 60–68. doi:10.1521/pedi.1991.5.1.60

Gunderson, J. G., & Pollack, W. (1985). Conceptual risks of the Axis I–II division. In H. Klar & L. J. Siever (Eds.), *Biologic response styles: Clinical implications* (pp. 82–95). Washington, DC: American Psychiatric Press.

Gunderson, J. G., Shea, M. T., Skodol, A. E., McGlashan, T. H., Morey, L. C., Stout, R. L., . . . Keller, M. B. (2000). The Collaborative Longitudinal Personality Disorders Study: Development, aims, design, and sample characteristics. *Journal of Personality Disorders, 14,* 300–315. doi:10.1521/pedi.2000.14.4.300

Hoch, P., & Polatin, P. (1949). Pseudoneurotic forms of schizophrenia. *Psychiatric Quarterly, 23,* 248–276. doi:10.1007/BF01563119

Jang, K. L., McCrae, R. R., Angleitner, A., Reimann, R., & Livesley, W. J. (1998). Heritability of facet-level traits in a cross-cultural twin sample: Support for a hierarchical model of personality. *Journal of Personality and Social Psychology, 74,* 1556–1565. doi:10.1037/0022-3514.74.6.1556

Kandel, E. R. (1998). A new intellectual framework for psychiatry. *The American Journal of Psychiatry, 155*, 457–469.

Kernberg, O. (1967). Borderline personality organization. *Journal of the American Psychoanalytic Association, 15*, 641–685. doi:10.1177/000306516701500309

Kernberg, O. F. (1970). A psychoanalytic classification of character pathology. *Journal of the American Psychoanalytic Association, 18*, 800–822. doi:10.1177/000306517001800403

Klerman, G. L., Vaillant, G. E., Spitzer, R. L., & Michels, R. (1984). A debate on *DSM–III. The American Journal of Psychiatry, 141*, 539–553.

Krueger, R. F., & Eaton, N. R. (2010). Personality traits and the classification of mental disorders: Toward a more complete integration in *DSM–5* and an empirical model of psychopathology. *Personality Disorders: Theory, Research, and Treatment, 1*, 97–118. doi:10.1037/a0018990

Krueger, R. F., Eaton, N. R., Clark, L. A., Watson, D., Markon, K. E., Derringer, J., . . . Livesley, W. J. (2011). Deriving and empirical structure of personality pathology for *DSM–5. Journal of Personality Disorders, 25*, 170–191. doi:10.1521/pedi.2011.25.2.170

Krueger, R. F., Skodol, A. E., Livesley, W. J., Shrout, P. E., & Huang, Y. (2007). Synthesizing dimensional and categorical approaches to personality disorders: Refining the research agenda for *DSM–V* Axis II. *International Journal of Methods in Psychiatric Research, 16*(Suppl. 1), S65–S73. doi:10.1002/mpr.212

Leichsenring, F., Leibing, E., Kruse, J., New, A. S., & Leweke, F. (2011, January 1). Borderline personality disorder. *The Lancet, 377*, 74–84. doi:10.1016/S0140-6736(10)61422-5

Levenson, J. C., Wallace, M. L., Fournier, J. C., Rucci, P., & Frank, E. (2012). The role of personality pathology in depression treatment outcome with psychotherapy and pharmacotherapy. *Journal of Consulting and Clinical Psychology, 80*, 719–729. doi:10.1037/a0029396

Lieb, K., Zanarini, M. C., Schmahl, C., Linehan, M. M., & Bohus, M. (2004, July 31). Borderline personality disorder. *The Lancet, 364*, 453–461. doi:10.1016/S0140-6736(04)16770-6

Livesley, W. J. (2011). An empirically-based classification of personality disorder. *Journal of Personality Disorders, 25*, 397–420. doi:10.1521/pedi.2011.25.3.397

Marjoribanks, J., Farquhar, C., Roberts, H., & Lethaby, A. (2012). Long term hormone therapy for perimenopausal and postmenopausal women. *Cochrane Database of Systematic Reviews, 2012*(7). doi:10.1002/14651858.CD004143.pub4

Merriam-Webster's collegiate dictionary (11th ed.). (2003). Springfield, MA: Merriam-Webster.

Morey, L. C., Krueger, R. F., & Skodol, A. E. (2013). The hierarchical structure of clinician ratings of proposed *DSM–5* pathological personality traits. *Journal of Abnormal Psychology, 122*, 836–841. doi:10.1037/a0034003

Morey, L. C., & Skodol, A. E. (2013). Convergence between *DSM–IV* and *DSM–5* diagnostic models for personality disorder: Evaluation of strategies for establishing diagnostic thresholds. *Journal of Psychiatric Practice, 19,* 179–193. doi:10.1097/01.pra.0000430502.78833.06

New, A. S., Triebwasser, J., & Charney, D. S. (2008). The case for shifting borderline personality disorder to Axis I. *Biological Psychiatry, 64,* 653–659. doi:10.1016/j.biopsych.2008.04.020

Oldham, J. M., & Skodol, A. E. (2000). Charting the future of Axis II. *Journal of Personality Disorders, 14,* 17–29. doi:10.1521/pedi.2000.14.1.17

Oleski, J., Cox, B. J., Robinson, J., & Grant, B. (2012). The predictive validity of Cluster C personality disorders on the persistence of major depression in the national epidemiologic survey on alcohol and related conditions. *Journal of Personality Disorders, 26,* 322–333. doi:10.1521/pedi.2012.26.3.322

Paris, J. (2011). Endophenotypes and the diagnosis of personality disorders. *Journal of Personality Disorders, 25,* 260–268. doi:10.1521/pedi.2011.25.2.260

Pincus, A. L. (2011). Some comments on nomology, diagnostic process, and narcissistic personality disorder in the *DSM–5* proposal for personality and personality disorders. *Personality Disorders: Theory, Research, and Treatment, 2,* 41–53. doi:10.1037/a0021191

Pinto, A., Liebowitz, M. R., Foa, E. B., & Simpson, H. B. (2011). Obsessive compulsive personality disorder as a predictor of exposure and ritual prevention outcome for obsessive compulsive disorder. *Behaviour Research and Therapy, 49,* 453–458. doi:10.1016/j.brat.2011.04.004

Plakun, E. M. (1996). Treatment of personality disorders in an era of limited resources. *Psychiatric Services, 47,* 128–130.

Qaseem, A., Barry, M. J., Denberg, T. D., Owens, D. K., Shekelle, P., & Clinical Guidelines Committee of the American College of Physicians. (2013). Screening for prostate cancer: A guidance statement from the Clinical Guidelines Committee of the American College of Physicians. *Annals of Internal Medicine, 158,* 761–769. doi:10.7326/0003-4819-158-10-201305210-00633

Rakowska, J. M. (2011). Brief strategic therapy in patients with social phobia with or without personality disorder. *Psychotherapy Research, 21,* 462–471. doi:10.1080/10503307.2011.581707

Ronningstam, E. (2011). Narcissistic personality disorder in *DSM–V:* In support of retaining a significant diagnosis. *Journal of Personality Disorders, 25,* 248–259. doi:10.1521/pedi.2011.25.2.248

Ronningstam, E. (2013). An update on narcissistic personality disorder. *Current Opinion in Psychiatry, 26,* 102–106. doi:10.1097/YCO.0b013e328359979c

Rottman, B. M., Ahn, W., Sanislow, C. A., & Kim, N. S. (2009). Can clinicians recognize *DSM–IV* personality disorders from five-factor model descriptions of patient cases? *American Journal of Psychiatry, 166,* 427–433. doi:10.1176/appi.ajp.2008.08070972

Shedler, J., Beck, A., Fonagy, P., Gabbard, G. O., Gunderson, J., Kernberg, O., . . . Westen, D. (2010). Personality disorders in *DSM–5. The American Journal of Psychiatry, 167,* 1026–1028. doi:10.1176/appi.ajp.2010.10050746

Siever, L. J., & Davis, K. L. (1991). A psychobiological perspective on the personality disorders. *American Journal of Psychiatry, 148,* 1647–1658.

Silk, K. R. (2010). The quality of depression in borderline personality disorder and the diagnostic process. *Journal of Personality Disorders, 24,* 25–37. doi:10.1521/pedi.2010.24.1.25

Silk, K. R. (2012, May). Unintended and nonpsychiatric consequences of a change in diagnosis. In J. Reich (Chair), *Clinical and administrative aspects of the* DSM–5 *personality disorders.* Symposium conducted at the meeting of the American Psychiatric Association, Philadelphia, PA.

Skodol, A. E., Bender, D. S., Morey, L. S., Clark, L. A., Oldham, J. O., Alarcon, R. D., . . . Siever, L. J. (2011). Personality disorder types proposed for *DSM–5. Journal of Personality Disorders, 25,* 136–169. doi:10.1521/pedi.2011.25.2.136

Skodol, A. E., Clark, L. A., Bender, D. S., Krueger, R. F., Morey, L. C., Verheul, R., . . . Oldham, J. M. (2011). Proposed changes in personality and personality disorder assessment and diagnosis for *DSM–5* Part I: Description and rationale. *Personality Disorders: Theory, Research, and Treatment, 2,* 4–22. doi:10.1037/a0021891

Skodol, A. E., Gunderson, J. G., Shea, M. T., McGlashan, T. H., Morey, L. C., Sanislow, C. A., . . . Stout, R. L. (2005). The Collaborative Longitudinal Personality Disorders Study (CLPS): Overview and implications. *Journal of Personality Disorders, 19,* 487–504. doi:10.1521/pedi.2005.19.5.487

Skodol, A. E., Siever, L. J., Livesley, W. J., Gunderson, J. G., Pfohl, B., & Widiger, T. A. (2002). The borderline diagnosis II: Biology, genetics, and clinical course. *Biological Psychiatry, 51,* 951–963. doi:10.1016/S0006-3223(02)01325-2

South, S. C., & DeYoung, N. J. (2013). Behavior genetics of personality disorders: Informing classification and conceptualization on *DSM–5. Personality Disorders: Theory, Research, and Treatment, 4,* 270–283. doi:10.1037/a0026255

Strack, S., & Millon, T. (2007). Contributions to the dimensional assessment of personality disorders using Millon's model and the Millon Clinical Multiaxial Inventory (MCMI–III). *Journal of Personality Assessment, 89,* 56–69. doi:10.1080/00223890701357217

Trull, T. J. (2005). Dimensional models of personality disorder: Coverage and cutoffs. *Journal of Personality Disorders, 19,* 262–282. doi:10.1521/pedi.2005.19.3.262

Verheul, R., Bartak, A., & Widiger, T. (2007). Prevalence and construct validity of Personality Disorder Not Otherwise Specified (PDNOS). *Journal of Personality Disorders, 21,* 359–370. doi:10.1521/pedi.2007.21.4.359

Watson, D., Clark, L. A., & Chmielewski, M. (2008). Structures of personality and their relevance to psychopathology: II. Further articulation of a comprehensive unified trait structure. *Journal of Personality, 76,* 1545–1586. doi:10.1111/j.1467-6494.2008.00531.x

Westen, D., DeFife, J. A., Bradley, B., & Hilsenroth, M. J. (2010). Prototype personality diagnosis in clinical practice: A viable alternative for *DSM–5* and ICD–11. *Professional Psychology: Research and Practice, 41,* 482–487. doi:10.1037/a0021555

Westen, D., & Shedler, J. (1999). Revising and assessing Axis II, Part II: Toward an empirically based and clinically useful classification of personality disorders. *The American Journal of Psychiatry, 156,* 273–285.

Westen, D., & Shedler, J. (2000). A prototype matching approach to diagnosing personality disorders: Towards *DSM–V. Journal of Personality Disorders, 14,* 109–126. doi:10.1521/pedi.2000.14.2.109

Zimmerman, M. (2011). A critique of the proposed prototype rating system for personality disorders in *DSM–5. Journal of Personality Disorders, 25,* 206–221. doi:10.1521/pedi.2011.25.2.206

Zimmerman, M., Galione, J. N., Ruggero, C. J., Chelminski, I., Young, D., Dalrymple, K., & McGlinchey, J. B. (2010). Screening for bipolar disorder and finding borderline personality disorder. *Journal of Clinical Psychiatry, 71,* 1212–1217. doi:10.4088/JCP.09m05161yel

2

A CRITICAL EVALUATION OF RETAINING PERSONALITY CATEGORIES AND TYPES

DOUGLAS B. SAMUEL AND SARAH A. GRIFFIN

Mental and physical illnesses have been treated as categorical entities, with few exceptions, since the very beginning of medicine. This viewpoint logically leads to identifying those individuals who share common symptoms. Given this backdrop, it is unsurprising that personality disorder (PD) diagnoses have been constructed via categories or prototypes. In the earliest incarnations of what could be called a PD nomenclature, the French physician Philippe Pinel offered a description of a certain group of mental patients who lacked delusions, hallucinations, or impaired intellectual functioning and yet had significant impairments in functioning. He labeled this group with a category of *manie sans délire*—insanity without delusion (Pinel, 1801/1962). Although some have analogized this category to the current constructs of psychopathy or antisocial personality disorder (e.g., Millon, Simonsen, & Birket-Smith, 1998), Pinel's category was almost certainly more broad and included all aspects of personality pathology and what are now called mood

http://dx.doi.org/10.1037/14549-003
Personality Disorders: Toward Theoretical and Empirical Integration in Diagnosis and Assessment,
S. K. Huprich (Editor)

and anxiety disorders. Nonetheless, the progress of psychiatry over the past 200 years has proceeded primarily by further subdividing this single category into increasingly narrower segments.

For PDs, this subdivision has yielded approximately 10 specific categorical entities within the official nomenclature at any given point in time. But when considered cumulatively across official and unofficial diagnostic systems, the number of PD categories or types is much larger and limited only by the creativity of individual clinicians who generate the labels (Widiger & Corbitt, 1994). Given this long history within the PD field and across medicine, it is perhaps not surprising that the American Psychiatric Association (2013) has been reluctant to switch to alternative approaches, despite the demonstrable inadequacy of the existing categories (Trull & Durrett, 2005).

There are, of course, some benefits to categories, as laid out in Chapter 1 of this book. Nonetheless, there remain a number of significant limitations to a categorical system of PDs that far outweigh any advantages. Some limitations are applicable to categories or types in general, and others are more accurately applied to the specific categories within the *Diagnostic and Statistical Manual of Mental Disorders* (4th ed., text rev. [*DSM–IV–TR*]; American Psychiatric Association, 2000) that were repeated in the manual's fifth edition (*DSM–5*; American Psychiatric Association, 2013).

GENERAL LIMITATIONS OF CATEGORICAL MODELS OF PERSONALITY DISORDER

The most compelling reason to avoid categories is simple: They sacrifice valuable information. Markon, Chmielewski, and Miller (2011) conducted two separate meta-analyses of 58 published studies of psychopathology to examine the reliability and validity of categories. They found that dichotomizing variables to create discrete categories had significant costs to the information conveyed. When measures of psychopathology were examined, the categorical representations had 15% lower reliability and 37% lower validity than continuous dimensional scores on the same measures. The estimated reliability values were .711 for discrete categories and .820 for continuous measures, whereas the comparable validity estimates were .305 for discrete categories and .419 for continuous measures. It is not surprising that information is lost when dimensional scores are converted to categories, as dichotomizing eliminates data on specific levels of severity within each group. But what is striking about these results is just how much nontrivial diagnostic information is sacrificed. This strongly suggests that discrete categories are limited relative to continuous measures and constructs.

Thus, although there may well remain situations in which a categorical decision must be made, such as for treatment decisions (e.g., hospitalization vs. outpatient) or diagnostic coding (e.g., for insurance reimbursement), it would be preferable to make these decisions on the basis of continuous information (Kamphuis & Noordhof, 2009). A parallel is the typical diagnosis of arterial hypertension, whereby an individual's diastolic and systolic blood pressures are compared with norms and assigned to diagnostic groups (e.g., prehypertension, Stage 1 hypertension, Stage 2 hypertension) depending on their numerical deviance from the adaptive ranges. In fact, there is already an example of a dimensional representation being used for diagnosis within *DSM–5*. The diagnosis of intellectual developmental disorder is provided partially on the basis of one's score on a standardized measure of intellectual functioning.

In the context of PDs, it is important to note that the individual diagnoses could themselves be dimensionalized, such as by rating them on a 1-to-5 scale to indicate severity of the current PDs (Oldham & Skodol, 2000) or other types or categories developed (Westen, Shedler, & Bradley, 2006). Thus, this most general criticism of dichotomous indicators does not fully dismiss *DSM–5*'s categories. Nonetheless, there are quite a few criticisms that are specific to *DSM–5* instantiations of the PD categories.

SPECIFIC CRITICISMS OF THE *DSM–5* PERSONALITY DISORDER CATEGORICAL MODEL

The difficulties with the current categorical model of PDs have been well documented over the past 10 to 15 years; so much of what we write here is not new and is simply an organization and amplification of these ideas. Many deficiencies of the *DSM–IV* (and now *DSM–5*) categorical system were pointed out repeatedly during the development of *DSM–5* (e.g., Krueger & Eaton, 2010; Livesley, 2012; Skodol, 2012). Chief among them are (a) failure to "carve nature at its joints," (b) lack of a meaningful or well-validated boundary between normal and disordered personality, (c) excessive heterogeneity within diagnostic categories, (d) excessive diagnostic co-occurrence across categories, (e) inadequate coverage of the full range of personality difficulties seen in clinical practice, (f) questionable temporal stability of the diagnoses, (g) dissatisfaction among the clinicians, and (h) inadequate scientific foundation (Clark, 2007; Krueger, Skodol, Livesley, Shrout, & Huang, 2007; Trull & Durrett, 2005; Widiger & Samuel, 2005; Widiger & Trull, 2007). These are discussed next, in turn.

Failure to "Carve Nature at Its Joints"

Although *DSM–5* divides the universe of personality pathology into 10 discrete categories, we are not aware of any empirical literature that has supported this organization (e.g., Huprich, Schmitt, Richard, Chelminski, & Zimmerman, 2010; Sheets & Craighead, 2007). Structural analyses of the diagnostic criteria in individual studies have revealed a variety of solutions ranging from as few as two (Krueger, Markon, Patrick, & Iacono, 2005) to as many as eight (Blais & Malone, 2013) or even 10 components or factors (Huprich et al., 2010), but most commonly the number is four (Livesley, 1987) or five (O'Connor, 2005). More important, when considered meta-analytically, the factors within the universe of personality pathology are arranged hierarchically such that different models (i.e., numbers of factors) can be extracted (Markon, Krueger, & Watson, 2005; Wright et al., 2012). Nonetheless, it does appear that the five-factor model is the most important level of analysis (Markon et al., 2005) for a variety of reasons. First, this solution corresponds well with the five domains recovered from normal personality research (Widiger & Trull, 2007), which have a vast literature of basic science support. Second, these five domains have emerged more consistently across independent analyses (Harkness, Finn, McNulty, & Shields, 2012; Krueger, Derringer, Markon, Watson, & Skodol, 2012; Markon et al., 2005; O'Connor, 2005).

One possible explanation for the empirical literature's failure to support the existence of 10 PD categories that correspond to the *DSM–5* categorical system is that discrete categories do not exist within the universe of PD pathology. Eaton, Krueger, South, Simms, and Clark (2011) utilized an extremely large sample of individuals (> 8,500) from a variety of settings. When the results of a well-validated self-report measure of PD were examined, Eaton et al. found that although clusters of personality pathology could be located, they failed to replicate across samples. Thus, although there may be descriptive value to identifying clusters or subgroups within specific samples, the attempt to extrapolate these groups across samples is likely to fail. Additional research is clearly needed on the structure of ratings from other methods (beyond self-report), to determine if discrete categories emerge. Nonetheless, to avoid potential artifacts of any particular method, the ultimate support for the existence of PD categories or types would require replication across diagnostic sources, as well as samples.

Taxometric analyses of the *DSM–5* PD categories have also provided limited evidence to support the existence of categories. Taxometric analyses are a group of statistical procedures that are designed to test whether the latent structure of a construct is dimensional or taxonic. The primary logic of these methods is that taxa should evince increasing patterns of covariance among indicators at the locations of the continuum where discrete breaks occur. Thus, for example, if depression was taxonic, we would expect a greater covariance among features such as loss of pleasure and sleep disturbance as the amount of depression increased. Haslam, Holland, and Kuppens (2012) recently reviewed the taxometric evidence for PDs and noted that although the data tended to support schizotypy as being relatively taxonic (but see Rawlings, Williams, Haslam, & Claridge, 2008, for another perspective), the overwhelming majority of studies suggest that the remaining PD constructs are dimensional in nature. In other words, there do not appear to be any discrete breaks in the distributions of these latent constructs, so any attempts to demarcate cut points are inherently arbitrary.

Boundary With Normality

Considering the results of taxometric studies, it perhaps is not surprising that an additional problem for the *DSM–5* categories has been the lack of a meaningful distinction between normal-range personality and the PDs. One of the innovations of the third edition of the *Diagnostic and Statistical Manual of Mental Disorders* (*DSM–III*; American Psychiatric Association, 1980) was the provision of explicit diagnostic criteria, including a specified threshold for a disorder's diagnosis; however, the existing diagnostic thresholds lack a compelling rationale (Tyrer & Johnson, 1996). In fact, no explanation or justification has ever been provided for most of them (Samuel & Widiger, 2006b), the exceptions being *DSM–III* schizotypal and borderline PDs. The *DSM–III* requirements that the patient have four of eight features for the schizotypal diagnosis and five of eight features for the borderline diagnosis (American Psychiatric Association, 1980) were determined on the basis of maximizing agreement with similar diagnoses provided by clinicians (Spitzer, Endicott, & Gibbon, 1979). However, the current diagnostic criteria for these PDs have shifted notably such that the original empirical thresholds established for *DSM–III* are likely obsolete. For example, Blashfield, Blum, and Pfohl (1992) reported a kappa of only −.025 for the *DSM–III* and *DSM–III–R* Schizotypal personality disorders, with a reduction in prevalence from 11% to 1%. Needless to say, the official boundary between normal and abnormal personality remains largely arbitrary.

The primary distinction between normal and abnormal personality in the *DSM* is whether an individual meets the diagnostic threshold or falls one criterion short of the threshold established for PD diagnosis. To illustrate, a client who exhibits clinically significant self-harm, dissociation, self-damaging impulsivity, and unstable self-image, without meeting other criteria for any PD, would not be considered to have Borderline Personality Disorder (BPD). In contrast, if he or she met a single additional BPD criterion, the diagnosis would be warranted. This abrupt distinction fails not only to accurately reflect clinical reality but also to acknowledge that certain combinations of criteria, even when fewer in number, signify greater severity (e.g., Cooper & Balsis, 2009).

Heterogeneity Within Categories

Another important limitation of the current categorical system is that there are important differences among persons who share the same PD diagnosis. Patients with the same PD diagnosis will vary substantially with respect to which diagnostic criteria were used to make the diagnosis, and these differences are not trivial. For example, only a subset of persons who meet the *DSM–IV–TR* criteria for Antisocial Personality Disorder will have the prototypic features of the callous, ruthless, arrogant, charming, and scheming psychopath (Hare, 2003), and there are important differences among the persons who would be diagnosed as psychopathic (Brinkley, Newman, Widiger, & Lynam, 2004). Similar distinctions are made for other PDs, such as the differentiation within borderline psychopathology with respect to the dimensions of affective dysregulation, impulsivity, and behavioral disturbance (Sanislow et al., 2002) and the differentiation of dependent personality disorder into submissive, exploitable, and affectionate variants (Pincus & Wilson, 2001).

A classic example of this heterogeneity is the fact that there are 256 different "ways" to be diagnosed with BPD when one calculates all the possible combinations of meeting at least five of the nine diagnostic criteria. This example is neither trivial nor restricted to theoretical mathematics. Johansen, Karterud, Pedersen, Gude, and Falkum (2004) examined a large clinical sample and located 252 patients who met criteria for BPD. In that group, 136 different combinations of BPD criteria were represented. The problem is even more complicated for the diagnosis of obsessive–compulsive personality disorder (OCPD), which requires the presence of only four of eight possible criteria, making it possible for two individuals to have the same diagnosis but have no features in common. Additionally, the individual symptoms for OCPD are among the most heterogeneous of any PD, often yielding levels of internal consistency values around .50 or even lower (Samuel & Widiger, 2010).

This level of heterogeneity within the *DSM–5* categories seriously undermines their validity. Smith, McCarthy, and Zapolski (2009) have argued persuasively that unidimensional constructs are necessary for the valid assessment of psychopathology, as these are the only types of constructs that can represent definable psychological processes. Smith et al. agreed that broad heterogeneous constructs, such as PD categories or types, can have descriptive or theoretical value. Nonetheless, they noted that no multidimensional construct can be adequately described by a single score. This fact is intuitive and obvious from modern psychometric theory but has wide implications for the categorical nosology. Thus, they posited that the science of PDs (and psychopathology more generally) will only be advanced by the descriptions of the phenomena in terms of the fine-grained, homogeneous building blocks that can be assessed reliably and validly (e.g., Widiger & Samuel, 2005).

Excessive Diagnostic Co-Occurrence

Of all the problems with the *DSM–5* PD categories, perhaps the most widely criticized aspect is that they lack discriminant validity. Large-scale studies within clinical populations indicate that PDs are quite common (Zimmerman, Chelminski, & Young, 2008), and, most often, multiple diagnoses are applicable. For example, Zimmerman, Rothschild, and Chelminski (2005) noted that within a clinical epidemiological sample of 859 patients, 391 (45%) met criteria for a PD, and a majority (60%) of those individuals were diagnosed with more than one. This excessive diagnostic co-occurrence of PDs has been widely replicated (e.g., R. F. Bernstein, 1998; Lilienfeld, Waldman, & Israel, 1994). Suffice it to say that the maladaptive personality functioning of patients does not appear to be adequately described by a single diagnostic category. Indeed, no person is generally well described by just one word. This is particularly true when those terms are emotionally laden, are conflated with evaluative judgments, and describe a heterogeneous construct (e.g., BPD). Instead, each person is more accurately described by a constellation of personality traits (John & Srivastava, 1999) that fully captures the richness of that person's individuality.

This co-occurrence not only complicates efforts to help individual clients but also greatly impedes the development and validation of new therapies. Not only does the homogeneity make it difficult to ensure that two individuals with the same PD are actually similar, but the likelihood that one or both have additional diagnoses makes it almost impossible to locate a sample of individuals who are sufficiently similar for a study of treatment effectiveness. In this way, the empirical support for treatments relevant to PDs is more a testament to their fundamental disaggregation of core components, such as disruptions in emotion regulation and impulse control (i.e., dialectical behavior therapy) or undifferentiated affects and representations of self and other (i.e., mentalization-based psychotherapy or transference focused psychotherapy), than to the validity of the putative category (e.g., Borderline). This is a primary reason why the National Institute of Mental Health has moved away from funding research on diagnostic categories and shifted toward a dimensional framework (Insel, 2013; Sanislow et al., 2010).

Inadequate Coverage

Trull (2005) defined *coverage* as "the extent to which a model or system of personality pathology adequately represents those conditions or symptoms that are frequently encountered by clinicians and studied by psychopathologists" (p. 263). A perfect diagnostic system would then have adequate coverage of all possible forms of psychopathology seen within clinical practice. By this measure, there is wide agreement that the *DSM–5* categories fall short. Much research suggests that clinicians still are not able to select an appropriate category for most clients with PD. Westen and Arkowitz-Westen (1998) reported that, in a national random sample of therapists, only 39.4% of their 714 patients who were being seen for "enduring, maladaptive personality patterns" actually met the criteria for any *DSM–IV–TR* PD diagnosis (Westen & Arkowitz-Westen, 1998, p. 1767). The clinicians reported the treatment of commitment, intimacy, shyness, work inhibition, perfectionism, and devaluation of others that were not well described by any of the diagnostic categories. Clark, Watson, and Reynolds (1995) reported that many persons are diagnosed with Personality Disorder—Not Otherwise Specified (PDNOS), making this "wastebasket category" among the most commonly used diagnoses in clinical practice (Verheul & Widiger, 2004). Indeed, roughly one third of all individuals who meet criteria for a PD are assigned to PDNOS (Zimmerman et al., 2005). If so many individuals whose personality traits cause clinically significant impairment cannot be usefully categorized by the current system, the diagnostic nomenclature does not appear to be providing adequate coverage.

Questionable Temporal Stability

The general definition for a PD in *DSM–IV–TR*, which was retained for *DSM–5* Section II, is an "*enduring pattern* of inner experience and behavior that deviates markedly from the expectations of the individual's culture, is *pervasive* and inflexible, has an onset in adolescence in early adulthood, *is stable over time*, and leads to distress or impairment" (American Psychiatric Association, 2000, p. 685; emphasis added). Note that in three different places this definition references the enduring, stable, and pervasive nature of personality pathology. Indeed, it is this temporal component that often differentiates PD from other mental disorders (Shea & Yen, 2003). Nonetheless, over the past decade a number of longitudinal studies have suggested that categorical diagnoses are not nearly as stable as this definition implies (e.g., Skodol et al., 2005; Zanarini, Frankenburg, Hennen, Reich, & Silk, 2005). Instead, the primary finding from the largest and most detailed longitudinal study of PDs ever conducted, the Collaborative Longitudinal Personality Disorder Study

(CLPS; Gunderson et al., 2000), was the surprising rate of remission for PD diagnoses (Gunderson et al., 2003). Early results from CLPS suggested that fewer than half (44%) of the individuals retained their PD diagnosis through the first 12 months (Shea et al., 2002). This percentage was similar to that found at the 2-year follow-up (Grilo et al., 2004), suggesting that at least some of the first-year change may have reflected regression to the mean (Watson, 2004). Nevertheless, the number of remissions did continue to increase; by the 10-year follow-up, 85% of those initially diagnosed with a PD evinced a full remission, with few examples of relapse (Gunderson et al., 2011). These findings were consistent across other studies, such as the McLean Study of Adult Development (Zanarini et al., 2005), suggesting that categorical PD diagnoses are not nearly as stable as their definition implies.

Interestingly though, although categorical diagnoses and mean levels of PD symptoms decreased so significantly over periods as brief as 1 year (Shea et al., 2002), levels of psychosocial functioning within these samples remained substantially more durable (Zanarini, Frankenburg, Reich, & Fitzmaurice, 2010). Similarly, dimensional representations of the PDs obtained higher levels of rank-order stability, even over 10 years (Hopwood et al., 2013). The Schedule for Nonadaptive and Adaptive Personality—2 (SNAP–2; Clark, Simms, Wu, & Casillas, 2014), a self-report measure of the PD categories completed by CLPS participants, showed much greater temporal consistency. The average mean-level change over the first 2 years was only $d = -.21$ for the 10 diagnoses according to the SNAP–2, an effect size that would be considered small by Cohen (1992). Further, the mean rank-order stability coefficient across the 10 PDs was .69, a value that is higher than schizophrenia symptoms (.48; Reichenberg, Rieckmann, & Harvey, 2005), lower than intelligence (.85; Larsen, Hartmann, & Nyborg, 2008), and almost identical to normal range personality traits (.67; Morey et al., 2007).

In conclusion, it appears that the current empirical evidence regarding the stability of PD diagnoses is at odds with their general definition (Morey & Meyer, 2012). Nonetheless, the research supporting the durability of functional impairment and associated dimensional traits suggests that it is the specific DSM–5 categories and not the general definition that are deficient.

Clinician Dissatisfaction

Given the numerous flaws already noted, it is perhaps unsurprising that clinicians are quite dissatisfied with the current categorical model and have been for quite some time. In a survey of clinicians across 42 countries with respect to DSM–III–R, Maser, Kaelber, and Weise (1991) reported that "the personality disorders led the list of diagnostic categories with which respondents were dissatisfied" (p. 275). Even more recently, D. P. Bernstein, Iscan, and Maser (2007) conducted a multinational survey and found that 74% of the membership from the Association for Research in Personality Disorders and the International Society for the Study of Personality Disorders believed that the *DSM–IV* categorical approach to PDs should be replaced; 80% indicated "PDs are better understood as variants of normal personality than as categorical disease entities" (p. 542, Table 2). This finding presents compelling evidence for clinician dissatisfaction with the current model of PDs.

Although the opinions of clinicians should not be the sole decider for revising the diagnostic nomenclature, we agree with First et al. (2004) that this feedback should be considered carefully, as even the most valid diagnostic system will fail its purpose if clinicians do not use it in practice. A number of studies have since compared the current *DSM–5* categories with alternative systems in terms of their perceived clinical utility. These studies have regularly indicated that almost any alternative dimensional system (even those that include matching individuals to a prototype or type) would be preferable to the current categories (Lowe & Widiger, 2009; Mullins-Sweatt & Widiger, 2011; Samuel & Widiger, 2006a; Spitzer, First, Shedler, Westen, & Skodol, 2008). These findings, indicating clinicians' long-standing discontent with the current categorical system and their preference for a dimensional model, make it all the more surprising that such a system was not adopted for *DSM–5*.

Inadequate Scientific Foundation

A final limitation of the current categories is that despite remaining fully unchanged for 20 years (and mostly unchanged for much longer), their empirical foundation remains less than ideal. One important aspect of this problem is that no biomarker has yet been developed for any of the PDs (Skodol, 2012). *Biomarkers* are specific biological identifiers of a disease and can include specific genes, cells, hormones, enzymes, and antibodies or larger by-products of a physiological system. They are important because they identify a disease on the basis of a blood or tissue sample and thus aid in the identification of pathology, as well as potentially suggesting mechanisms of action and even treatments. For example, the amount of glucose in urine is an important biomarker for diabetes and white blood cell counts are an indicator of infection.

There is also scarce evidence for almost all PDs from molecular and behavioral genetic studies (South, Reichborn-Kjennerud, Eaton, & Krueger, 2012). What data do exist are primarily for borderline but also for antisocial and schizotypal PDs. What is clear from this research literature is that the specific *DSM–5* categories do not map well onto the genetic structure of psychopathology. This likely occurs for a variety of reasons, but chief among them are likely several of the concerns covered previously, such as heterogeneity within categories and co-occurrence within and outside the PDs. Given the extensive comorbidity that is found in psychopathology more generally, it is rather difficult to imagine that any single PD diagnosis could have a strong genetic loading that is not shared with a variety of other disorders as well (South et al., 2012).

Another relevant aspect of the empirical literature that does not favor the continued use of the current diagnostic categories is misuse by clinicians. A wide literature has well documented the fact that the median interrater reliability for specific PDs between treating clinicians using routine diagnostic methods is modest—in the range of .40—suggesting little overlap between the diagnoses assigned by two separate clinicians (Hesse & Thylstrup, 2008; Mellsop, Varghese, Joshua, & Hicks, 1982; Regier, Kaelber, Roper, & Rae, 1994). Further, unstructured diagnoses assigned by treating clinicians have limited convergence with self-report questionnaires (e.g., Hyler, Rieder, Williams, & Spitzer, 1989; Rossi, Van den Brande, Tobac, Sloore, & Hauben, 2003) or semistructured interviews (Fridell & Hesse, 2006; Tenney, Schotte, Denys, van Megen, & Westenberg, 2003).

More recent evidence from a sample of more than 300 individuals carefully diagnosed with PDs suggests that clinicians' unstructured PD diagnoses, even when recorded dimensionally with an established method of collecting prototype ratings (i.e., the Personality Assessment Form; Shea, Glass, Pilkonis, Watkins, & Docherty, 1987), have limited convergence with self-report and semistructured interviews (Samuel et al., 2013). More important, Samuel et al. (2013) noted that those dimensional prototype ratings by clinicians, even when based on more than a year of clinical contact, were less useful than self-report and semistructured interviews for predicting prospective psychosocial functioning over a 5-year period. This finding raises concern about the validity of unstructured PD diagnoses within clinical practice (Westen, 1997) and suggests that prototype matching approaches fail to remedy this concern.

In addition, clinicians' diagnoses of PD categories often exhibit gender bias (Anderson, Sankis, & Widiger, 2001). The PDs have wide gender differences in terms of the diagnostic rates, and analog studies have suggested these differences may reflect clinician bias. Vignettes portraying women are more likely to be diagnosed as histrionic, whereas male vignettes achieve higher ratings for antisocial and narcissistic PDs (Flanagan & Blashfield, 2003; Samuel & Widiger, 2009). In the case of histrionic PD, this may reflect a fundamental bias within the category itself (Lynam & Widiger, 2007; Sprock, 2000), but for others it might be attributable to application errors on the part of clinicians. Initial evidence suggests that dimensional trait models are less prone to errors of gender bias (Samuel & Widiger, 2009). This is likely because the evaluatively charged connotations of the PDs pull for global ratings based on specific cues and can be understood in the context of research demonstrating that clinicians tend to use global impressions when assigning PD diagnoses and that sometimes those diagnoses fail to agree with their own ratings of individuals' diagnostic criteria (Morey & Ochoa, 1989). Thus, it is quite possible that clinicians implicitly weight certain features of a PD more heavily than others (e.g., Kim & Ahn, 2002) and fail to apply the prescribed criteria correctly.

CONCLUSIONS AND FUTURE DIRECTIONS

With regard to the widespread and multiple problems with the current PD categories, we consider their perpetuation within *DSM–5* to be quite unfortunate and to represent a major missed opportunity to improve the diagnostic system. Nonetheless, the inclusion of a hybrid-dimensional model within *DSM–5* Section III sets the stage for a shift away from these troubled categories in the future. That dimensional system defines PD in terms of functional impairments and the presence of pathological traits. Other alternatives exist, such as the prototype matching system that was initially proposed for *DSM–5* but ultimately abandoned (i.e., Westen, DeFife, Bradley, & Hilsenroth, 2010). However, the basic framework of the *DSM–5* Section III model holds the promise of improving on or eliminating most of the flaws of the current nomenclature. Existing evidence from dimensional models, such as the five-factor model (Widiger & Trull, 2007), suggests that the Section III system would create a natural flow between normality and pathology, eliminate problematic heterogeneity, remove concerns about co-occurrence, improve coverage of all possible forms of pathology, bring temporal consistency in line with PD definitions, and be more useful to clinicians. Perhaps most important, the dimensional traits within the Section III model rest upon a bedrock of basic personality science embedded in trait psychology (Costa & McCrae, 2010).

Finally, as noted at the outset, these concerns with categories are long-standing and have been elaborated many times over. In this regard, we hope that this chapter will be among the last recounts of these failures of a current categorical PD system that need be written. We hope instead that future generations of clinicians will know about these failures only from their history classes and that their patients will benefit from an improved diagnostic system that better reflects the realities of PD pathology.

REFERENCES

American Psychiatric Association. (1980). *Diagnostic and statistical manual of mental disorders* (3rd ed.). Washington, DC: Author.

American Psychiatric Association. (2000). *Diagnostic and statistical manual of mental disorders* (4th ed., text rev.). Washington, DC: Author.

American Psychiatric Association. (2013). *Diagnostic and statistical manual of mental disorders* (5th ed.). Arlington, VA: Author.

Anderson, K. G., Sankis, L. M., & Widiger, T. A. (2001). Pathology versus statistical infrequency: Potential sources of gender bias in personality disorder criteria. *Journal of Nervous and Mental Disease, 189,* 661–668. doi:10.1097/00005053-200110000-00002

Bernstein, D. P., Iscan, C., & Maser, J. (2007). Opinions of personality disorder experts regarding the *DSM–IV* personality disorders classification system. *Journal of Personality Disorders, 21,* 536–551. doi:10.1521/pedi.2007.21.5.536

Bernstein, R. F. (1998). Reconceptualizing personality disorder diagnosis in the *DSM–V:* The discriminant validity challenge. *Clinical Psychology: Science and Practice, 5,* 333–343. doi:10.1111/j.1468-2850.1998.tb00153.x

Blais, M. A., & Malone, J. C. (2013). Structure of the *DSM–IV* personality disorders as revealed in clinician ratings. *Comprehensive Psychiatry, 54,* 326–333. doi:10.1016/j.comppsych.2012.10.014

Blashfield, R., Blum, N., & Pfohl, B. (1992). The effects of changing Axis II diagnostic criteria. *Comprehensive Psychiatry, 33,* 245–252. doi:10.1016/0010-440X(92)90048-U

Brinkley, C. A., Newman, J. P., Widiger, T. A., & Lynam, D. R. (2004). Two approaches to parsing the heterogeneity of psychopathy. *Clinical Psychology: Science and Practice, 11,* 69–94. doi:10.1093/clipsy.bph054

Clark, L. A. (2007). Assessment and diagnosis of personality disorder: Perennial issues and an emerging reconceptualization. *Annual Review of Psychology, 58,* 227–257. doi:10.1146/annurev.psych.57.102904.190200

Clark, L. A., Simms, L. J., Wu, K. D., & Casillas, A. (2014). *Manual for the Schedule for Nonadaptive and Adaptive Personality—2 (SNAP–2).* Minneapolis: University of Minnesota Press.

Clark, L. A., Watson, D., & Reynolds, S. (1995). Diagnosis and classification of psychopathology: Challenges to the current system and future directions. *Annual Review of Psychology, 46,* 121–153. doi:10.1146/annurev.ps.46.020195.001005

Cohen, J. (1992). A power primer. *Psychological Bulletin, 112,* 155–159. doi:10.1037/0033-2909.112.1.155

Cooper, L. D., & Balsis, S. (2009). When less is more: How fewer diagnostic criteria can indicate greater severity. *Psychological Assessment, 21,* 285–293. doi:10.1037/a0016698

Costa, P. T., Jr., & McCrae, R. R. (2010). Bridging the gap with the five-factor model. *Personality Disorders: Theory, Research, and Treatment, 1,* 127–130. doi:10.1037/a0020264

Eaton, N. R., Krueger, R. F., South, S. C., Simms, L. J., & Clark, L. A. (2011). Contrasting prototypes and dimensions in the classification of personality pathology: Evidence that dimensions, but not prototypes, are robust. *Psychological Medicine, 41,* 1151–1163. doi:10.1017/S0033291710001650

First, M. B., Pincus, H. A., Levine, J. B., Williams, J. B. W., Ustun, B., & Peele, R. (2004). Clinical utility as a criterion for revising psychiatric diagnoses. *The American Journal of Psychiatry*, *161*, 946–954. doi:10.1176/appi.ajp.161.6.946

Flanagan, E. H., & Blashfield, R. K. (2003). Gender bias in the diagnosis of personality disorders: The roles of base rates and social stereotypes. *Journal of Personality Disorders*, *17*, 431–446. doi:10.1521/pedi.17.5.431.22974

Fridell, M., & Hesse, M. (2006). Clinical diagnosis and SCID-II assessment of *DSM–III–R* personality disorders. *European Journal of Psychological Assessment*, *22*, 104–108. doi:10.1027/1015-5759.22.2.104

Grilo, C. M., Shea, M. T., Sanislow, C. A., Skodol, A. E., Gunderson, J. G., Stout, R. L., . . . McGlashan, T. H. (2004). Two-year stability and change of schizotypal, borderline, avoidant, and obsessive-compulsive personality disorders. *Journal of Consulting and Clinical Psychology*, *72*, 767–775. doi:10.1037/0022-006X.72.5.767

Gunderson, J. G., Bender, D., Sanislow, C., Yen, S., Rettew, J. B., Dolan-Sewell, R., . . . Skodol, A. E. (2003). Plausibility and possible determinants of sudden "remissions" in borderline patients. *Psychiatry: Interpersonal and Biological Processes*, *66*, 111–119. doi:10.1521/psyc.66.2.111.20614

Gunderson, J. G., Shea, M. T., Skodol, A. E., McGlashan, T. H., Morey, L. C., Stout, R. L., . . . Keller, M. B. (2000). The Collaborative Longitudinal Personality Disorders Study: Development, aims, design, and sample characteristics. *Journal of Personality Disorders*, *14*, 300–315. doi:10.1521/pedi.2000.14.4.300

Gunderson, J. G., Stout, R. L., McGlashan, T. H., Shea, T., Morey, L. C., Grilo, C. M., . . . Skodol, A. E. (2011). Ten-year course of borderline personality disorder psychopathology and function from the Collaborative Longitudinal Personality Disorders Study. *Archives of General Psychiatry*, *68*, 827–837. doi:10.1001/archgenpsychiatry.2011.37

Hare, R. D. (2003). *Manual for the Revised Psychopathology Checklist* (2nd ed.). Toronto, Ontario, Canada: Multi-Health Systems.

Harkness, A. R., Finn, J. A., McNulty, J. L., & Shields, S. M. (2012). The Personality Psychopathology—Five (PSY–5): Recent constructive replication and assessment literature review. *Psychological Assessment*, *24*, 432–443. doi:10.1037/a0025830

Haslam, N., Holland, E., & Kuppens, P. (2012). Categories versus dimensions in personality and psychopathology: A quantitative review of taxometric research. *Psychological Medicine*, *42*, 903–920. doi:10.1017/S0033291711001966

Hesse, M., & Thylstrup, B. (2008). Inter-rater agreement of comorbid *DSM–IV* personality disorders in substance abusers. *BMC Psychiatry*, *8*, Article 37. doi:10.1186/1471-244x-8-37

Hopwood, C. J., Morey, L. C., Donnellan, M. B., Samuel, D. B., Grilo, C. M., McGlashan, T. H., . . . Skodol, A. E. (2013). Ten-year rank-order stability of personality traits and disorders in a clinical sample. *Journal of Personality*, *81*, 335–344. doi:10.1111/j.1467-6494.2012.00801.x

Huprich, S. K., Schmitt, T. A., Richard, D. C. S., Chelminski, I., & Zimmerman, M. A. (2010). Comparing factor analytic models of the *DSM–IV* personality disorders. *Personality Disorders: Theory, Research, and Treatment, 1*, 22–37. doi:10.1037/a0018245

Hyler, S. E., Rieder, R. O., Williams, J. B., & Spitzer, R. L. (1989). A comparison of clinical and self-report diagnoses of *DSM–III* personality disorders in 552 patients. *Comprehensive Psychiatry, 30*, 170–178. doi:10.1016/0010-440X(89)90070-9

Insel, T. (2013, April 29). Transforming diagnosis [web log message]. Retrieved from http://www.nimh.nih.gov/about/director/2013/transforming-diagnosis.shtml

Johansen, M., Karterud, S., Pedersen, G., Gude, T., & Falkum, E. (2004). An investigation of the prototype validity of the borderline *DSM–IV* construct. *Acta Psychiatrica Scandinavica, 109*, 289–298. doi:10.1046/j.1600-0447.2003.00268.x

John, O. P., & Srivastava, S. (1999). The Big Five trait taxonomy: History, measurement, and theoretical perspectives. In L. A. Pervin & O. P. John (Eds.), *Handbook of personality: Theory and research* (Vol. 2, pp. 102–138). New York, NY: Guilford Press.

Kamphuis, J. H., & Noordhof, A. (2009). On categorical diagnoses in *DSM–V*: Cutting dimensions at useful points? *Psychological Assessment, 21*, 294–301. doi:10.1037/a0016697

Kim, N. S., & Ahn, W. K. (2002). The influence of naive causal theories on lay concepts of mental illness. *The American Journal of Psychology, 115*, 33–65. doi:10.2307/1423673

Krueger, R. F., Derringer, J., Markon, K. E., Watson, D., & Skodol, A. E. (2012). Initial construction of a maladaptive personality trait model and inventory for *DSM–5*. *Psychological Medicine, 42*, 1879–1890. doi:10.1017/S0033291711002674

Krueger, R. F., & Eaton, N. R. (2010). Personality traits and the classification of mental disorders: Toward a more complete integration in *DSM–5* and an empirical model of psychopathology. *Personality Disorders: Theory, Research, and Treatment, 1*, 97–118. doi:10.1037/A0018990

Krueger, R. F., Markon, K. E., Patrick, C. J., & Iacono, W. G. (2005). Externalizing psychopathology in adulthood: A dimensional-spectrum conceptualization and its implications for *DSM–V*. *Journal of Abnormal Psychology, 114*, 537–550. doi:10.1037/0021-843X.114.4.537

Krueger, R. F., Skodol, A. E., Livesley, W. J., Shrout, P. E., & Huang, Y. Q. (2007). Synthesizing dimensional and categorical approaches to personality disorders: Refining the research agenda for *DSM–V* Axis II. *International Journal of Methods in Psychiatric Research, 16*, S65–S73. doi:10.1002/mpr.212

Larsen, L., Hartmann, P., & Nyborg, H. (2008). The stability of general intelligence from early adulthood to middle-age. *Intelligence, 36*, 29–34. doi:10.1016/j.intell.2007.01.001

Lilienfeld, S. O., Waldman, I. D., & Israel, A. C. (1994). A critical examination of the use of the term and concept of comorbidity in psychopathology research.

Clinical Psychology: Science and Practice, 1, 71–83. doi:10.1111/j.1468-2850.1994. tb00007.x

Livesley, W. J. (1987). A systematic approach to the delineation of personality disorders. *The American Journal of Psychiatry, 144,* 772–777.

Livesley, W. J. (2012). Tradition versus empiricism in the current *DSM–5* proposal for revising the classification of personality disorders. *Criminal Behaviour and Mental Health, 22,* 81–90. doi:10.1002/cbm.1826

Lowe, J. R., & Widiger, T. A. (2009). Clinicians' judgments of clinical utility: A comparison of *DSM–IV* with dimensional models of general personality. *Journal of Personality Disorders, 23,* 211–229. doi:10.1521/pedi.2009.23.3.211

Lynam, D. R., & Widiger, T. A. (2007). Using a general model of personality to understand sex differences in the personality disorders. *Journal of Personality Disorders, 21,* 583–602. doi:10.1521/pedi.2007.21.6.583

Markon, K. E., Chmielewski, M., & Miller, C. J. (2011). The reliability and validity of discrete and continuous measures of psychopathology: A quantitative review. *Psychological Bulletin, 137,* 856–879. doi:10.1037/a0023678

Markon, K. E., Krueger, R. F., & Watson, D. (2005). Delineating the structure of normal and abnormal personality: An integrative hierarchical approach. *Journal of Personality and Social Psychology, 88,* 139–157. doi:10.1037/0022-3514.88.1.139

Maser, J. D., Kaelber, C., & Weise, R. E. (1991). International use and attitudes toward *DSM–III* and *DSM–III–R:* Growing consensus in psychiatric classification. *Journal of Abnormal Psychology, 100,* 271–279. doi:10.1037/0021-843X.100.3.271

Mellsop, G., Varghese, F., Joshua, S., & Hicks, A. (1982). The reliability of Axis II of *DSM–III. The American Journal of Psychiatry, 139,* 1360–1361.

Millon, T., Simonsen, E., & Birket-Smith, M. (1998). Historical conceptions of psychopathy in the United States and Europe. In T. Millon, E. Simonsen, M. Birket-Smith, & R. D. Davis (Eds.), *Psychopathy: Antisocial, criminal, and violent behavior* (pp. 3–31). New York, NY: Guilford Press.

Morey, L. C., Hopwood, C. J., Gunderson, J. G., Skodol, A. E., Shea, M. T., Yen, S., . . . McGlashan, T. H. (2007). Comparison of alternative models for personality disorders. *Psychological Medicine, 37,* 983–994. doi:10.1017/S0033291706009482

Morey, L. C., & Meyer, J. K. (2012). Course of personality disorder. In T. A. Widiger (Ed.), *The Oxford handbook of personality disorders* (pp. 275–287). New York, NY: Oxford University Press.

Morey, L. C., & Ochoa, E. S. (1989). An investigation of adherence to diagnostic criteria: Clinical diagnosis of the *DSM–III* personality disorders. *Journal of Personality Disorders, 3,* 180–192. doi:10.1521/pedi.1989.3.3.180

Mullins-Sweatt, S. N., & Widiger, T. A. (2011). Clinician's judgments of the utility of the *DSM–IV* and five-factor models for personality disordered patients. *Journal of Personality Disorders, 25,* 463–477. doi:10.1521/pedi.2011.25.4.463

O'Connor, B. P. (2005). A search for consensus on the dimensional structure of personality disorders. *Journal of Clinical Psychology, 61*, 323–345. doi:10.1002/jclp.20017

Oldham, J. M., & Skodol, A. E. (2000). Charting the future of Axis II. *Journal of Personality Disorders, 14*, 17–29. doi:10.1521/pedi.2000.14.1.17

Pincus, A. L., & Wilson, K. R. (2001). Interpersonal variability in dependent personality. *Journal of Personality, 69*, 223–251. doi:10.1111/1467-6494/00143

Pinel, P. (1962). *A treatise on insanity* (D. Davis, Trans.). New York, NY: Hafner. (Original work published 1801)

Rawlings, D., Williams, B., Haslam, N., & Claridge, G. (2008). Taxometric analysis supports a dimensional latent structure for schizotypy. *Personality and Individual Differences, 44*, 1640–1651. doi:10.1016/j.paid.2007.06.005

Regier, D. A., Kaelber, C. T., Roper, M. T., & Rae, D. S. (1994). The *ICD–10* clinical field trial for mental and behavioral disorders: Results in Canada and the United States. *The American Journal of Psychiatry, 151*, 1340–1350.

Reichenberg, A., Rieckmann, N., & Harvey, P. D. (2005). Stability in schizophrenia symptoms over time: Findings from the Mount Sinai Pilgrim Psychiatric Center longitudinal study. *Journal of Abnormal Psychology, 114*, 363–372. doi:10.1037/0021-843X.114.3.363

Rossi, G., Van den Brande, I., Tobac, A., Sloore, H., & Hauben, C. (2003). Convergent validity of the MCMI-III personality disorder scales and the MMPI-2 scales. *Journal of Personality Disorders, 17*, 330–340. doi:10.1521/pedi.17.4.330.23970

Samuel, D. B., Sanislow, C. A., Hopwood, C. J., Shea, M. T., Skodol, A. E., Morey, L. C., . . . Grilo, C. M. (2013). Convergent and incremental predictive validity of clinician, self-report, and diagnostic interview assessment methods for personality disorders over 5 years. *Journal of Consulting and Clinical Psychology, 81*, 650–659. doi:10.1037/a0032813

Samuel, D. B., & Widiger, T. A. (2006a). Clinicians' judgments of clinical utility: A comparison of the *DSM–IV* and five-factor models. *Journal of Abnormal Psychology, 115*, 298–308. doi:10.1037/0021-843X.115.2.298

Samuel, D. B., & Widiger, T. A. (2006b). Differentiating normal and abnormal personality from the perspective of the *DSM*. In S. Strack (Ed.), *Differentiating normal and abnormal personality* (2nd ed., pp. 165–183). New York, NY: Springer.

Samuel, D. B., & Widiger, T. A. (2009). Comparative gender biases in models of personality disorder. *Personality and Mental Health, 3*, 12–25. doi:10.1002/pmh.61

Samuel, D. B., & Widiger, T. A. (2010). A comparison of obsessive-compulsive personality disorder scales. *Journal of Personality Assessment, 92*, 232–240. doi:10.1080/00223891003670182

Sanislow, C. A., Grilo, C. M., Morey, L. C., Bender, D. S., Skodol, A. E., Gunderson, J. G., . . . McGlashan, T. H. (2002). Confirmatory factor analysis of *DSM–IV* criteria for borderline personality disorder: Findings from the Collaborative

Longitudinal Personality Disorders Study. *The American Journal of Psychiatry, 159*, 284–290. doi:10.1176/appi.ajp.159.2.284

Sanislow, C. A., Pine, D. S., Quinn, K. J., Kozak, M. J., Garvey, M. A., Heinssen, R. K., . . . Cuthbert, B. N. (2010). Developing constructs for psychopathology research: Research domain criteria. *Journal of Abnormal Psychology, 119*, 631–639. doi:10.1037/a0020909

Shea, M. T., Glass, D. R., Pilkonis, P. A., Watkins, J. T., & Docherty, J. P. (1987). Frequency and implications of personality disorders in a sample of depressed outpatients. *Journal of Personality Disorders, 1*, 27–42. doi:10.1521/pedi.1987.1.1.27

Shea, M. T., Stout, R., Gunderson, J., Morey, L. C., Grilo, C. M., McGlashan, T., . . . Keller, M. B. (2002). Short-term diagnostic stability of schizotypal, borderline, avoidant, and obsessive-compulsive personality disorders. *The American Journal of Psychiatry, 159*, 2036–2041. doi:10.1176/appi.ajp.159.12.2036

Shea, M. T., & Yen, S. (2003). Stability as a distinction between Axis I and Axis II disorders. *Journal of Personality Disorders, 17*, 373–386. doi:10.1521/pedi.17.5.373.22973

Sheets, E., & Craighead, W. E. (2007). Toward an empirically based classification of personality pathology. *Clinical Psychology: Science and Practice, 14*, 77–93. doi:10.1111/j.1468-2850.2007.00065.x

Skodol, A. E. (2012). Personality disorders in *DSM–5*. *Annual Review of Clinical Psychology, 8*, 317–344. doi:10.1146/annurev-clinpsy-032511-143131

Skodol, A. E., Gunderson, J. G., Shea, M. T., McGlashan, T. H., Morey, L. C., Sanislow, C. A., . . . Stout, R. L. (2005). The Collaborative Longitudinal Personality Disorders Study (CLPS): Overview and implications. *Journal of Personality Disorders, 19*, 487–504. doi:10.1521/pedi.2005.19.5.487

Smith, G. T., McCarthy, D. M., & Zapolski, T. C. B. (2009). On the value of homogeneous constructs for construct validation, theory testing, and the description of psychopathology. *Psychological Assessment, 21*, 272–284. doi:10.1037/a0016699

South, S. C., Reichborn-Kjennerud, T., Eaton, N. R., & Krueger, R. F. (2012). Behavior and molecular genetics of personality disorders. In T. A. Widiger (Ed.), *The Oxford handbook of personality disorders* (pp. 143–165). New York, NY: Oxford Press.

Spitzer, R. L., Endicott, J., & Gibbon, M. (1979). Crossing the border into borderline personality and borderline schizophrenia: Development of criteria. *Archives of General Psychiatry, 36*, 17–24. doi:10.1001/archpsyc.1979.01780010023001

Spitzer, R. L., First, M. B., Shedler, J., Westen, D., & Skodol, A. E. (2008). Clinical utility of five dimensional systems for personality diagnosis: A "consumer preference" study. *Journal of Nervous and Mental Disease, 196*, 356–374. doi:10.1097/NMD.0b013e3181710950

Sprock, J. (2000). Gender-typed behavioral examples of histrionic personality disorder. *Journal of Psychopathology and Behavioral Assessment, 22*, 107–122. doi:10.1023/A:1007514522708

Tenney, N. H., Schotte, C. K. W., Denys, D. A. J. P., van Megen, H. J. G. M., & Westenberg, H. G. M. (2003). Assessment of *DSM–IV* personality disorders in obsessive-compulsive disorder: Comparison of clinical diagnosis, self-report questionnaire, and semi-structured interview. *Journal of Personality Disorders, 17,* 550–561. doi:10.1521/pedi.17.6.550.25352

Trull, T. J. (2005). Dimensional models of personality disorder: Coverage and cutoffs. *Journal of Personality Disorders, 19,* 262–282. doi:10.1521/pedi.2005.19.3.262

Trull, T. J., & Durrett, C. A. (2005). Categorical and dimensional models of personality disorder. *Annual Review of Clinical Psychology, 1,* 355–380. doi:10.1146/annurev.clinpsy.1.102803.144009

Tyrer, P., & Johnson, T. (1996). Establishing the severity of personality disorder. *The American Journal of Psychiatry, 153,* 1593–1597.

Verheul, R., & Widiger, T. A. (2004). A meta-analysis of the prevalence and usage of the personality disorder not otherwise specified (PDNOS) diagnosis. *Journal of Personality Disorders, 18,* 309–319.

Watson, D. (2004). Stability versus change, dependability versus error: Issues in the assessment of personality over time. *Journal of Research in Personality, 38,* 319–350. doi:10.1016/j.jrp.2004.03.001

Westen, D. (1997). Divergences between clinical and research methods for assessing personality disorders: Implications for research and the evolution of Axis II. *The American Journal of Psychiatry, 154,* 895–903.

Westen, D., & Arkowitz-Westen, L. (1998). Limitations of Axis II in diagnosing personality pathology in clinical practice. *The American Journal of Psychiatry, 155,* 1767–1771.

Westen, D., DeFife, J. A., Bradley, B., & Hilsenroth, M. J. (2010). Prototype personality diagnosis in clinical practice: A viable alternative for *DSM–5* and *ICD–11. Professional Psychology: Research and Practice, 41,* 482–487. doi:10.1037/a0021555

Westen, D., Shedler, J., & Bradley, R. (2006). A prototype approach to personality disorder diagnosis. *The American Journal of Psychiatry, 163,* 846–856. doi:10.1176/appi.ajp.163.5.846

Widiger, T. A., & Corbitt, E. (1994). Normal versus abnormal personality from the perspective of the DSM. In S. Strack & M. Lorr (Eds.), *Differentiating normal and abnormal personality* (pp. 158–175). New York, NY: Springer.

Widiger, T. A., & Samuel, D. B. (2005). Diagnostic categories or dimensions? A question for the *Diagnostic and Statistical Manual of Mental Disorders—Fifth Edition. Journal of Abnormal Psychology, 114,* 494–504. doi:10.1037/0021-843X.114.4.494

Widiger, T. A., & Trull, T. J. (2007). Plate tectonics in the classification of personality disorder: Shifting to a dimensional model. *American Psychologist, 62,* 71–83. doi:10.1037/0003-066X.62.2.71

Wright, A. G. C., Thomas, K. M., Hopwood, C. J., Markon, K. E., Pincus, A. L., & Krueger, R. F. (2012). The hierarchical structure of *DSM–5* pathological personality traits. *Journal of Abnormal Psychology, 121,* 951–957. doi:10.1037/a0027669

Zanarini, M. C., Frankenburg, F. R., Hennen, J., Reich, D. B., & Silk, K. R. (2005). The McLean Study of Adult Development (MSAD): Overview and implications of the first six years of prospective follow-up. *Journal of Personality Disorders, 19*, 505–523. doi:10.1521/pedi.2005.19.5.505

Zanarini, M. C., Frankenburg, F. R., Reich, D. B., & Fitzmaurice, G. (2010). The 10-year course of psychosocial functioning among patients with borderline personality disorder and Axis II comparison subjects. *Acta Psychiatrica Scandinavica, 122*, 103–109. doi:10.1111/j.1600-0447.2010.01543.x

Zimmerman, M., Chelminski, I., & Young, D. (2008). The frequency of personality disorders in psychiatric patients. *Psychiatric Clinics of North America, 31*, 405–420. doi:10.1016/j.psc.2008.03.015

Zimmerman, M., Rothschild, L., & Chelminski, I. (2005). The prevalence of DSM–IV personality disorders in psychiatric outpatients. *The American Journal of Psychiatry, 162*, 1911–1918. doi:10.1176/appi.ajp.162.10.1911

3

THE ROLE OF TRAITS IN DESCRIBING, ASSESSING, AND UNDERSTANDING PERSONALITY PATHOLOGY

KRISTIAN E. MARKON AND KATHERINE G. JONAS

Although trait models of personality pathology have been proposed for some time, their formal recognition recently in authoritative nosologies—for example, the *Diagnostic and Statistical Manual of Mental Disorders* (5th ed. [*DSM–5*]; American Psychiatric Association, 2013) and the 11th revision of the *International Classification of Diseases* (*ICD–11*) draft—has greatly increased their salience to researchers, clinicians, and the general public. *DSM–5*, for example, includes within Section III the trait model proposed by the *DSM–5* Personality Disorders Workgroup (American Psychiatric Association, 2013); the *ICD–11* draft currently comprises a trait model as well (Tyrer et al., 2011). This chapter reviews reasons for the movement toward trait models, beginning with a discussion of what trait models are, including some select examples of trait models, before reviewing theoretical and empirical arguments in favor of trait models.

http://dx.doi.org/10.1037/14549-004
Personality Disorders: Toward Theoretical and Empirical Integration in Diagnosis and Assessment,
S. K. Huprich (Editor)

WHAT IS A TRAIT MODEL? A DEFINITION BY WAY OF EXAMPLES

In order to understand the movement toward trait models, it is necessary to understand what traits and trait models are. Although this may seem obvious to some, the increasing prominence of trait models in the literature and official nomenclature has led to confusion about what these paradigms actually are.

Paraphrasing Tellegen (1991), a *trait* may be defined as a variable underlying a relatively stable disposition toward particular behavioral patterns. Aspects of this definition can be interpreted more or less flexibly—for example, the definition of "relatively stable" is intentionally vague and debatable—but the general idea is that a trait is some construct or structure that accounts for the tendency of a person to behave in predictable ways across time. When someone is relatively aggressive, for example, it is implied that the individual is more likely than others to interpret ambiguous social cues as being hostile, is more likely to attend to power dynamics in relationships, is more likely to respond to stress with behaviors that harm others, and so forth (James & LeBreton, 2010). Aggressiveness, similarly, is the variable used to quantify or describe tendencies toward these behavioral patterns.

As Johnson (1997) suggested, in a trait model, different traits are used together as building blocks to characterize someone's personality functioning. That is, to satisfactorily characterize someone's personality functioning within a trait model, it is necessary to characterize his or her standing on all the traits within the model, implicitly or explicitly. In a model comprising three traits—for example, negative emotionality, positive emotionality, and disinhibition—one would assess an individual's standing on all three traits in order to provide a generally complete description of that individual's personality functioning. This would be true of nonclinical as well as clinical populations, although nonclinical trait levels might not be a focus of communication in clinical settings (see Hopwood, 2011, for an expanded discussion of this issue).

In recent years, confusion has arisen about certain aspects of trait models. For example, although most trait models do assume, with empirical support, that traits vary continuously in the population, smoothly from low to moderate to high standing on the trait, this is not necessary within a trait model. A trait might exhibit a number of distributions, including various non-normal distributions (e.g., Ferrando, 2003; Jonas & Markon, 2013; Woods & Lin, 2009). Moreover, the phenotypic expression of a trait as a unitary construct does not necessarily imply that it is subtended by a single psychological or neural structure. A single unitary trait might result from a distributed structure, such as a network of brain regions or cognitions, that is dynamically linked in such a way as to behave as a larger unit. In such cases, a trait might be thought of as reflecting the status of an underlying distributed structure considered as a whole.

BIG TRAIT MODELS

The best-known trait models are arguably the Big Trait models: the Big Two (Digman, 1997), Big Three (e.g., Eysenck & Eysenck, 1976; Tellegen, 2000), Big Four (e.g., Austin & Deary, 2000; Livesley, Jang, & Vernon, 1998; O'Connor & Dyce, 1998), and Big Five (e.g., Goldberg, 1993) models. The Big Two traits, for example, include a trait reflecting general overall emotional and behavioral control, especially under stress, and another trait reflecting positive emotion and a general approach orientation to the environment. Big Three models generally bifurcate the stability trait of the Big Two into neuroticism or negative emotionality trait on the one hand and disinhibition on the other, retaining the positive emotionality or extroversion trait. The Big Four models are similar, but they bifurcate the disinhibition trait into two traits: one related to aggression or disagreeableness and the other related to unconscientiousness or impulsivity. The Big Five, arguably the best known of the Big Trait models (and arguably of all trait models), retains the Big Four structure, except that it distinguishes between extraversion and a trait related to ideational flexibility, imagination, absorption, and cognitive ability, variously interpreted as openness to experience, intellectual engagement, or psychotic liability (DeYoung, Grazioplene, & Peterson, 2012; Saucier, 1992; Trapnell, 1994). The Big Trait models can be treated as being related to one another within a single hierarchical framework (Digman, 1997; Markon, Krueger, & Watson, 2005), in that Big Trait models with more traits can be thought of as representing personality variation in greater detail than those with fewer traits, rather than representing different traits altogether. For example, Big Four or Big Five disagreeableness and unconscientiousness generally can be thought of as subfactors or subtraits of Big Three disinhibition; disagreeableness and unconscientiousness are not absent from the Big Three but are subsumed within the higher order disinhibition trait within that model.

The Big Trait models generally posit that personality pathology reflects the extremes of trait continua, so that the difference between normal and abnormal personality is one of degree rather than kind. Through this approach, the Big Trait models have been shown to account empirically for patterns of individual differences in personality disorder (PD; e.g., Samuel & Widiger, 2008). Often, both extremes of a trait are assumed to be associated with personality pathology (e.g., extreme introversion as well as extraversion are assumed to be associated with pathology), although this is currently a matter of debate (e.g., Samuel, 2011; Widiger, Lynam, Miller, & Oltmanns, 2012).

Trait models have also recently been introduced into official nomenclature through the *DSM–5* and *ICD*. The *DSM–5* trait model was part of the Personality and Personality Disorders Work Group proposal and appears in Section III. In many ways, at the domain level, the *DSM–5* trait model can be thought of as a variant of the Big Five: Negative affectivity represents a variant of neuroticism; detachment, a variant of extroversion; antagonism, a variety of disagreeableness; disinhibition, a variety of unconscientiousness; and psychoticism, a variant of openness (see also Harkness, Finn, McNulty, & Shields, 2012). Although there is debate over whether psychoticism reflects the same trait as openness (e.g., DeYoung et al., 2012; Watson, Clark, & Chmielewski, 2008), emerging evidence suggests the former can be thought of as an extreme, maladaptive variant of the latter, especially in the presence of relatively poor cognitive functioning (DeYoung et al., 2012; Nusbaum & Silvia, 2011).

Although the *DSM–5* trait model is relatively new in a certain sense, it is not in other ways, as it is essentially a variant of well-established models in the literature (e.g., Goldberg, 1993; Harkness et al., 2012). The *DSM–5* model, moreover, has already demonstrated considerable support in the literature. For example, the *DSM–5* traits account for substantial variance in *Diagnostic and Statistical Manual of Mental Disorders* (4th ed.; *DSM–IV*; American Psychiatric Association, 1994) PD symptom counts (Hopwood, Thomas, Markon, Wright, & Krueger, 2012), and they show predicted relationships with Big Five (e.g., Thomas et al., 2013) and other constructs (e.g., Anderson et al., 2013; Strickland, Drislane, Lucy, Krueger, & Patrick, 2013; Watson, Stasik, Ro, & Clark, 2013). Measures of the *DSM–5* trait model demonstrate self-informant convergent validity (Markon, Quilty, Bagby, & Krueger, 2013), have been studied in multiple cultural settings and age groups (e.g., De Clercq et al., 2014), and show utility in understanding psychotherapeutic constructs (e.g., in predicting cognitive biases and beliefs associated with and targeted by cognitive–behavioral therapy for PDs; Hopwood, Schade, Krueger, Wright, & Markon, 2013).

The *ICD* trait model is currently in draft form and, therefore, may change (Tyrer et al., 2011). However, in its current form, the *ICD* proposal comprises five traits, resembling the Big Four with an additional emotional instability trait, roughly corresponding to borderline PD. Therefore, although the *ICD* proposal also includes five traits, one of these traits does not correspond well to traditional Big Trait models (although the emotional stability trait might be seen as a very abstract trait corresponding to the first of the Big Two traits, at a different level from the other four; e.g., Digman, 1997).

Both the *DSM* and *ICD* proposals for PD assessment include two fundamental elements of a diagnosis: a specification of overall level of impairment or severity and a specification of which trait elevations are implicated in clinically significant impairment, if there is such impairment. The proposals resemble the criteria for intellectual developmental disability in this regard (American Psychiatric Association, 2013), in that elevation or extreme standing on a trait is assumed to result in some form of impairment. One important area for future research is how traits and impairment are actually related. For example, can traits and impairment be empirically distinguished? Are both ends of a trait continuum related to impairment (e.g., is extreme extraversion as well as extreme introversion related to impairment; Samuel, 2011)?

PSYCHOMETRIC ARGUMENTS FOR TRAIT MODELS: RELIABILITY AND VALIDITY

Given the long history of arguments in favor of trait models (e.g., Eysenck, 1970; A. Lewis, 1938; Mapother, 1926; Strauss, 1973), it is somewhat surprising that trait paradigms did not appear in official PD nosology earlier (see Frances, 1980, for perspective on this issue). A number of arguments, theoretical as well as empirical, can be made in favor of trait models of personality pathology and of psychopathology in general.

One of the most fundamental arguments in favor of trait models, for example, is that they tend to beget measures that are more reliable and valid (in a predictive or criterion-related sense) than those begotten by typological models (Clark, 1999; Markon, Chmielewski, & Miller, 2011; Widiger, 1992). This follows from the assumption that the traits are continuous, which leads to continuous or quasi-continuous measures of those constructs. A large body of psychometric literature has demonstrated that, all other things being equal, continuous measures are generally more reliable and produce larger observed correlations than do discrete measures of the same constructs. This is so because when an underlying construct is actually continuous, discretizing the construct through its measurement results in a loss of information (e.g., MacCallum, Zhang, Preacher, & Rucker, 2002). Individuals who are similar on the trait but near the point of discretization may be classified differently, and individuals who are different on the trait but on the same side of the discretization point may be classified in the same way. Information about the trait level is lost, resulting in a much coarser level of measurement and lower reliabilities and validities. Conversely, if a trait or construct is actually discrete, retaining a continuous level of measurement is unlikely to lose information, resulting in equally reliable and valid measures as a discrete measure. In this way, continuous measures will be at least as reliable and valid as discrete measures and generally will be more reliable and valid (MacCallum et al., 2002).

Empirical studies comparing continuous and discrete measures of personality pathology constructs support psychometric theory, in that continuous measures tend to outperform discrete measures. In various systematic reviews, for example, continuous measures of personality pathology have been found to be more reliable than discrete measures of the same constructs (Clark, 1999; Widiger, 1992). More generally, meta-analyses have shown that, on average, continuous measures of various forms of psychopathology are 15% more reliable and 37% more valid (in a correlation metric) than discrete measures (Markon et al., 2011). In these meta-analyses, continuous and categorical measures of the same construct were compared with regard to different forms of reliability (e.g., cross-interviewer and test–retest reliability) and criterion-related validity. These meta-analyses demonstrate that the superiority of continuous measures with regard to reliability and validity does not appear to vary across type of psychopathology or setting, and they suggest that similar gains will be seen with measures of personality pathology (Markon et al., 2011).

As was noted, trait models do not need to assume continuous traits or use continuous measures of those traits. Conversely, continuous measures can be used within typological frameworks, as when a continuous measure is used to quantify how many features of a type an individual possesses (Morey et al., 2007, 2012; Skodol et al., 2005). However, in general, most common trait models do assume that traits are continuous and are associated with continuous indicators. Also, typological measures essentially by definition have as an ultimate goal some discrete classification, which implies some discretization at some point even if a continuous indicator is used. As such, trait models allow for measures that are more reliable and produce greater predictive and concurrent validities.

INCREASING INCREMENTAL VALIDITY THROUGH THE HOMOGENEITY OF EXPLANATORY UNITS

Traits function as building blocks, or explanatory units, in accounting for patterns of individual differences in behavior (Johnson, 1997). As such, they are generally posited to be relatively unidimensional in nature, in the sense of being dominated by a single factor. For example, although measures of neuroticism can be thought of in terms of more specific subtraits such as depressivity or emotional lability (DeYoung, Quilty, & Peterson, 2007), they nevertheless are all highly correlated enough to be accounted for by a single broad trait reflecting negative emotionality or avoidance-related processing. In this sense, neuroticism is unidimensional and relatively homogeneous in the context of other personality characteristics such as extroversion.

Many typological models, in contrast, comprise constructs that are more heterogeneous. For example, PDs listed in the third edition of the *Diagnostic and Statistical Manual of Mental Disorders* (3rd ed.; *DSM–III*; American Psychiatric Association, 1980) and *DSM–IV* include overlapping criteria (e.g., antisocial and borderline disorders both include impulsivity as a criterion), and structural analyses have demonstrated that symptom areas span multiple personality types (e.g., Austin & Deary, 2000; Livesley et al., 1998; O'Connor & Dyce, 1998). To the extent that types represent forms of individual differences in behavior in a typological paradigm, they are less unidimensional in nature.

Although, in a theoretical sense, this unidimensionality is not necessary, it has the advantage of increasing the incremental validity of the explanatory units with regard to some outcome or criterion. That is, each trait will add to another trait in the prediction of external criteria more than more heterogeneous constructs would. This is related to issues of collinearity in regression and correlations among predictors, in that correlations among predictors decrease their incremental validity. Although traits can be correlated, for any given set of measures, they will be less correlated than a construct that is more heterogeneous with regard to that set of measures. For example, knowing an individual meets criteria for two disorders such as Avoidant and Schizotypal Personality Disorders may be less informative, given the overlap between their characteristics, than knowing the same individual's standing on two traits such as detachment and psychoticism, which are more distinct. In this sense, each trait provides a more differentiated quantum of information in communicating about or predicting individual differences in behavior.

As an example, for this chapter, we examined the incremental validity of trait and type scorings of the SCID-II PDs screening questionnaire (First, Gibbon, Spitzer, William, & Benjamin, 1997) in the 2000 British Office for National Statistics (ONS) Survey of Psychiatric Morbidity (ONSPM; Jenkins et al., 2003; Singleton, Bumpstead, O'Brien, Lee, & Meltzer, 2003). The 2000 ONSPM is part of a set of population-representative psychiatric epidemiological surveys conducted in Great Britain during recent decades (Jenkins et al., 1997). Individuals in the 2000 ONSPM were recruited via a stratified multistage random probability sample strategy, resulting in data on 8,405 individuals (44.7% were male, 55.3% were female, and the average age was 46.0 years). The SCID personality screening inventory is a 116-item measure of personality pathology designed to screen for *DSM–IV* PDs. We scored this instrument in two ways: using sum scores reflecting *DSM–IV* symptom counts for each diagnosis and using trait sum scores (in which trait scores were based on the items' largest loadings in a seven-factor exploratory factor analysis of the *DSM–IV* items with promax rotation; cf. Austin & Deary, 2000).[1]

To determine the average incremental validity of traits and type scores, we randomly sampled either two trait or two type scores and entered them sequentially to predict a criterion using hierarchical regression. We did this 1,000 times with both the trait and type scores and each time calculated the increase in R^2 associated with the second score. We also examined two outcome criteria: internalizing psychopathology, as reflected in the sum of Revised Clinical Interview Schedule scale scores (G. Lewis & Pelosi, 1990; G. Lewis, Pelosi, Araya, & Dunne, 1992), and substance use problems, as reflected in a sum of number of substance dependence criteria met during the previous year. In these analyses, the increase in variance accounted for with the addition of a trait score or a type score could be interpreted as the average incremental validity of a trait relative to other traits and the average incremental validity of types relative to other types.

As predicted, the trait scores demonstrated greater incremental validity than the type scores for both criterion variables. For the internalizing criterion, the mean increase in R^2 with the addition of the trait scores was .073 and with the addition of the type scores was .064. (Note that the average total R^2 for the trait and type scores were .178 and .169, respectively.) For the substance use criterion, the increase in R^2 with the addition of the trait scores was .038 and with the addition of the type scores was .025. (Note that the average total R^2 for the trait and type scores were .086 and .061, respectively.) In general, the use of relatively unidimensional variables, such as are found in trait paradigms, increased the incremental validity of those variables relative to what would be observed with the use of more heterogeneous variables. From this point of view, trait measures are more differentiated and provide more differentiated information (predictively speaking) than do typological measures, even when both are assessed continuously.

EMPIRICAL EVIDENCE FOR CONTINUITY IN PERSONALITY PATHOLOGY

As has been noted, although trait models do not need to assume continuousness, they generally do, and typological models do necessarily imply some level of discreteness in the distribution. In this regard, statistical tests of

---

[1]Seven factors were retained on the basis of their interpretability and similarity to factors reported by Austin and Deary (2000) using the same instrument. The factors reflected social anxiety, antisociality, attention seeking, introversion, eccentricity, compulsivity, and emotional lability. These are very similar (although not identical) to those identified by Austin and Deary. Moreover, as was reported by Austin and Deary, a four-factor higher order exploratory analysis of the seven factors yields the Big Four traits.

the continuousness versus discreteness of personality variation provide direct empirical evidence regarding the appropriateness of trait models.

In general, the continuousness of personality variation has been examined statistically in two ways: psychometric or phenomenological continuity. *Psychometric continuity* refers to continuity in the distribution of a variable itself, in terms of its shape, such as whether it is bimodal or shows other signs of discreteness. *Phenomenological continuity* refers to continuity in how a variable relates to other criteria, in terms of whether or not there are discontinuities in relationships, such as sudden changes in personality pathology as risk factors increase, or sudden changes in consequences of personality pathology as trait levels increase.

Empirical Evidence From Psychometric Continuity Models

Tests of psychometric continuity statistically compare continuous and discrete accounts of how a personality characteristic is distributed in the population. As a simplified example, a personality trait such as narcissism could be normally distributed in the population, or it could be bimodal, reflecting distinct groups of individuals. To formally compare these two possibilities, researchers have generally used either taxometric procedures or latent variable models. Both methods have largely found symptoms of personality pathology to be continuously distributed.

Taxometric procedures developed by Golden and Meehl (Golden, 1982; Meehl, 1973) search for zones of rarity in the distribution of symptoms. This method was first used to identify a latent taxon of schizoid characteristics (Golden & Meehl, 1979) and was later applied to symptoms of Borderline, Schizotypal, and Antisocial Personality Disorders, which were interpreted in one initial qualitative review as generally supportive of taxonicity (Haslam, 2003). More recently, however, taxometric analyses have found support for dimensional models of narcissism and Avoidant, Dependent, Obsessive-Compulsive, Depressive, Borderline, and Paranoid Personality Disorders (Arntz et al., 2009; Foster & Campbell, 2007; Olatunji, Williams, Haslam, Abramowitz, & Tolin, 2008; Rothschild, Cleland, Haslam, & Zimmerman, 2003).

Although early taxometric analyses tended to support discrete models, more recent findings have tended to support dimensional accounts. This discrepancy has been shown to be partly attributable to methodological differences (Haslam, Holland, & Kuppens, 2012). Early taxometric analyses depended on visual inspection of plots by the researcher, who then decided whether the graphs were more reflective of dimensionality or taxonicity. A more stringent variation of taxometric analysis, developed by Ruscio, Ruscio, and Meron (2007), compares the observed data to simulated data generated from dimensional and discrete models and generates an empirical measure of model fit. An example of the contrast between subjective and empirical taxometric analysis can be seen in the domain of antisocial behavior and psychopathy. Early studies argued for a discrete taxon of antisocial individuals (e.g., Skilling, Harris, Rice, & Quinsey, 2002), but the taxonic model has been countered by a plethora of studies that used the methods of Ruscio et al. (2007) and that support a dimensional model (e.g., Guay, Ruscio, Knight, & Hare, 2007; Marcus, Lilienfeld, Edens, & Poythress, 2006). As a rule, studies using empirical measures of fit support dimensional models of personality pathology (Haslam et al., 2012). The one exception to the trend of psychometric dimensionality, in the domain of schizotypy, may again be attributable to differences in statistical methods, as studies using visual inspection (e.g., Fossati, Raine, Borroni, & Maffei, 2007) find evidence of taxonicity, but all studies reporting empirical fit support a dimensional model (e.g., Daneluzzo et al., 2009).

Psychometric studies employing latent variable methods are less common, and further use of these methods in the domain of personality pathology is necessary. In this approach, continuous latent variable models are directly compared to discrete latent variable models using standard inferential methods (e.g., Bayesian or frequentist model selection statistics or inferential tests, such as the Akaike information criterion or the Bayesian information criterion). Studies comparing discrete and continuous latent variable models in this way generally support a trait model of personality pathology, insofar as they suggest formal PD criteria have underlying continuous distributions. For example, Fossati et al.'s (1999) latent class analysis of Borderline Personality Disorder symptoms identified three latent classes, each with a progressively higher probability of symptom endorsement. Similarly, latent class analyses of Antisocial Personality Disorder have consistently resulted in numerous classes ordered by severity (Bucholz, Hesselbrock, Heath, Kramer, & Schuckit, 2000; Kovac, Mérette, Legault, Dongier, & Palmour, 2002). When the fits of continuous and discrete latent variable models are explicitly compared, continuous latent variable models are preferred in describing externalizing pathology, which includes antisocial personality pathology (Markon & Krueger, 2005). Comparisons between continuous and discrete latent variable models have supported continuous latent variable models of schizotypy as well (Ahmed et al., 2013).

Empirical Evidence From Phenomenological Continuity Models

Even if symptoms of psychopathology are distributed continuously, they may be discontinuous in their relationships with other constructs (Flett, Vredenburg, & Krames, 1997). For example, pathological personality traits may suddenly increase at some point along a risk dimension, even if the traits are themselves normally distributed (e.g., levels of emotional lability might suddenly increase at a certain level of trauma exposure). Alternatively, personality pathology might suddenly increase risk of certain outcomes beyond some point (e.g., risk of unemployment might accelerate at some level of impulsivity).

When personality characteristics for phenomenological discontinuities are studied, impairment is a particularly important construct to examine, as psychological phenomena are generally considered pathological only when associated with distress, harm, or impairment. If a trait is phenomenologically continuous with regard to impairment, change along the dimension of the trait will be associated with equivalent changes in distress and impairment. Though limited, the existing research on this topic suggests this relationship holds true.

Studies of personality, impairment, and psychosocial functioning, for example, are generally consistent with the broader literature in showing that continuous measures demonstrate greater criterion-related validity than do discrete measures (Markon et al., 2011). Continuous measures of PD criteria account for variance in psychosocial functioning, disability, and treatment seeking beyond that explained by a categorical diagnosis of the same symptoms (Ahmed et al., 2013; Skodol et al., 2005), but the inverse is not true: Categorical diagnoses do not provide information about psychosocial functioning in excess of that provided by dimensional measures. In the assessment of criminality, dimensional measures have again been shown to be superior to categorical measures. In one study, categorical diagnosis correctly classified 61.6% of individuals as either criminal offenders or controls, and dimensional assessment correctly identified 89.2% of cases (Ullrich, Borkenau, & Marneros, 2001).

Studies quantifying impairment associated with varying degrees of symptom severity have found that, across diagnostic categories, control, subthreshold, and suprathreshold patients demonstrate increasing degrees of impairment (Nakao et al., 1992). Such findings are consistent with analyses of *DSM–IV* PD criteria (Nestadt et al., 2006) showing that dimensions of personality pathology were generally associated with impaired functioning (the exception being compulsivity, which may have improved functioning up to a point). Furthermore, consecutive quintiles of "avoidant," "callous," and "egocentric" factors were associated with an increasing number of days of disability.

New methods, such as mixture structural equation models, have the ability to describe the relationship between psychopathology and impairment across all points of those dimensions (Bauer, 2005). Although these methods have not yet been applied to the study of personality pathology, they have shown internalizing and psychosis to be linearly related to impairment (Markon, 2010, and Jonas & Markon, 2013, respectively). To the extent that these constructs are closely related to personality pathology, the same findings may be expected in that domain. More research is clearly needed.

TRAITS AS FUNDAMENTAL ELEMENTS OF PERSONALITY THEORY

Although traits function as building blocks in describing individual differences in behavior, they also serve as fundamental explanatory elements of personality theory. A set of traits in combination can be used provide a comprehensive description of how an individual is functioning in his or her personality (e.g., a person is at a certain percentile of negative emotionality, another percentile of positive emotionality, another percentile of disinhibition, and so forth), but the set also can be used to elaborate theories about why individuals differ. In some sense, in fact, it might be argued that traits are necessary in elaborating theories about why individuals exhibit stable differences in personality and behavior.

Consider the definition of a trait we presented earlier (following Tellegen, 1991): "a variable underlying a relatively stable disposition toward particular behavioral patterns." As many, if not most, theories of individual differences posit propensities toward particular behavior patterns that are stable over some time frame, they will necessarily imply traits, by definition. Individual differences in those dispositions are represented by traits, with each trait reflecting variability in the tendency to exhibit a particular behavioral pattern, as well as variability in the underlying structures involved (e.g., etiologic network, physical structure). A given trait represents variation in a single psychological structure that forms a part of the numerous structures that account for individual differences in behavior.

Even type theories often implicitly incorporate traits as part of their structure. Consider, for example, a theory of borderline personality disorder (BPD) that accounts for the disorder partially in terms of emotional dysregulation and impulsivity, resulting from inconsistent attachment experiences during development and other factors (e.g., genetic liability; Levy, 2005; Nigg, Silk, Stavro, & Miller, 2005; Skodol et al., 2002). In an important sense, any given deficit in emotional dysregulation or impulsivity reflects one end of a trait that ranges from a healthy state, through normative states, to disordered states. Because BPD comprises a number of such variables—including those related to impulsivity, dissociative phenomena, and identity—it might be argued that the borderline personality type is implicitly defined in terms of a confluence of traits.

The *DSM–5* PD proposal, now in Section III of the *DSM*, recognizes this by defining PD types partly in terms of trait status (American Psychiatric Association, 2013). Together with characteristic forms of psychosocial impairment, each PD is defined in terms of a characteristic set of trait abnormalities. Schizotypal Personality Disorder, for example, is defined in terms of significant cognitive dysregulation, unusual beliefs, eccentricity, restricted affectivity, withdrawal, and suspiciousness. In this way, traits form the elemental units or building blocks in defining types.

Some authors have approached the relationship between traits and types by distinguishing traits and types as variable-centered versus person-centered approaches, respectively, in describing and explaining personality differences between individuals (Mervielde & Asendorpf, 2000). Trait paradigms are focused on the structures that vary and constitute sources of differences across individuals; type paradigms focus on descriptions of the persons themselves, in terms of how a person with a given combination of trait values would appear psychologically.

BRIDGING IDIOGRAPHIC AND NOMOTHETIC PERSPECTIVES ON PERSONALITY

The problem of how to integrate idiographic and nomothetic perspectives on personality—that is, perspectives derived from within the framework of an individual versus those derived from within the framework of comparisons among individuals (Allport, 1962)—is long-standing and common in applied clinical work. Clinicians are typically faced with integrating scientific findings, which are almost always nomothetic summaries of patterns in groups of individuals, with idiographic problems as they present in each client. This is a core issue in clinical decision making, creating problems such as defining the appropriate population from which a client is assumed to come and identifying when exceptions are to be made in making predictions (i.e., the "broken leg problem"; Dawes, Faust, & Meehl, 1989; Grove & Meehl, 1996). The fundamental question is, how unique is an individual and in what respects?

Although most common trait models are inherently nomothetic in nature, it might be argued that traits help bridge idiographic and nomothetic perspectives on personality. Traits provide a framework that is common to all persons; within this framework, persons are individuated by their standing on the traits and the intersection of their standings on all the traits. The profile implied by an individual's standing on all the traits considered together defines a relatively specific description of a person (as a hypothetical example, consider that if five traits each can take on 10 values, this still implies 100,000 different possible profiles; with more specific traits and more values, the number of possible profiles increases even more). These profile differences are strictly speaking nomothetic in nature, but they do help bring a clinician or other assessor closer to a fully idiographic approach, if for no other reason than that they provide a very detailed, individuating description of personality. This is especially true relative to type approaches, which reduce idiographic variation among individuals to small sets of types.

Trait models facilitate idiographic approaches to personality in other ways. Some authors, for example, have argued that even when two individuals have the same level of a trait, they may express that trait level in very different ways, leading to idiographic expressions of traits (Nesselroade, Gerstorf, Hardy, & Ram, 2007). One individual, for example, may be emotionally manipulative in close relationships, while another individual may express manipulativeness in the workplace, perhaps by undermining others' efforts. Others have argued for idiographic traits themselves; that is, relatively stable behavioral environment-response patterns that are nevertheless unique to a single person (e.g., Allport, 1965; Molenaar, 2004). A specific individual may exhibit relatively stable patterns of behavior that vary in strength over time, such as a certain type of coping behavior in response to a certain type of stressor, that are specific to that individual. Although it can be difficult to interpret idiographic traits or expressions of traits vis-à-vis nomothetic constructs—how can one understand patterns of behavior that are truly unique to a single person?—some have suggested that patterns of associations with and among idiographic factors are what inherently define the meanings of those factors, in the sense of an idiographic nomological network. For example, if some idiographic pattern reflects anxiety, it should increase in response to situations that typically provoke anxiety, decrease in response to situations that are generally calming, and be related to other expressions of negative emotion such as depression (e.g., Nesselroade et al., 2007; see also Haynes, Mumma, & Pinson, 2009, for a discussion of idiographic assessment in clinical contexts, which merits a great deal of further research).

As traits become more specific in nature, they are able to accommodate a more idiographic understanding of an individual's functioning. A framework involving a relatively large number of specific, more narrowly defined traits is able to describe idiosyncrasies of personality through the sheer number of available profiles. As these traits become more specific in expression or become more specific to the point of being specific to a given individual, a more fully idiographic approach is made possible. Of course, as these traits become more idiographic or specific in nature, it becomes more likely that they are less generalizable to the entire population. As such, it becomes necessary to identify an optimal balance between breadth and generalizability on the one hand and specificity and lack of generalizability on the other.

CONCLUSION

With a rich history in personality theory and assessment, trait models are now being introduced into official nomenclature. There are a number of reasons for this, theoretical as well as empirical and practical. Traits represent fundamental elements of frameworks for explaining and describing individual differences, and they have tremendous utility in constructing comprehensive theories of personality variation. They help to bridge relatively nomothetic approaches to personality with more idiographic approaches. Empirical evidence supports the continuity of traits and trait measures, which have greater reliability and criterion-related validity than do discrete, typological approaches to personality assessment.

As research on personality and personality pathology moves forward, more research is needed to address questions related to the processes underlying traits and how they manifest in specific individuals. What, for example, are the core processes—neural, genetic, environmental, social—underlying traits such as emotional lability or disorganized thinking? How are the explanations provided at different levels of analysis related to one another? How might these processes manifest differently in different individuals across time? These and other questions, motivated by trait theory, hold great promise in better describing, assessing, and understanding the psychological challenges that individuals face across their life span.

REFERENCES

Ahmed, A. O., Green, B. A., Goodrum, N. M., Doane, N. J., Birgenheir, D., & Buckley, P. F. (2013). Does a latent class underlie schizotypal personality disorder? Implications for schizophrenia. *Journal of Abnormal Psychology, 122,* 475–491. doi:10.1037/a0032713

Allport, G. W. (1962). The general and the unique in psychological science. *Journal of Personality, 30,* 405–422. doi:10.1111/j.1467-6494.1962.tb02313.x

Allport, G. W. (1965). *Letters from Jenny.* New York, NY: Harcourt.

American Psychiatric Association. (1980). *Diagnostic and statistical manual of mental disorders* (3rd ed.). Washington, DC: Author.

American Psychiatric Association. (1994). *Diagnostic and statistical manual of mental disorders* (4th ed.). Washington, DC: Author.

American Psychiatric Association. (2013). *Diagnostic and statistical manual of mental disorders* (5th ed.). Arlington, VA: Author.

Anderson, J. L., Sellbom, M., Bagby, R. M., Quilty, L. C., Veltri, C. O. C., Markon, K. E., & Krueger, R. F. (2013). On the convergence between PSY–5 domains and PID–5 domains and facets: Implications for assessment of *DSM–5* personality traits. *Assessment, 20,* 286–284. doi:10.1177/1073191112471141

Arntz, A., Bernstein, D., Gielen, D., van Nieuwenhuyzen, M., Penders, K., Haslam, N., & Ruscio, J. (2009). Taxometric evidence for the dimensional structure of Cluster-C, paranoid, and borderline personality disorders. *Journal of Personality Disorders, 23,* 606–628. doi:10.1521/pedi.2009.23.6.606

Austin, E. J., & Deary, I. J. (2000). The "four As": A common framework for normal and abnormal personality? *Personality and Individual Differences, 28,* 977–995. doi:10.1016/S0191-8869(99)00154-3

Bauer, D. (2005). A semiparametric approach to modeling nonlinear relations among latent variables. *Structural Equation Modeling, 12,* 513–535. doi:10.1207/s15328007sem1204_1

Bucholz, K. K., Hesselbrock, V. M., Heath, A. C., Kramer, J. R., & Schuckit, M. A. (2000). A latent class analysis of antisocial personality disorder symptom data from a multi-centre family study of alcoholism. *Addiction, 95,* 553–567. doi:10.1046/j.1360-0443.2000.9545537.x

Clark, L. A. (1999). Dimensional approaches to personality disorder assessment and diagnosis. In C. R. Cloninger (Ed.), *Personality and psychopathology* (pp. 219–244). Arlington, VA: American Psychiatric Press.

Daneluzzo, E., Stratta, P., Di Tommaso, S., Pacifico, R., Riccardi, I., & Rossi, A. (2009). Dimensional, non-taxonic latent structure of psychotic symptoms in a student sample. *Social Psychiatry and Psychiatric Epidemiology, 44,* 911–916. doi:10.1007/s00127-009-0028-2

Dawes, R. M., Faust, D., & Meehl, P. E. (1989, March 31). Clinical versus actuarial judgment. *Science, 243,* 1668–1674. doi:10.1126/science.2648573

De Clercq, B., De Fruyt, F., De Bolle, M., Van Hiel, A., Markon, K. E., & Krueger, R. F. (2014). The hierarchical structure and construct validity of the PID-5 trait measure in adolescence. *Journal of Personality, 82,* 158–169. doi:10.1111/jpoy.12042

DeYoung, C. G., Grazioplene, R. G., & Peterson, J. B. (2012). From madness to genius: The openness/intellect trait domain as a paradoxical simplex. *Journal of Research in Personality, 46,* 63–78. doi:10.1016/j.jrp.2011.12.003

DeYoung, C. G., Quilty, L. C., & Peterson, J. B. (2007). Between facets and domains: 10 aspects of the Big Five. *Journal of Personality and Social Psychology, 93,* 880–896. doi:10.1037/0022-3514.93.5.880

Digman, J. M. (1997). Higher-order factors of the Big Five. *Journal of Personality and Social Psychology, 73,* 1246–1256. doi:10.1037/0022-3514.73.6.1246

Eysenck, H. J. (1970). The classification of depressive illnesses. *British Journal of Psychiatry, 117,* 241–250. doi:10.1192/bjp.117.538.241

Eysenck, H. J., & Eysenck, S. B. G. (1976). *Psychoticism as a dimension of personality.* New York, NY: Crane, Russak.

Ferrando, P. J. (2003). The accuracy of the E, N and P trait estimates: An empirical study using the EPQ-R. *Personality and Individual Differences, 34*, 665–679. doi:10.1016/S0191-8869(02)00053-3

First, M. B., Gibbon, M., Spitzer, R. L., William, J. B. W., & Benjamin, L. (1997). *Structured Clinical Interview for DSM–IV Axis II Personality Disorders.* Washington, DC: American Psychiatric Press.

Flett, G. L., Vredenburg, K., & Krames, L. (1997). The continuity of depression in clinical and nonclinical samples. *Psychological Bulletin, 121*, 395–416. doi:10.1037/0033-2909.121.3.395

Fossati, A., Maffei, C., Bagnato, M., Donati, D., Namia, C., & Novella, L. (1999). Latent structure analysis of DSM–IV borderline personality disorder criteria. *Comprehensive Psychiatry, 40*, 72–79. doi:10.1016/S0010-440X(99)90080-9

Fossati, A., Raine, A., Borroni, S., & Maffei, C. (2007). Taxonic structure of schizotypal personality in nonclinical subjects: Issues of replicability and age consistency. *Psychiatry Research, 152*, 103–112. doi:10.1016/j.psychres.2004.04.019

Foster, J. D., & Campbell, W. K. (2007). Are there such things as "Narcissists" in social psychology? A taxometric analysis of the Narcissistic Personality Inventory. *Personality and Individual Differences, 43*, 1321–1332. doi:10.1016/j.paid.2007.04.003

Frances, A. (1980). The *DSM–III* personality disorders section: A commentary. *American Journal of Psychiatry, 137*, 1050–1054.

Goldberg, L. R. (1993). The structure of phenotypic personality traits. *American Psychologist, 48*, 26–34. doi:10.1037/0003-066X.48.1.26

Golden, R. R. (1982). A taxometric model for the detection of a conjectured latent taxon. *Multivariate Behavioral Research, 17*, 389–416. doi:10.1207/s15327906mbr1703_6

Golden, R. R., & Meehl, P. E. (1979). Detection of the schizoid taxon with MMPI indicators. *Journal of Abnormal Psychology, 88*, 217–233. doi:10.1037/0021-843X.88.3.217

Grove, W. M., & Meehl, P. E. (1996). Comparative efficiency of informal (subjective, impressionistic) and formal (mechanical, algorithmic) prediction procedures: The clinical–statistical controversy. *Psychology, Public Policy, and Law, 2*, 293–323. doi:10.1037/1076-8971.2.2.293

Guay, J.-P., Ruscio, J., Knight, R. A., & Hare, R. D. (2007). A taxometric analysis of the latent structure of psychopathy: Evidence for dimensionality. *Journal of Abnormal Psychology, 116*, 701–716. doi:10.1037/0021-843X.116.4.701

Harkness, A. R., Finn, J. A., McNulty, J. L., & Shields, S. M. (2012). The Personality Psychopathology—Five (PSY–5): Recent constructive replication and assessment literature review. *Psychological Assessment, 24*, 432–443. doi:10.1037/a0025830

Haslam, N. (2003). Categorical versus dimensional models of mental disorder: The taxometric evidence. *Australian and New Zealand Journal of Psychiatry, 37*, 696–704. doi:10.1080/j.1440-1614.2003.01258.x

Haslam, N., Holland, E., & Kuppens, P. (2012). Categories versus dimensions in personality and psychopathology: A quantitative review of taxometric research. *Psychological Medicine, 42*, 903–920. doi:10.1017/S0033291711001966

Haynes, S. N., Mumma, G. H., & Pinson, C. (2009). Idiographic assessment: Conceptual and psychometric foundations of individualized behavioral assessment. *Clinical Psychology Review, 29*, 179–191. doi:10.1016/j.cpr.2008.12.003

Hopwood, C. J. (2011). Personality traits in the *DSM–5*. *Journal of Personality Assessment, 93*, 398–405. doi:10.1080/00223891.2011.577472

Hopwood, C. J., Schade, N., Krueger, R. F., Wright, A. G. C., & Markon, K. E. (2013). Connecting *DSM–5* personality traits and pathological beliefs: Toward a unifying model. *Journal of Psychopathology and Behavioral Assessment, 35*, 162–172. doi:10.1007/s10862-012-9332-3

Hopwood, C. J., Thomas, K. M., Markon, K. E., Wright, A. G. C., & Krueger, R. F. (2012). *DSM–5* personality traits and *DSM–IV* personality disorders. *Journal of Abnormal Psychology, 121*, 424–432. doi:10.1037/a0026656

James, L. R., & LeBreton, J. M. (2010). Assessing aggression using conditional reasoning. *Current Directions in Psychological Science, 19*, 30–35. doi:10.1177/0963721409359279

Jenkins, R., Bebbington, P., Brugha, T., Farrell, M., Gill, B., Lewis, G., . . . Petticrew, M. (1997). The National Psychiatric Morbidity Surveys of Great Britain—Strategy and methods. *Psychological Medicine, 27*, 765–774. doi:10.1017/S003329179700531X

Jenkins, R., Bebbington, P., Brugha, T., Farrell, M., Gill, B., Lewis, G., . . . Petticrew, M. (2003). The National Psychiatric Morbidity Surveys of Great Britain—Strategy and methods. *International Review of Psychiatry, 15*, 5–13. doi:10.1080/0954026021000045895

Johnson, J. A. (1997). Units of analysis for the description and explanation of personality. In R. Hogan, J. A. Johnson, & S. Briggs (Eds.), *Handbook of personality* (pp. 73–93). San Diego, CA: Academic Press.

Jonas, K. G., & Markon, K. E. (2013). A model of psychosis and its relationship with impairment. *Social Psychiatry and Psychiatric Epidemiology, 48*, 1367–1375. doi:10.1007/s00127-012-0642-2

Kovac, I., Mérette, C., Legault, L., Dongier, M., & Palmour, R. M. (2002). Evidence in an international sample of alcohol-dependent subjects of subgroups with specific symptom patterns of antisocial personality disorder. *Alcoholism: Clinical and Experimental Research, 26*, 1088–1096. doi:10.1111/j.1530-0277.2002.tb02643.x

Levy, K. N. (2005). The implications of attachment theory and research for understanding borderline personality disorder. *Development and Psychopathology, 17*, 959–986. doi:10.1017/S0954579405050455

Lewis, A. (1938). States of depression: Their clinical and aetiological differentiation. *British Medical Journal, 2*, 875–878. doi:10.1136/bmj.2.4060.875

Lewis, G., & Pelosi, A. J. (1990). *Manual of the Revised Clinical Interview Schedule*. London, England: Institute of Psychiatry.

Lewis, G., Pelosi, A. J., Araya, R. C., & Dunne, G. (1992). Measuring psychiatric disorder in the community: A standardized assessment for use by lay interviewers. *Psychological Medicine, 22*, 465–486. doi:10.1017/S0033291700030415

Livesley, W. J., Jang, K. L., & Vernon, P. A. (1998). Phenotypic and genetic structure of traits delineating personality disorder. *Archives of General Psychiatry, 55*, 941–948. doi:10.1001/archpsyc.55.10.941

MacCallum, R. C., Zhang, S., Preacher, K. J., & Rucker, D. D. (2002). On the practice of dichotomization of quantitative variables. *Psychological Methods, 7*, 19–40. doi:10.1037/1082-989X.7.1.19

Mapother, E. (1926). Discussion on manic-depressive psychosis. *British Medical Journal, 2*, 872–879. doi:10.1136/bmj.2.3436.872

Marcus, D. K., Lilienfeld, S. O., Edens, J. F., & Poythress, N. G. (2006). Is antisocial personality disorder continuous or categorical? A taxometric analysis. *Psychological Medicine, 36*, 1571–1581. doi:10.1017/S0033291706008245

Markon, K. E. (2010). How things fall apart: Understanding the nature of internalizing through its relationship with impairment. *Journal of Abnormal Psychology, 119*, 447–458. doi:10.1037/a0019707

Markon, K. E., Chmielewski, M., & Miller, C. (2011). The reliability and validity of discrete and continuous measures of psychopathology: A quantitative review. *Psychological Bulletin, 137*, 856–879. doi:10.1037/a0023678

Markon, K. E., & Krueger, R. F. (2005). Categorical and continuous models of liability to externalizing disorders: A direct comparison in NESARC. *Archives of General Psychiatry, 62*, 1352–1359. doi:10.1001/archpsyc.62.12.1352

Markon, K. E., Krueger, R. F., & Watson, D. (2005). Delineating the structure of normal and abnormal personality: An integrative hierarchical approach. *Journal of Personality and Social Psychology, 88*, 139–157. doi:10.1037/0022-3514.88.1.139

Markon, K. E., Quilty, L. C., Bagby, R. M., & Krueger, R. F. (2013). The development and psychometric properties of an informant-report form of the Personality Inventory for *DSM–5* (PID–5). *Assessment, 20*, 370–383. doi:10.1177/1073191113486513

Meehl, P. E. (1973). MAXCOV-HITMAX: A taxonomic search method for loose genetic syndromes. In P. E. Meehl (Ed.), *Psychodiagnosis: Selected papers* (pp. 200–224). Minneapolis: University of Minnesota Press.

Mervielde, I., & Asendorpf, J. B. (2000). Variable-centered and person-centered approaches to childhood personality. In S. E. Hampson (Ed.), *Advances in personality psychology* (Vol. 1, pp. 37–76). Philadelphia, PA: Psychology Press.

Molenaar, P. C. M. (2004). A manifesto on psychology as idiographic science: Bringing the person back into scientific psychology, this time forever. *Measurement: Interdisciplinary Research and Perspectives, 2*, 201–218. doi:10.1207/s15366359mea0204_1

Morey, L. C., Hopwood, C. J., Gunderson, J. G., Skodol, A. E., Shea, M. T., Yen, S., . . . McGlashan, T. H. (2007). Comparison of alternative models for personality disorders. *Psychological Medicine, 37*, 983–994. doi:10.1017/S003329 1706009482

Morey, L. C., Hopwood, C. J., Markowitz, J. C., Gunderson, J. G., Grilo, C. M., McGlashan, T. H., . . . Skodol, A. E. (2012). Comparison of alternative models for personality disorders, II: 6-, 8- and 10-year follow-up. *Psychological Medicine, 42*, 1705–1713. doi:10.1017/S0033291711002601

Nakao, K., Gunderson, J. G., Phillips, K. A., Tanaka, N., Yorifuji, K., Takaishi, J., & Nishimura, T. (1992). Functional impairment in personality disorders. *Journal of Personality Disorders, 6*, 24–33. doi:10.1521/pedi.1992.6.1.24

Nesselroade, J. R., Gerstorf, D., Hardy, S. A., & Ram, N. (2007). Idiographic filters for psychological constructs. *Measurement: Interdisciplinary Research and Perspectives, 5*, 217–235. doi:10.1080/15366360701741807

Nestadt, G., Hsu, F.-C., Samuels, J., Bienvenu, O. J., Reti, I., Costa, P. T., Jr., & Eaton, W. W. (2006). Latent structure of the *Diagnostic and Statistical Manual of Mental Disorders, Fourth Edition* personality disorder criteria. *Comprehensive Psychiatry, 47*, 54–62. doi:10.1016/j.comppsych.2005.03.005

Nigg, J. T., Silk, K. R., Stavro, G., & Miller, T. (2005). Disinhibition and borderline personality disorder. *Development and Psychopathology, 17*, 1129–1149. doi:10.1017/S0954579405050534

Nusbaum, E. C., & Silvia, P. J. (2011). Are openness and intellect distinct aspects of openness to experience? A test of the O/I model. *Personality and Individual Differences, 51*, 571–574. doi:10.1016/j.paid.2011.05.013

O'Connor, B. P., & Dyce, J. A. (1998). A test of models of personality disorder configuration. *Journal of Abnormal Psychology, 107*, 3–16. doi:10.1037/0021-843X.107.1.3

Olatunji, B. O., Williams, B. J., Haslam, N., Abramowitz, J. S., & Tolin, D. F. (2008). The latent structure of obsessive-compulsive symptoms: A taxometric study. *Depression and Anxiety, 25*, 956–968. doi:10.1002/da.20387

Rothschild, L., Cleland, C., Haslam, N., & Zimmerman, M. (2003). A taxometric study of borderline personality disorder. *Journal of Abnormal Psychology, 112*, 657–666. doi:10.1037/0021-843X.112.4.657

Ruscio, J., Ruscio, A. M., & Meron, M. (2007). Applying the bootstrap to taxometric analysis: Generating empirical sampling distributions to help interpret results. *Multivariate Behavioral Research, 42*, 349–386. doi:10.1080/002731707 01360795

Samuel, D. B. (2011). Assessing personality in the *DSM–5*: The utility of bipolar constructs. *Journal of Personality Assessment, 93*, 390–397. doi:10.1080/002238 91.2011.577476

Samuel, D. B., & Widiger, T. A. (2008). A meta-analytic review of the relationships between the five-factor model and *DSM–IV–TR* personality disorders:

A facet level analysis. *Clinical Psychology Review, 28,* 1326–1342. doi:10.1016/j.cpr.2008.07.002

Saucier, G. (1992). Openness versus intellect: Much ado about nothing? *European Journal of Personality, 6,* 381–386. doi:10.1002/per.2410060506

Singleton, N., Bumpstead, R., O'Brien, M., Lee, A., & Meltzer, H. (2003). Psychiatric morbidity among adults living in private households, 2000. *International Review of Psychiatry, 15,* 65–73. doi:10.1080/0954026021000045967

Skilling, T. A., Harris, G. T., Rice, M. E., & Quinsey, V. L. (2002). Identifying persistently antisocial offenders using the Hare Psychopathy Checklist and *DSM* antisocial personality disorder criteria. *Psychological Assessment, 14,* 27–38. doi:10.1037/1040-3590.14.1.27

Skodol, A. E., Oldham, J. M., Bender, D. S., Dyck, I. R., Stout, R. L., Morey, L. C., . . . Gunderson, J. G. (2005). Dimensional representations of *DSM–IV* personality disorders: Relationships to functional impairment. *American Journal of Psychiatry, 162,* 1919–1925. doi:10.1176/appi.ajp.162.10.1919

Skodol, A. E., Siever, L. J., Livesley, W. J., Gunderson, J. G., Pfohl, B., & Widiger, T. A. (2002). The borderline diagnosis II: Biology, genetics, and clinical course. *Biological Psychiatry, 51,* 951–963. doi:10.1016/S0006-3223(02)01325-2

Strauss, J. S. (1973). Diagnostic models and the nature of psychiatric disorder. *Archives of General Psychiatry, 29,* 445–449. doi:10.1001/archpsyc.1973.04200040005001

Strickland, C. M., Drislane, L. E., Lucy, M., Krueger, R. F., & Patrick, C. J. (2013). Characterizing psychopathy using *DSM–5* personality traits. *Assessment, 20,* 327–338. doi:10.1177/1073191113486691

Tellegen, A. (1991). Personality traits: Issues of definition, evidence, and assessment. In D. Cicchetti & W. M. Grove (Eds.), *Thinking clearly about psychology: Vol. 2. Personality and psychopathology* (pp. 10–35). Minneapolis: University of Minnesota Press.

Tellegen, A. (2000). *Manual of the Multidimensional Personality Questionnaire.* Minneapolis: University of Minnesota Press.

Thomas, K. M., Yalch, M. M., Krueger, R. F., Wright, A. G. C., Markon, K. E., & Hopwood, C. J. (2013). The convergent structure of *DSM–5* personality trait facets and five-factor model trait domains. *Assessment, 20,* 308–311. doi:10.1177/1073191112457589

Trapnell, P. D. (1994). Openness versus intellect: A lexical left turn. *European Journal of Personality, 8,* 273–290. doi:10.1002/per.2410080405

Tyrer, P., Crawford, M., Mulder, R., Blashfield, R., Farnam, A., Fossati, A., . . . Reed, G. M. (2011). The rationale for the reclassification of personality disorder in the 11th revision of the *International Classification of Diseases (ICD–11). Personality and Mental Health, 5,* 246–259. doi:10.1002/pmh.190

Ullrich, S., Borkenau, P., & Marneros, A. (2001). Personality disorders in offenders: Categorical versus dimensional approaches. *Journal of Personality Disorders, 15,* 442–449. doi:10.1521/pedi.15.5.442.19199

Watson, D., Clark, L. A., & Chmielewski, M. (2008). Structures of personality and their relevance to psychopathology: II. Further articulation of a comprehensive unified trait structure. *Journal of Personality, 76,* 1545–1586. doi:10.1111/j.1467-6494.2008.00531.x

Watson, D., Stasik, S. M., Ro, E., & Clark, L. A. (2013). Integrating normal and pathological personality: Relating the *DSM–5* trait-dimensional model to general traits of personality. *Assessment, 20,* 312–326. doi:10.1177/1073191113485810

Widiger, T. (1992). Categorical versus dimensional classification: Implications from and for research. *Journal of Personality Disorders, 6,* 287–300. doi:10.1521/pedi.1992.6.4.287

Widiger, T. A., Lynam, D. R., Miller, J. D., & Oltmanns, T. F. (2012). Measures to assess maladaptive variants of the five-factor model. *Journal of Personality Assessment, 94,* 450–455. doi:10.1080/00223891.2012.677887

Woods, C. M., & Lin, N. (2009). Item response theory with estimation of the latent density using Davidian curves. *Applied Psychological Measurement, 33,* 102–117. doi:10.1177/0146621608319512

4

A CRITICAL EVALUATION OF MOVING TOWARD A TRAIT SYSTEM FOR PERSONALITY DISORDER ASSESSMENT

KEVIN B. MEEHAN AND JOHN F. CLARKIN

Personality disorders (PDs) are serious, chronic psychiatric illnesses that commonly occur in the general population, with a prevalence of 9.1% for any PD (American Psychiatric Association, 2013). Further, those with PDs tend to be quite impaired in terms of work, social functioning, and self-care (Lenzenweger, Lane, Loranger, & Kessler, 2007), and they tend to utilize both medical and psychiatric treatment services at high rates (Bender et al., 2001; Moran, Rendu, Jenkins, Tylee, & Mann, 2001), making the costs of these disorders considerable.

It is essential to accurately categorize and diagnose PDs in order to study and treat them. However, there has been considerable debate as to how well the *Diagnostic and Statistical Manual for Mental Disorders*, now in its fifth edition (*DSM–5*; American Psychiatric Association, 2013), does with regard to this task. Though there have been significant commentary and contrasting opinions about what future personality diagnosis in the *DSM* should look like

http://dx.doi.org/10.1037/14549-005
Personality Disorders: Toward Theoretical and Empirical Integration in Diagnosis and Assessment,
S. K. Huprich (Editor)

(Shedler et al., 2010), most agree that the taxonomy from the *Diagnostic and Statistical Manual of Mental Disorders, Fourth Edition, Text Revision* (*DSM–IV–TR*; American Psychiatric Association, 2000), now retained in *DSM–5* is problematic (Shedler & Westen, 2004b). Much has been written about problems with the diagnostic criteria for PDs in the *DSM*. Such problems are only briefly reviewed here, as more detailed accounts can be found elsewhere (e.g., Shedler & Westen, 2004b; see also the Introduction and Chapter 1, this volume). Most notable for the current discussion, the *DSM–IV–TR* PD categories tend to be quite heterogeneous. For example, Clarkin (1999) and Clarkin, Levy, Lenzenweger, and Kernberg (2004) have argued that because of the polythetic nature of the criteria for Borderline Personality Disorder (BPD), patients may have strikingly different symptom profiles with pertinent prognostic implications (i.e., suicidality), and yet each meets criteria for the disorder. There is considerable comorbidity both among the PDs and between Axis I and II disorders (Lenzenweger et al., 2007). Further, problems with differential diagnosis as well as concerns about stigma may lead clinicians to diagnose Axis I but not PDs (Paris, 2007).

The Personality and Personality Disorders Workgroup (PPDWG) was acutely aware of these problems and sought to address them in a novel diagnostic system (Krueger, 2013). Though ultimately not adopted, Section III's "Alternative *DSM–5* Model for Personality Disorders" offers an intriguing hybrid model that combines an assessment of personality functioning with personality traits (American Psychiatric Association, 2013). This chapter seeks to contribute to the dialogue regarding how the field moves forward in diagnosing personality pathology by reviewing and evaluating the latter trait system for diagnosing personality pathology. First, we briefly review the history of trait models of personality pathology that led to the proposed *DSM–5* model; more detailed accounts of this can be found elsewhere (Krueger, Skodol, Livesley, Shrout, & Huang, 2007; Widiger & Mullins-Sweatt, 2009; see also Chapter 3, this volume). Next, we critique various aspects of the trait model as a diagnostic system, including concerns with clinical utility as well as the nature of trait expression in healthy populations versus those with PDs. Last, we make some suggestions for future diagnostic models.

TRAIT MODELS OF PERSONALITY FOR PERSONALITY DISORDER ASSESSMENT

The Five-Factor Model and Personality Pathology

Traits are conceptualized as enduring dispositions that express themselves in relatively consistent ways across contexts and time, providing the building blocks of personality (McCrae & Costa, 1997). Though personality dispositions are wide ranging and diverse, a psycholexical approach has traditionally been used to cull the basic dimensions of personality (Allport & Odbert, 1936). This approach assumes that the total adjective descriptors naturally found in language systems (identified primarily from English-language dictionaries) broadly reflect the diversity of complex human attributes. The taxonomy of personality is, therefore, represented by the latent structure of adjective descriptors, which has been mostly consistently summarized in factor analytic studies with five factors. The five-factor model (FFM) is thought to represent the basic dimensions of personality (neuroticism, extraversion, conscientiousness, agreeableness, openness), with relative consistency in this factor structure found cross culturally (Allik, 2005; McCrae & Costa, 1997).

Therefore, in the FFM, personality is operationalized as dimensions along self-reported lexical attributes, with the interaction among these trait dimensions describing complex dispositions that are relatively stable across time and context. In trait models there is no assumption about the etiology or processes that underlie these dispositions; rather, these trait dimensions are thought to be broad and comprehensive descriptors of complex human attributes.

The clinical application of the FFM posits that personality pathology reflects extremes on these trait dimensions (Trull, 2012; Widiger & Mullins-Sweatt, 2009). For example, Avoidant Personality Disorder may be conceptualized in terms of pathologically low extraversion; Obsessive-Compulsive Personality Disorder may be conceptualized in terms of pathologically high conscientiousness. In fact, Trull (2012) argued that current *DSM* PD criteria could be thought of as already representing either direct traits (e.g., impulsivity, a symptom of BPD, is itself a facet of low conscientiousness) or indirect indicators of traits (e.g., self-harm, also a symptom of BPD, is a behavioral manifestation of low conscientiousness). Thus, the argument goes, the FFM structure is latent in the *DSM* already, albeit not always directly or comprehensively (Trull, 2012).

The *DSM–5* Trait Model for Personality Disorder Assessment

Although the trait system represented in the "Alternative *DSM–5* Model for Personality Disorders" is based in large part on the FFM, it is not itself an FFM system (Krueger et al., 2007; Livesley, 2007). The *DSM–5* model culls the major dimensions of personality from the FFM as well as a number of related dimensional models of personality pathology (Widiger & Simonsen, 2005). However, there was recognition of the fact that measures of the FFM (i.e., the Revised NEO Personality Inventory, or NEO-PI–R; Costa & McCrae, 1992) may not reflect a level of severity that captures the full range of personality pathology (Krueger et al., 2011). Thus, the five proposed trait domains can be broadly conceptualized as representing pathological variants of the basic FFM dimensions: Negative affectivity reflects pathologically high neuroticism, detachment reflects pathologically low extraversion, disinhibition reflects pathologically low conscientiousness (whereas compulsivity reflects pathologically high conscientiousness), antagonism reflects pathologically low agreeableness, and psychoticism reflects pathologically high openness. In the proposed *DSM–5* model these five trait domains, as well as 25 trait facets within these domains, would each be rated dimensionally (American Psychiatric Association, 2013). PDs would reflect relative elevations across trait dimensions (e.g., BPD would be characterized by high negative affectivity, disinhibition, and antagonism).

The evaluation of these pathological trait dimensions has been operationalized by Krueger, Derringer, Markon, Watson, and Skodol (2012) with the Personality Inventory for *DSM–5* (PID-5), which may function as both a research tool and a clinical compendium. Because the measure was developed only recently, the evidence base for the PID-5 is still in its infancy. Some have argued that the PID-5 is a natural extension of the FFM model, and thus they tether their evidence bases together in considering the empirical support for this model (see Chapter 3, this volume). Others, such as Trull (2012), have argued that when the FFM dimensions were converted into pathological variants and integrated with other models, some coverage of trait facets was lost. Further, it is not clear that PID-5 dimensions are simply pathological variants of FFM dimensions. For example, there are now substantial data that psychoticism has a more complex relationship to trait openness than previously recognized (DeYoung, Grazioplene, & Peterson, 2012; Quilty, Ayearst, Chmielewski, Pollock, & Bagby, 2013; Watson, Stasik, Ro, & Clark, 2013).

Further, although data on the PID-5 thus far are quite promising, they show the measure's youthful age in that the majority of the empirical base for the PID-5 has so far involved primarily nonclinical samples using self-report data. With regard to the use of nonclinical participants, most studies employing the PID-5 have used large undergraduate samples (Anderson et al., 2013; De Fruyt et al., 2013; Gore & Widiger, 2013; Hopwood, Schade, Krueger, Wright, & Markon, 2013; Hopwood, Thomas, Markon, Wright, & Krueger, 2012; Samuel, Mullins-Sweatt, & Widiger, 2013; Wright et al., 2012, 2013) or community samples recruited through online research platforms (solely or in combination with undergraduate samples; Markon, Quilty, Bagby, & Krueger, 2013; Miller, Gentile, Wilson, & Campbell, 2013; Strickland, Drislane, Lucy, Krueger, & Patrick, 2013; Thomas et al., 2013). In a recent special issue of *Assessment* on the PID-5, eight of 10 studies used undergraduate samples. Further, the two studies that used clinical samples were each quite limited, in that the PID-5 was compared only to other self-report trait measures (Quilty et al., 2013; Watson et al., 2013). In each study, convergent validity was found to be stronger than discriminant validity: PID-5 facets related to their FFM (or Big Three) counterparts but not exclusively so, raising a question of specificity. The use of nonclinical samples is not a problem in and of itself. In fact, this may sometimes be a necessary first step in a program of research that then extends findings to clinical populations. However, to date the PID-5 literature has not fully advanced to clinical populations. This will be a necessary step in its advancement as a clinical diagnostic tool.

EVALUATING CORE ASSUMPTIONS OF TRAIT MODELS

A number of essential questions that arise from the assumptions made in trait models must be considered before these models are applied to PD assessment. Is it best to assess and characterize PDs at the level of self-identified attributes? Should an assessment system emphasize the characterization of manifest attributes and deemphasize the processes that give rise to such attributes? Do trait dimensions capture the essential domains of dysfunction relevant to personality pathology? Do trait factors such as those in the FFM represent dimensions of both normal and abnormal personality?

Research has largely confirmed the five-factor structure as related to PD pathology (Widiger & Mullins-Sweatt, 2009) but with a very important caveat. The five factors of the FFM have been consistently replicated with regard to the PDs using FFM instruments (usually the NEO-PI–R; Samuel & Widiger, 2008). However, if these factors are latent variables found in nature, they presumably should appear in the factor structure of any reasonably comprehensive collection of personality descriptors. Does the FFM structure emerge when non-FFM measures are used? Shedler and Westen (2004a) tested this question directly by having 530 clinicians rate their patients with PD with a set of clinically relevant personality descriptors (Shedler–Westen Assessment Procedure, or SWAP-200; see Chapter 9, for more details) and then Q factor analyzing both the full set of 200 descriptors and a subset of 60 descriptors that represented only FFM dimensions. They found that when only the 60 FFM descriptors were included, the five-factor solution indeed emerged. But when the full 200 descriptors were included, a total of 12 factors emerged that represented pathological types (i.e., psychopathy, narcissism) only loosely related to DSM categories and not related to FFM trait dimensions. Further, these 12 factors were found to have stronger convergent and discriminant validity than the five-factor solution. In another study, Huprich, Schmitt, Richard, Chelminski, and Zimmerman (2010) factored the PD symptoms from structured DSM–IV–TR interviews and found the best fit to be a 10-factor solution loosely related to DSM categories. A five-factor model had only adequate fit and showed notable differences from the FFM. Thus it may be the case that when FFM descriptors alone are used to characterize PD samples, the FFM structure emerges, but when a wider range of personality descriptors and symptoms is used, neither the FFM nor the DSM structures are fully supported.

Further, the empirical foundation for trait models of personality pathology is overwhelmingly based on the use of self-report data (Huprich, 2011a). To date, there is no clinical interview version of the PID-5. Although a good structured interview has been developed for the FFM (Structured Interview for the Five-Factor Model of Personality; Trull & Widiger, 1997), it has not been widely used in comparison to the ubiquitous NEO-PI–R self-report measure (Costa & McCrae, 1992). The problems with excessive reliance on self-report data, particularly as applied to populations with PD, are well known (Bornstein, 2003; Huprich, 2011a). Often incumbent to the nature of PDs is limited insight into one's own pathology. The adage that people "don't know what they don't know" about themselves is particularly apt when it comes to this population. Further, self-report scales may not be able to distinguish between low scores reflecting health versus low scores reflecting a defensive denial of distress (Shedler, Mayman, & Manis, 1993). Again, the use of self-report is not a problem in and of itself. However, to date this tool has not been supplemented with performance-based measures to allow for a fuller exploration of the complexity of the personality phenomena in question (Bornstein, 2002; Huprich, 2011b).

In a recent study that did not rely on excessive use of self-report or nonclinical samples but rather related trait dimensions to structured clinical interview and behavioral outcome data in a rigorously assessed sample of patients with PD, trait dimensions did not emerge as a primary predictor of personality dysfunction. Hopwood et al. (2011) evaluated diagnostic data from the Collaborative Longitudinal Personality Disorders Study (CLPS) in terms of the contribution of personality pathology type (i.e., factors of PD symptoms), severity (i.e., total number of any PD symptom met), and trait dimensions (i.e., NEO-PI–R, Costa & McCrae, 1992; Schedule for Nonadaptive and Adaptive Personality, Clark, 1993) in predicting concurrent and prospective dysfunction. Although the evaluations of trait dimensions were significant predictors, they were tertiary to the evaluation of clinician-assessed personality type and severity in predicting impairment in social and occupational functioning 3 years later. Self-reported traits did not relate to personality types as expected; Hopwood et al. (2011) noted, "Results also suggest that personality traits relate mostly to severity and are less useful for depicting individual differences in stylistic features of PDs [personality disorders]" (p. 314). Although self-reported traits made a contribution in terms of incremental validity, it was only a modest contribution above and beyond the clinician's assessment of severity and was not sufficient to characterize the type of presenting pathology.

In summary, self-reported trait dimensions are clearly of value in contextualizing the assessing personality pathology, but data are not sufficient at this time to suggest these models can supplant other models as the diagnostic system for PDs. The modest incremental validity demonstrated by the studies discussed above certainly suggests a role for trait assessment, but it may be of secondary (or tertiary) importance to other information needed to diagnose these disorders.

IS THERE CLINICAL UTILITY OF A TRAIT SYSTEM FOR PERSONALITY DISORDER ASSESSMENT?

A diagnostic system must not only be psychometrically sound but also useful to the average clinician for the purposes of assessment and treatment planning (Clarkin & Huprich, 2011). First et al. (2004) articulated a set of widely accepted indicators of clinical utility (Verheul, 2005). They noted that an effective diagnostic system must have a set of coherently defined entities mutually recognized between clinicians that facilitate the communication of clinical information. Further, an effective diagnostic system must help the clinician discriminate between clinical conditions in order to correctly characterize the presenting pathology and apply this knowledge toward choosing appropriate clinical interventions and/or management tools.

The development of a new PD assessment system may be starting with a low bar, as many have argued that the *DSM–IV–TR* system (now readopted in *DSM–5*) struggles to meet many of these benchmarks (Livesley, 1998; Mullins-Sweatt & Lengel, 2012; Verheul, 2005). As we have noted, excessive comorbidity reflects the fact that the current PD categories may not be sufficiently distinctive; yet, the necessity to independently assess disorders with shared pathology often results in redundant assessment efforts. This excessive comorbidity also suggests that the *DSM* categories may not be coherently defined. Livesley (2007) noted that "*DSM–IV–TR* diagnoses are not natural kinds that 'carve nature at its joints'" (p. 200). Further, given the heterogeneity of disorders such as BPD, the specificity of the clinical communication when these diagnostic labels are used may be called into question (Widiger & Samuel, 2005).

Proponents of the FFM and PID-5 trait models argue that such systems address many of the aforementioned shortcomings. For instance, Trull (2012) argued that *DSM* criteria could be thought of as redundant, as different levels of analysis (i.e., trait impulsivity, behavioral self-harm) are being used to evaluate the same latent structure (i.e., disinhibition). The added advantage of diagnosing PDs from a trait framework is that its (mostly) orthogonal dimensions would reduce redundant evaluation of pathology while adding other dimensions that are not captured in the current *DSM* criteria (Widiger & Mullins-Sweatt, 2009). Further, if the heterogeneity of PDs stems from the fact that they are not empirically driven but rather represent a consolidation of clinical observation over time, an FFM framework may afford more taxometrically distinctive classifications (Meehl, 1995). Further, the dimensional nature of trait assessment allows for an implicit measure of severity while also more closely resembling the nature of personality (Widiger & Samuel, 2005).

We are in strong agreement as to the problems articulated with the current *DSM* system and share in the sense of urgency to see PD diagnosis have stronger clinical utility. However, more data and experience with trait models may be necessary before we conclude that these systems reconcile the problems they purport to reconcile. Do trait systems adequately address the functions of a clinically relevant diagnostic system, as defined by First et al. (2004)?

As noted, a diagnostic system should aid in conceptualizing the entity (First et al., 2004). Because the *DSM* has no theoretical or empirical underpinning, it has a relative weakness in its capacity to aid in conceptualizing personality pathology (Krueger, 2013; Widiger & Samuel, 2005). Trait models have an advantage over the *DSM* in that they have a strong empirical basis for describing complex attributes. However, there are also disadvantages to conceptualizing and evaluating PDs solely at the level of self-identified attributes. There is often significant clinical value in evaluating the same facet of pathology (i.e., disinhibition) at different levels of analysis (i.e., trait attribution, behavioral manifestation), as discrepancies between the two often provide valuable information about the level of personality organization (Bornstein, 2002; Clarkin, Yeomans, & Kernberg, 2006). For example, a greater disparity between self-attribution (i.e., "I am a victim") and interpersonal behaviors (i.e., verbally aggression toward others) may suggest poor integration, an important indicator of pathological severity. Trait models cannot account for the dynamic processes that give rise to such discrepancies in personality functioning (Luyten & Blatt, 2011). Evaluating the pathology at only one level of analysis—self-identified traits—may detract from the conceptual complexity of personality pathology.

Second, a diagnostic system should aid in communicating clinical information to relevant others (First et al., 2004). While it is true that the heterogeneity of some PDs, such as BPD, detracts from specificity when communicating a diagnosis (Widiger & Samuel, 2005), it is not clear that trait models improve on this. Clinicians do not tend to use the language of traits when thinking and communicating about a patient (Shedler et al., 2010). Although trait-based descriptors may contextualize clinical communication of diagnosis, Huprich and Bornstein (2007) noted that it is unlikely the categorical labels for PDs will fall out of use and that, with increased use, trait language may itself become canned descriptors (as is often the fate of common parlance).

Third, patients do not use the language of traits when describing a presenting problem to a clinician. A diagnostic system should also aid in clinical interviewing and differential diagnosis (First et al., 2004). There appears to be a gap between the language of traits and the language of chief complaints used by patients. As Shedler and Westen (2004a, 2004b; see also Chapter 9, this volume) have noted, most clinicians approach diagnostic interviewing in terms of the degree of fit to a prototype. Clinicians ask patients to describe their chief complaints, which usually take the form of temporally and contextually unstable feelings and behaviors (i.e., "for the past 2 weeks I've been really moody and snapping at people") rather than static trait attributes (i.e., "I'm generally too outgoing"); such attributes may be of interest but do not address why the patient has decided to seek clinical attention right now. Clinicians ask differential questions about these complaints in terms of "if/then" precipitants (Huprich, 2011a, 2011b) rather than trait dimensions (such as asking about time frames and precipitants in differentiating between mood lability in mania versus BPD). Clinicians then ask about other symptoms not yet discussed but consistent with the emerging profile, in the service of matching the patient to an internalized prototype (Shedler & Westen, 2004a, 2004b; Westen, 2006). Finally, clinicians communicate to both the patient and other clinicians the type of problem in need of clinical attention. Trait dimensions are characteristic ways of describing normal personalities, but they are not the characteristic ways that patients communicate problems to clinicians or that clinicians communicate to each other. Further, because subtle distinctions between clinical concerns usually hinge on temporal and contextual factors, failure to evaluate such contingencies may result in a loss of complexity in differential diagnosis.

Fourth, a diagnostic system should aid one in choosing clinical interventions (First et al., 2004). Whereas a diagnostic label such as BPD has immediate and specific prescriptive implications (i.e., a structured treatment such as mentalization-based therapy [MBT], dialectical behavior therapy [DBT], or transference-focused psychotherapy), trait dimensions (i.e., high negative affectivity, disinhibition, and antagonism) do not necessarily suggest a treatment approach. Further, when one looks at treatment literature for PDs, trait dimensions do not seem to be generally conceptualized as the target of therapeutic intervention per se. For example, none of the major empirically supported treatments for BPD target pathological trait dimensions as their primary mechanism of change. MBT (Bateman & Fonagy, 1999) targets the hyperarousal of the attachment system that impedes the capacity of patients with BPD to reflect on the mental states of self and other. Although negative affectivity may be a manifestation of attachment arousal, evaluation for MBT focuses on interview-based measures of attachment organization and mentalization, and interventions focus on the regulation of those domains. Transference-focused psychotherapy (TFP; Clarkin et al., 2006) targets unintegrated mental representations of self and other that lead to distortions in the way the patient's identity and relationships to others are perceived. Although antagonism may be an outgrowth of polarized representations of self and other, evaluation for and interventions in TFP focus on the experience of these relational distortions, including in the transference with Therapist. DBT (Linehan, 1998) comes closest to using a trait model in its focus on negative affectivity and disinhibition, but the treatment targets behavioral contingencies arising from these dispositions, not the dispositions themselves. Whereas behaviors such as self-harm may be an outgrowth of disinhibition, interventions focus on helping patients to identify triggers of and management skills for behaviors in spite of their dispositional disinhibition. These three treatments posit very different mechanisms of change, and therefore it is telling that none of them emphasize evaluating patients on self-reported trait facets or making these the primary target of therapeutic intervention.

Fifth, a diagnostic system should aid in predicting future clinical management needs (First et al., 2004). Longitudinal studies of BPD over a 10-year period suggest that though the more impulsivity-driven symptoms may remit over time, levels of interpersonal and occupational impairment tend to remain high (Choi-Kain, Zanarini, Frankenburg, Fitzmaurice, & Reich, 2010; Zanarini et al., 2007). This suggests that if a diagnostic system is to be informative in the future clinical management needs of patients with PD, it must rigorously assess the patients' impairment in relational functioning and the capacity to work. Although it is true that the dimensional assessment of traits provides some indication of the level of pathological severity, it may not be the strongest indicator of severity (for example, as compared to total *DSM* symptoms; Hopwood et al., 2011). Functional impairments in the capacity to love and work are not well represented in trait models.

Last, we note that data on clinical utility of FFM models for diagnosing PDs are mixed but mostly lean against this approach. Samuel and Widiger (2006) found that clinicians rated the FFM as superior to the *DSM* for diagnostically characterizing vignettes of unknown patients. In contrast, when Spitzer, First, Shedler, Westen, and Skodol (2008) asked clinicians to diagnostically characterize their own established patients, they rated the FFM as less clinically useful than rating *DSM–IV–TR* criteria. They also reported that it was difficult to use and failed to cover the range of severe psychopathology. Rottman, Ahn, Sanislow, and Kim (2009) also found that clinicians preferred *DSM* to FFM profiles for rating patient vignettes and that they were more accurate in using the *DSM* than the FFM in arriving at the correct diagnosis. Rhadigan and Huprich (2012) found that clinicians were less accurate with FFM vignettes than with *DSM*-based vignettes that were adapted to specify "if . . . then" triggers of pathological behaviors, based on a cognitive-affective processing system (CAPS) model (Mischel, 2004; see also Chapter 16, this volume). It is important to note that each of these studies precedes the PID-5, which may do a better job of capturing more severe personality pathology. However, the data from the FFM suggest that on average clinicians like it less than DSM-based systems for diagnosis, and clinicians may be less accurate in applying it to case formulations.

ILLUSTRATION OF THE CLINICAL APPLICATION OF TRAIT MODELS FOR NARCISSISTIC PERSONALITY DISORDER

To illustrate the possible limitations of trait assessment of PDs, we will use the example of diagnosing Narcissistic Personality Disorder (NPD). Despite its once being slated for removal from the DSM–5, there has been growing clinical interest in the diagnosis and treatment of patients with NPD (Diamond & Meehan, 2013). There is wide agreement that NPD is not well characterized in the DSM system, as it reflects a grandiose presentation at the expense of capturing more vulnerable dimensions of the disorder (Cain, Pincus, & Ansell, 2008; Levy, Meehan, Cain, & Ellison, 2013). It should be noted that the choice of NPD is not a "straw man"; in fact, NPD has received among the most attention of the PDs using the PID-5 model (Miller et al., 2013; Wright et al., 2013), and proponents of this system have cited NPD as an example of how a trait system can better the current approach (Krueger, 2013).

So, does a trait system do a better job of characterizing these patients? What does a clinician look for when evaluating NPD from a trait perspective? A number of recent studies in both nonclinical undergraduate samples (Hopwood et al., 2013; Wright et al., 2013) and community samples (Amazon's Mechanical Turk; Miller et al., 2013) suggest that narcissistic pathology is most strongly represented by trait Antagonism on the PID-5. In fact, the other four higher order trait domains made minimal to no contribution to the narcissistic profile above and beyond Antagonism, thus giving that domain strong discriminant validity (Wright et al., 2013).

To what degree does high trait Antagonism alone provide the average clinician with a distinctive profile in discriminating NPD from among the other PDs? What is notable when looking at the various PDs at a trait level is how similar some that are conceptualized as phenomenologically quite different look at the domain level. For example, in terms of the five trait domains, NPD is distinguished from Obsessive-Compulsive Personality Disorder (OCPD) only by its score on Antagonism; they otherwise each have no elevation on other domains (Hopwood et al., 2012). (In fact, OCPD has no elevation on any of the domains and thus no distinctive profile on the

PID-5.) Across the 25 lower-order facets, NPD is only distinguished from OCPD by being high on the lower-order facets of Grandiosity and Attention Seeking, whereas OCPD is high on the Rigid Perfectionism facet. To be sure, these two disorders share some clinical characteristics, but clinically they are much more distinctive personality styles than their trait dimensions would imply. This observation seems to be consistent with data suggesting that trait dimensions may not be particularly good at distinguishing between personality styles (Hopwood et al., 2011).

To what degree does the trait system aid in characterizing both grandiose and vulnerable dimensions of NPD? Wright et al. (2013) found that grandiosity was well represented by the Antagonism domain and a number of its facets. In contrast, vulnerability had modest relationships to all of the PID-5 domains, resulting in a relatively indistinctive profile. Miller et al. (2013) found that, unlike the highly specific grandiose profile, the vulnerable profile was surprisingly unspecific in that it correlated with most PD types as well as most PID-5 traits. Therefore, it seems that this system does not substantially improve upon the lacking characterization of vulnerable dimensions in the diagnosis of NPD.

Does high trait Antagonism capture the full clinical presentation of NPD? Although narcissistic patients can certainly be antagonistic, what is often quite distinctive clinically is not antagonism as a static trait but rather relationally bound fluctuations between antagonistic/domineering and hypersensitive/submissive presentations (Pincus & Lukowitsky, 2010). Trait models fail to capture vacillation between personality presentations (Luyten & Blatt, 2011) and the situational "if/then" precipitants that lead to movement between the two (Huprich, 2011a, 2011b). It may also be particularly important in NPD for clinicians to evaluate the same facet of pathology (i.e., antagonism) at different levels of analysis (i.e., trait attribution, behavioral manifestation). Patients with NPD often have striking disparities between self-attribution (i.e., "She's lucky to have me") and observer report (i.e., resentful partner), which would not be captured in this system. Further, the severity of the antagonism score tells us little about the patient's level of impairment, as there is no indication of the negative implications of antagonism in terms of diminished interpersonal and occupational functioning.

What are the treatment implications of high trait Antagonism? Although there are more robust literatures on related constructs, such as the treatment implications of dismissive attachment (Levy, Meehan, Temes, & Yeomans, 2012), little is known about treating antagonism. To be fair, the treatment literature on NPD is still quite limited. No randomized clinical trials of any kind exist for this disorder, although there are extensive clinical literatures on treating narcissistic pathologies (Diamond & Meehan, 2013; Ronningstam, 2010). Further, it is unclear whether the implication of a trait model is to then address the trait deficit as the target of clinical attention and, if so, what interventions would be effective for Antagonism.

Is there value in the clinical assessment of traits for NPD? Yes, of course trait dimensions add valuable information that may contextualize the clinical presentation, but it appears of lesser importance than other information needed to diagnose NPD. Though not yet investigated, trait dimensions may also demonstrate value as a putative client variable in predicting treatment outcome (Clarkin & Levy, 2004). Although the present research base demonstrates the value of trait models in contextualizing diagnosis, it does not appear to be fully capable of being a replacement diagnostic system.

CONCEPTUAL ISSUES IN PERSONALITY PHENOTYPES

In evaluating trait systems for PD assessment, it is also important to evaluate the underlying assumptions in these models about the phenotypic presentation of personality and personality pathology. There is no doubt that traits are essential descriptors of complex personality attributes. Further, there is no doubt that trait research has been useful in teasing apart the component dimensions of personality phenotypes. However, there is an implicit assumption that the opposite process is equally useful: that these components are then useful for identifying personality phenotypes. Lenzenweger (2010a, 2010b) has written cogently about the importance of recognizing PDs as emergent phenomena. He noted,

> In this model, PDs are described as emergent because the disorders arise from the underlying neurobehavioral systems in interaction with one another and with environmental forces (e.g., severe childhood sexual trauma) to create a configural phenotype. This configural phenotype is considered to be emergent in nature as it is not readily reducible to individual input components (neurobehavioral systems, trauma, and so on), although the necessary individual components can be known. (Lenzenweger, 2010b, pp. 761–762)

Personality phenotypes are the product of a complex interaction of underlying genetic, epigenetic, and trait dimensions (reflecting underlying neurobehavioral systems) that are contextualized by individuals' personal histories (Depue & Lenzenweger, 2005). The interaction of those neurobehavioral systems with the environment gives rise to the individuals' characteristic ways of thinking, feeling, behaving, and relating. Although trait dimensions, understood in this model as reflecting the activity of neurobehavioral systems, can be studied and understood, this process has given rise to a more complex phenotype that is not merely the sum of its constituent parts.

A parallel point is often emphasized in the philosophy of mind literature through the concept of supervenience (Kim, 1993). Although supervenience has been primarily applied to the mind–body problem, it has direct implications for personality assessment. This concept posits that properties understood in their dependence upon one another only then become intelligible. A classic example is fine art; the constituent properties in isolation (colors, shapes, textures) belie the representational meaning and affective resonance of the work. In this light, personality can be conceptualized as supervenient on its trait properties: Trait dimensions give rise to personality, but personality cannot be reduced back to its constituent traits without a loss of the influence of the supervenient cognitive-affective representational structures. Although trait-based dispositions may contribute to the larger personality organization, that organizational structure subsequently influences the experience and expression of those traits, such that observing them in the absence of the larger structure belie their cognitive-affective meaning.

The organization of our internal representational structures is central to how we experience our personality (Blatt, 1995; Kernberg, 1975). In normal personality development, the infant's early experience is relatively undifferentiated and organized around moments of pain and pleasure. Through developmental experiences in interaction with trait-based dispositions, increasingly differentiated and hierarchically integrated cognitive-affective representational structures of self and others emerge. The quality and organization of our personality structure subsequently influence the experience and expression of those trait-based dispositions in dynamic and affectively rich ways. Healthy personality functioning is based in cognitive-affective representational structures that are coherent enough to create a sense of identity that is relatively stable across time and contexts, while being flexible enough to regulate affect and adapt to changing circumstances. Thus, the expression of trait-based dispositions, while predictable enough to afford a sense of continuity in self-definition, is also flexibly applied in relational contexts in a manner that promotes affiliation. In contrast, personality pathology is based in cognitive-affective representational structures that are diffusely organized, limited in breadth, and rigidly applied. In struggling to flexibly process and respond to affectively valenced information, an individual with such a personality organization is likely to feel unmoored by novel contexts and to respond to them as if they are old ones, leading to discontinuity in self-definition and relational ruptures. Thus, the expression of trait-based dispositions is likely to be of limited variability, to be affectively reactive, and to be inflexible to contextual constraints (Blatt & Levy, 2003).

A cognitive-affective model of personality helps to explain why the expression of trait-based dispositions will vary considerably in the context of personality pathology (Mischel, 2004; Mischel & Shoda, 1995). Mischel (2004) wrote,

> If different situations acquire different meanings for the same individual, as they surely do, the kinds of appraisals, expectations and beliefs, affects, goals, and behavioral scripts that are likely to become activated in relation to particular situations will vary. Therefore, there is no theoretical reason to expect the individual to display similar behavior in relation to different psychological situations unless they are functionally equivalent in meaning. (p. 5)

In healthy personality functioning, cognitive-affective representational structures are quickly and flexibly able to sort through affectively encoded memory systems to make highly differentiated appraisals, arrive at a refined meaning of the situation, and respond appropriately.

Pathological personality functioning, by contrast, reflects cognitive-affective representational structures that rigidly apply appraisals with little distinction between contexts to arrive at the same meaning each time (e.g., the patient with BPD who continually thinks "this means I'm being abandoned"), leaving the individual beholden to automatic response tendencies (Mischel, 2004). The expression of trait-based dispositions will, therefore, vary as a function of the personality organization and style. To give an example, the trait facet Suspiciousness will be elevated in patients with Paranoid Personality Disorder across most relational contexts, whereas in patients with BPD suspiciousness will be elevated in more meaning-specific relational contexts (i.e., abandonment). In contrast, an individual with healthy personality functioning will make a highly nuanced analysis of the context to arrive at an uncommon conclusion of suspicion.

Therefore, as can be seen, trait dimensions must be understood in the context of their superordinate cognitive-affective representational structures. Although trait-based dispositions may influence the process of development of the personality structure, that cognitive-affective structure subsequently influences the experience and expression of those traits, such that the traits cannot be easily identified and understood in the absence of that structure. The problem this creates for diagnosis, by way of analogy, is that if one wants to identify "purple" in nature one should not go looking for "red" and "blue."

CONCLUDING REMARKS

Livesley (1998) described the presence of a PD as when "the structure of personality prevents the person from achieving adaptive solutions to the universal life tasks of establishing a self-system, attachment and intimacy, and cooperativeness and prosocial behavior" (p. 141). We seek to help our patients achieve a sturdy sense of self-definition and the capacity for relatedness, as they are the key ingredients for adaptation to life's challenges (Blatt, 1995). One of the more heartening aspects of Section III's "Alternative DSM–5 Model for Personality Disorders" is the inclusion of an assessment of self and interpersonal functioning (DSM–5); we hope to see such considerations at the forefront of any future system for assessing PDs. Traits have significant value as complex descriptors of personality attributes. However, we need to keep at the forefront of our diagnostic thinking the superordinate identity around which those attributes come to be organized (Kernberg & Caligor, 2005). From a coherent identity stems the capacity for love and intimacy, investment in work and community, and personal growth. In breaking down the component structure of personality pathology we can lose sight of the fact that as clinicians what we want most for our patients is, in Freud's famous words, "to love and to work" (Erikson, 1950, p. 265).

REFERENCES

Allik, J. (2005). Personality dimensions across cultures. *Journal of Personality Disorders, 19*, 212–232. doi:10.1521/pedi.2005.19.3.212

Allport, G. W., & Odbert, H. S. (1936). Trait-names: A psycho-lexical study. *Psychological Monographs, 47*(1), i–171. doi:10.1037/h0093360

American Psychiatric Association. (2000). *Diagnostic and statistical manual of mental disorders* (4th ed., text rev.). Washington, DC: Author.

American Psychiatric Association. (2013). *Diagnostic and statistical manual of mental disorders* (5th ed.). Arlington, VA: American Psychiatric Publishing.

Anderson, J. L., Sellbom, M., Bagby, R. M., Quilty, L. C., Veltri, C. O. C., Markon, K. E., & Krueger, R. F. (2013). On the convergence between PSY-5 domains and PID-5 domains and facets: Implications for assessment of DSM–5 personality traits. *Assessment, 20*, 286–294. doi:10.1177/1073191112471141

Bateman, A., & Fonagy, P. (1999). Effectiveness of partial hospitalization in the treatment of borderline personality disorder: A randomized control trial. *The American Journal of Psychiatry, 156*, 1563–1569.

Bender, D. S., Dolan, R. T., Skodol, A. E., Sanislow, C. A., Dyck, I. R., McGlashan, T. H., . . . Gunderson, J. G. (2001). Treatment utilization by patients with personality disorders. *The American Journal of Psychiatry, 158*, 295–302. doi:10.1176/appi.ajp.158.2.295

Blatt, S. J. (1995). Representational structures in psychopathology. In D. Cicchetti & S. L. Toth (Eds.), *Rochester Symposium on Developmental Psychopathology: Vol. 6. Emotion, cognition, and representation* (pp. 1–33). Rochester, NY: University of Rochester Press.

Blatt, S. J., & Levy, K. N. (2003). Attachment theory, psychoanalysis, personality development, and psychopathology. *Psychoanalytic Inquiry, 23*, 102–150. doi:10.1080/07351692309349028

Bornstein, R. F. (2002). A process dissociation approach to objective–projective test score interrelationships. *Journal of Personality Assessment, 78*, 47–68. doi:10.1207/S15327752JPA7801_04

Bornstein, R. F. (2003). Behaviorally referenced experimentation and symptom validation: A paradigm for 21st-century personality disorder research. *Journal of Personality Disorders, 17*, 1–18. doi:10.1521/pedi.17.1.1.24056

Cain, N. M., Pincus, A. L., & Ansell, E. B. (2008). Narcissism at the crossroads: Phenotypic description of pathological narcissism across clinical theory, social/personality psychology, and psychiatric diagnosis. *Clinical Psychology Review, 28*, 638–656. doi:10.1016/j.cpr.2007.09.006

Choi-Kain, L. W., Zanarini, M. C., Frankenburg, F. R., Fitzmaurice, G. M., & Reich, D. B. (2010). A longitudinal study of the 10-year course of interpersonal features in borderline personality disorder. *Journal of Personality Disorders, 24*, 365–376. doi:10.1521/pedi.2010.24.3.365

Clark, L. A. (1993). *Manual for the Schedule of Nonadaptive and Adaptive Personality.* Minneapolis: University of Minnesota Press.

Clarkin, J. F. (1999). Research findings on the personality disorders. *In Session: Psychotherapy in Practice, 4*, 91–102. doi:10.1002/(SICI)1520-6572(199924)4:4<91::AID-SESS7>3.0.CO;2-U

Clarkin, J. F., & Huprich, S. K. (2011). Do the *DSM–5* proposals for personality disorders meet the criteria for clinical utility? *Journal of Personality Disorders, 25*, 192–205. doi:10.1521/pedi.2011.25.2.192

Clarkin, J. F., & Levy, K. N. (2004). The influence of client variables on psychotherapy. In M. J. Lambert (Ed.), *Bergin and Garfield's handbook of psychotherapy and behavior change* (5th ed., pp. 194–226). New York, NY: Wiley.

Clarkin, J. F., Levy, K. N., Lenzenweger, M. F., & Kernberg, O. F. (2004). The Personality Disorders Institute/Borderline Personality Disorder Research Foundation randomized control trial for borderline personality disorder. *Journal of Personality Disorders, 18*, 52–72. doi:10.1521/pedi.18.1.52.32769

Clarkin, J. F., Yeomans, F., & Kernberg, O. F. (2006). *Psychotherapy of borderline personality: Focusing on object relations.* Washington, DC: American Psychiatric Publishing.

Costa, P. T., Jr., & McCrae, R. R. (1992). *Revised NEO Personality Inventory (NEO-PI–R) and NEO Five-Factor Inventory (NEO-FFI) professional manual.* Odessa, FL: Psychological Assessment Resources.

De Fruyt, F., De Clercq, B., De Bolle, M., Wille, B., Markon, K., & Krueger, R. F. (2013). General and maladaptive traits in a five-factor framework for *DSM–5* in a university student sample. *Assessment, 20*, 295–307. doi:10.1177/1073191113475808

Depue, R. A., & Lenzenweger, M. F. (2005). A neurobehavioral model of personality disturbance. In M. F. Lenzenweger & J. F. Clarkin (Eds.), *Major theories of personality disorder* (2nd ed., pp. 391–453). New York, NY: Guilford Press.

DeYoung, C. G., Grazioplene, R. G., & Peterson, J. B. (2012). From madness to genius: The Openness/Intellect trait domain as a paradoxical simplex. *Journal of Research in Personality, 46*, 63–78. doi:10.1016/j.jrp.2011.12.003

Diamond, D., & Meehan, K. B. (2013). Attachment and object relations in patients with narcissistic personality disorder: Implications for therapeutic process and outcome. *Journal of Clinical Psychology, 69*, 1148–1159. doi:10.1002/jclp.22042

Erikson, E. H. (1950). *Childhood and society.* New York, NY: Norton.

First, M. B., Pincus, H. A., Levine, J. B., Williams, J. B. W., Ustun, B., & Peele, R. (2004). Clinical utility as a criterion for revising psychiatric diagnoses. *The American Journal of Psychiatry, 161*, 946–954. doi:10.1176/appi.ajp.161.6.946

Gore, W. L., & Widiger, T. A. (2013). The *DSM–5* dimensional trait model and five-factor models of general personality. *Journal of Abnormal Psychology, 122*, 816–821. doi:10.1037/a0032822

Hopwood, C. J., Malone, J. C., Ansell, E. B., Sanislow, C. A., Grilo, C. M., McGlashan, T. H., . . . Morey, L. C. (2011). Personality assessment in *DSM–5*: Empirical support for rating severity, style, and traits. *Journal of Personality Disorders, 25*, 305–320. doi:10.1521/pedi.2011.25.3.305

Hopwood, C. J., Schade, N., Krueger, R. F., Wright, A. G. C., & Markon, K. E. (2013). Connecting *DSM–5* personality traits and pathological beliefs: Toward a unifying model. *Journal of Psychopathology and Behavioral Assessment, 35*, 162–172. doi:10.1007/s10862-012-9332-3

Hopwood, C. J., Thomas, K. M., Markon, K. E., Wright, A. G. C., & Krueger, R. F. (2012). *DSM–5* personality traits and *DSM–IV* personality disorders. *Journal of Abnormal Psychology, 121*, 424–432. doi:10.1037/a0026656

Huprich, S. K. (2011a). Contributions from personality and psychodynamically-oriented assessment for the development of *DSM–5* personality disorders. *Journal of Personality Assessment, 93*, 354–361. doi:10.1080/00223891.2011.577473

Huprich, S. K. (2011b). Reclaiming the value of assessing unconscious and subjective psychological experience. *Journal of Personality Assessment, 93*, 151–160. doi:10.1080/00223891.2010.542531

Huprich, S. K., & Bornstein, R. F. (2007). An overview of issues related to categorical and dimensional models of personality disorder assessment. *Journal of Personality Assessment, 89*, 3–15. doi:10.1080/00223890701356904

Huprich, S. K., Schmitt, T. A., Richard, D. C., Chelminski, I., & Zimmerman, M. A. (2010). Comparing factor analytic models of the *DSM–IV* personality disorders. *Personality Disorders: Theory, Research, and Treatment, 1*, 22–37. doi:10.1037/a0018245

Kernberg, O. F. (1975). *Borderline conditions and pathological narcissism.* New Haven, CT: Yale University Press.

Kernberg, O. F., & Caligor, E. (2005). A psychoanalytic theory of personality disorders. In M. F. Lenzenweger & J. F. Clarkin (Eds.), *Major theories of personality disorder* (2nd ed., pp. 114–156). New York, NY: Guilford Press.

Kim, J. (1993). *Supervenience and mind: Selected philosophical essays.* Cambridge, England: Cambridge University Press.

Krueger, R. F. (2013). Personality disorders are the vanguard of the post-*DSM–5.0* era. *Personality Disorders: Theory, Research, and Treatment, 4*, 355–362. doi:10.1037/per0000028

Krueger, R. F., Derringer, J., Markon, K. E., Watson, D., & Skodol, A. E. (2012). Initial construction of a maladaptive personality trait model and inventory for *DSM–5*. *Psychological Medicine, 42*, 1879–1890. doi:10.1017/S0033291711002674

Krueger, R. F., Eaton, N. R., Clark, L. A., Watson, D., Markon, K. E., Derringer, J., . . . Livesley, W. J. (2011). Deriving an empirical structure of personality pathology for *DSM–5*. *Journal of Personality Disorders, 25*, 170–191. doi:10.1521/pedi.2011.25.2.170

Krueger, R. F., Skodol, A. E., Livesley, W. J., Shrout, P. E., & Huang, Y. (2007). Synthesizing dimensional and categorical approaches to personality disorders: Refining the research agenda for *DSM–V* Axis II. *International Journal of Methods in Psychiatric Research, 16*(Suppl. 1), S65–S73. doi:10.1002/mpr.212

Lenzenweger, M. F. (2010a). Current status of the scientific study of the personality disorders: An overview of epidemiological, longitudinal, experimental psychopathology, and neurobehavioral perspectives. *Journal of the American Psychoanalytic Association, 58*, 741–778. doi:10.1177/0003065110386111

Lenzenweger, M. F. (2010b). *Schizotypy and schizophrenia: The view from experimental psychopathology.* New York, NY: Guilford Press.

Lenzenweger, M. F., Lane, M. C., Loranger, A. W., & Kessler, R. C. (2007). *DSM–IV* personality disorders in the National Comorbidity Study replication. *Biological Psychiatry, 62*, 553–564. doi:10.1016/j.biopsych.2006.09.019

Levy, K. N., Meehan, K. B., Cain, N. M., & Ellison, W. D. (2013). Narcissism in the DSM. In J. S. Ogrodniczuk (Ed.), *Understanding and treating pathological narcissism* (pp. 45–62).Washington, DC: American Psychological Association.

Levy, K. N., Meehan, K. B., Temes, C. M., & Yeomans, F. E. (2012). Attachment theory and research: Implications for psychodynamic psychotherapy. In R. Levy, J. S. Ablon, & H. Kaechele (Eds.), *Psychodynamic psychotherapy research: Evidence-based practice and practice-based evidence* (pp. 401–416). New York, NY: Springer.

Linehan, M. M. (1998). An illustration of dialectical behavior therapy. *In Session: Psychotherapy in Practice, 4*, 21–44. doi:10.1002/(SICI)1520-6572(199822)4:2<21::AID-SESS3>3.0.CO;2-B

Livesley, W. J. (1998). Suggestions for a framework for an empirically based classification of personality disorder. *Canadian Journal of Psychiatry/Revue canadienne de psychiatrie, 43*, 137–147.

Livesley, W. J. (2007). A framework for integrating dimensional and categorical classifications of personality disorder. *Journal of Personality Disorders, 21*, 199–224. doi:10.1521/pedi.2007.21.2.199

Luyten, P., & Blatt, S. J. (2011). Integrating theory-driven and empirically-derived models of personality development and psychopathology: A proposal for *DSM V. Clinical Psychology Review, 31*, 52–68. doi:10.1016/j.cpr.2010.09.003

Markon, K. E., Quilty, L. C., Bagby, R. M., & Krueger, R. F. (2013). The development and psychometric properties of an informant-report form of the Personality Inventory for DSM–5 (PID-5). *Assessment, 20*, 370–383. doi:10.1177/1073191113486513

McCrae, R. R., & Costa, P. T., Jr. (1997). Personality trait structure as a human universal. *American Psychologist, 52*, 509–516. doi:10.1037/0003-066X.52.5.509

Meehl, P. E. (1995). Bootstraps taxometrics: Solving the classification problem in psychopathology. *American Psychologist, 50*, 266–275. doi:10.1037/0003-066X.50.4.266

Miller, J. D., Gentile, B., Wilson, L., & Campbell, W. K. (2013). Grandiose and vulnerable narcissism and the *DSM–5* pathological personality trait model. *Journal of Personality Assessment, 95*, 284–290. doi:10.1080/00223891.2012.685907

Mischel, W. (2004). Toward an integrative science of the person. *Annual Review of Psychology, 55*, 1–22. doi:10.1146/annurev.psych.55.042902.130709

Mischel, W., & Shoda, Y. (1995). A cognitive-affective system theory of personality: Reconceptualizing situations, dispositions, dynamics, and invariance in personality structure. *Psychological Review, 102*, 246–268. doi:10.1037/0033-295X.102.2.246

Moran, P., Rendu, A., Jenkins, R., Tylee, A., & Mann, A. (2001). The impact of personality disorder in UK primary care: A 1-year follow-up of attenders. *Psychological Medicine, 31*, 1447–1454. doi:10.1017/S003329170105450z

Mullins-Sweatt, S. N., & Lengel, G. L. (2012). Clinical utility of the five-factor model of personality disorder. *Journal of Personality, 80*, 1615–1639. doi:10.1111/j.1467-6494.2012.00774.x

Paris, J. (2007). Why psychiatrists are reluctant to diagnose: Borderline personality disorder. *Psychiatry, 4*(1), 35–39.

Pincus, A. L., & Lukowitsky, M. R. (2010). Pathological narcissism and narcissistic personality disorder. *Annual Review of Clinical Psychology, 6*, 421–446. doi:10.1146/annurev.clinpsy.121208.131215

Quilty, L. C., Ayearst, L., Chmielewski, M., Pollock, B. G., & Bagby, R. M. (2013). The psychometric properties of the Personality Inventory for *DSM–5* in an APA *DSM–5* field trial sample. *Assessment, 20*, 362–369. doi:10.1177/1073191113486183

Rhadigan, C., & Huprich, S. K. (2012). The utility of the cognitive-affective processing system in the diagnosis of personality disorders: Some preliminary evidence. *Journal of Personality Disorders, 26*, 162–178. doi:10.1521/pedi.2012.26.2.162

Ronningstam, E. (2010). Narcissistic personality disorder: A current review. *Current Psychiatry Reports, 12*, 68–75. doi:10.1007/s11920-009-0084-z

Rottman, B. M., Ahn, W., Sanislow, C. A., & Kim, N. S. (2009). Can clinicians recognize *DSM–IV* personality disorders from five-factor model descriptions of patient cases? *The American Journal of Psychiatry, 166*, 427–433. doi:10.1176/appi.ajp.2008.08070972

Samuel, D. B., Mullins-Sweatt, S. N., & Widiger, T. A. (2013). An investigation of the factor structure and convergent validity of the Five-Factor Model Rating Form. *Assessment, 20*, 24–35. doi:10.1177/1073191112455455

Samuel, D. B., & Widiger, T. A. (2006). Clinicians' judgments of clinical utility: A comparison of the *DSM–IV* and five-factor models. *Journal of Abnormal Psychology, 115*, 298–308. doi:10.1037/0021-843X.115.2.298

Samuel, D. B., & Widiger, T. A. (2008). A meta-analytic review of the relationships between the five-factor model and *DSM–IV–TR* personality disorders: A facet level analysis. *Clinical Psychology Review, 28*, 1326–1342. doi:10.1016/j.cpr.2008.07.002

Shedler, J., Beck, A., Fonagy, P., Gabbard, G. O., Gunderson, J., Kernberg, O., . . . Westen, D. (2010). Personality disorders in *DSM–5*. *The American Journal of Psychiatry, 167*, 1026–1028. doi:10.1176/appi.ajp.2010.10050746

Shedler, J., Mayman, M., & Manis, M. (1993). The illusion of mental health. *American Psychologist, 48*, 1117–1131. doi:10.1037/0003-066X.48.11.1117

Shedler, J., & Westen, D. (2004a). Dimensions of personality pathology: An alternative to the five-factor model. *The American Journal of Psychiatry, 161*, 1743–1754. doi:10.1176/appi.ajp.161.10.1743

Shedler, J., & Westen, D. (2004b). Refining *DSM–IV* personality disorder diagnosis: Integrating science and practice. *The American Journal of Psychiatry, 161*, 1350–1365. doi:10.1176/appi.ajp.161.8.1350

Spitzer, R. L., First, M. B., Shedler, J., Westen, D., & Skodol, A. (2008). Clinical utility of five dimensional systems for personality diagnosis. *Journal of Nervous and Mental Disease, 196*, 356–374. doi:10.1097/NMD.0b013e3181710950

Strickland, C. M., Drislane, L. E., Lucy, M., Krueger, R. F., & Patrick, C. J. (2013). Characterizing psychopathy using *DSM–5* personality traits. *Assessment, 20*, 327–338. doi:10.1177/1073191113486691

Thomas, K. M., Yalch, M. M., Krueger, R. F., Wright, A. G. C., Markon, K. E., & Hopwood, C. J. (2013). The convergent structure of *DSM–5* personality trait facets and five-factor model trait domains. *Assessment, 20*, 308–311. doi:10.1177/1073191112457589

Trull, T. J. (2012). The five-factor model of personality disorder and *DSM–5*. *Journal of Personality, 80*, 1697–1720. doi:10.1111/j.1467-6494.2012.00771.x

Trull, T. J., & Widiger, T. A. (1997). *Structured Interview for the Five-Factor Model of Personality*. Odessa, FL: Psychological Assessment Resources.

Verheul, R. (2005). Clinical utility of dimensional models for personality pathology. *Journal of Personality Disorders, 19*, 283–302. doi:10.1521/pedi.2005.19.3.283

Watson, D., Stasik, S. M., Ro, E., & Clark, L. A. (2013). Integrating normal and pathological personality: Relating the *DSM–5* trait-dimensional model to general traits of personality. *Assessment, 20,* 312–326. doi:10.1177/1073191113485810

Westen, D. (2006). Commentary on Trull: Drizzling on the 5 + 3 factor parade. In T. A. Widiger, E. Simonsen, P. J. Sirovatka, & D. A. Regier (Eds.), *Dimensional models of personality disorders: Refining the research agenda for* DSM–V (pp. 189–194). Washington, DC: American Psychiatric Publishing.

Widiger, T. A., & Mullins-Sweatt, S. N. (2009). Five-factor model of personality disorder: A proposal for *DSM–V. Annual Review of Clinical Psychology, 5,* 197–220. doi:10.1146/annurev.clinpsy.032408.153542

Widiger, T. A., & Samuel, D. B. (2005). Evidence-based assessment of personality disorders. *Psychological Assessment, 17,* 278–287. doi:10.1037/1040-3590.17.3.278

Widiger, T. A., & Simonsen, E. (2005). Alternative dimensional models of personality disorder: Finding a common ground. *Journal of Personality Disorders, 19,* 110–130. doi:10.1521/pedi.19.2.110.62628

Wright, A. G. C., Pincus, A. L., Thomas, K. M., Hopwood, C. J., Markon, K. E., & Krueger, R. F. (2013). Conceptions of narcissism and the *DSM–5* pathological personality traits. *Assessment, 20,* 339–352. doi:10.1177/1073191113486692

Wright, A. G. C., Thomas, K. M., Hopwood, C. J., Markon, K. E., Pincus, A. L., & Krueger, R. F. (2012). The hierarchical structure of *DSM–5* pathological personality traits. *Journal of Abnormal Psychology, 121,* 951–957. doi:10.1037/a0027669

Zanarini, M. C., Frankenburg, F. R., Reich, D. B., Silk, K. R., Hudson, J. I., & McSweeney, L. B. (2007). The subsyndromal phenomenology of borderline personality disorder: A 10-year follow-up study. *The American Journal of Psychiatry, 164,* 929–935. doi:10.1176/appi.ajp.164.6.929

II

RESEARCH AND
ASSESSMENT STRATEGIES

5

AT THE NEXUS OF SCIENCE AND PRACTICE: ANSWERING BASIC CLINICAL QUESTIONS IN PERSONALITY DISORDER ASSESSMENT AND DIAGNOSIS WITH QUANTITATIVE MODELING TECHNIQUES

AIDAN G. C. WRIGHT AND JOHANNES ZIMMERMANN

Rigorous science and effective treatment both rest on a foundation of valid and reliable assessment and diagnosis. In the consulting room, assessment and diagnosis should provide useful information for clear communication among professionals and to patients, establishing prognosis and ultimately deciding whether and, if so, how to treat. In the laboratory, assessment and diagnosis are necessary to decide which participants to include and exclude from studies, while also providing data of interest to examine as predictors and outcomes. In turn, assessment and diagnosis are predicated on the understanding of the nature and structure of the target phenomenon, in this case personality disorder (PD). Thoroughly and accurately assessing and diagnosing PD can be a demanding enterprise. Patients with severe PDs often lead chaotic lives and have a fragmented or diffuse sense of self that can become embodied in a frenzied assessment process and a muddled clinical picture. In contrast, milder but nevertheless impairing personality pathology

http://dx.doi.org/10.1037/14549-006
Personality Disorders: Toward Theoretical and Empirical Integration in Diagnosis and Assessment,
S. K. Huprich (Editor)

often becomes apparent only as a clinician learns the patient's characteristic manner of perceiving and responding to others and set ways of regulating self and affect. These difficulties in the assessment process are understandable and to be expected, given the nature of the pathology.

However, a further challenge to this enterprise is that the current diagnostic framework more often than not serves to obfuscate as opposed to clarify clinical description. For more than 30 years, the modern era of the *Diagnostic and Statistical Manual of Mental Disorders* has furthered a model of personality pathology in which patients can receive one of 10 putatively discrete, categorical PD diagnoses or a diagnosis of PD not otherwise specified (PD-NOS).[1] Despite a growing body of scientific work that calls its fundamental structure into question (Widiger & Trull, 2007), this remains the model for the foreseeable future as it has been imported virtually verbatim from the *DSM*'s fourth edition (*DSM–IV*; American Psychiatric Association, 1994) to its fifth edition (*DSM–5*; American Psychiatric Association, 2013). Here we highlight a number of key questions that emerge when the extant PD model is applied in clinical practice, and we demonstrate how they are directly amenable to investigation using contemporary quantitative methodology.

First, why do so many patients meet the criteria for multiple PDs or no specific PD (i.e., PD-NOS)? When diagnostic rules are followed, the modal number of diagnoses a patient with one PD receives is considerably higher than one (Widiger & Rogers, 1989). At the same time, one of the most frequent (and correct, given the characterization of PD) diagnoses is PD-NOS (Verheul & Widiger, 2004). As a result, clinicians most often must provide a cumbersome polydiagnosis or an ambiguous catchall diagnosis, making the official diagnostic categories largely uninformative for individual case formulation and treatment planning (Krueger, 2013).

Second, is personality pathology dimensional, categorical, or some hybrid of the two? Clinical theory suggests that discrete lines cannot be drawn between individuals with and without PDs as espoused in the *DSM* (e.g., Clarkin, Yeomans, & Kernberg, 2006). Nonetheless, it would be a mistake to follow the psychiatric nosology or clinical theory by fiat without subjecting each assertion to a test.

Third, regardless of whether PD is strictly dimensional, categorical, or a hybrid, a practical issue must be addressed: What is a reasonable diagnostic threshold for PD(s)? Clinicians have long recognized that individuals just one (or more) criterion shy of a diagnosis still experience significant

---

[1]We recognize that there have been modest changes across editions of the *DSM* related to aspects of the PD models such as the exact wording of the diagnostic criteria, the exact number necessary to achieve diagnostic threshold, and even the number of included disorders. However, the core of the model has remained fundamentally unchanged since *DSM–III*, as have the constructs and their operationalization. Moreover, this model persists in the *DSM–5*.

impairment, and they frequently decide to treat as a result (Blagov, Bradley, & Westen, 2007; Westen & Arkowitz-Westen, 1998). Given the importance of decisions that arise from diagnostic decisions (e.g., explanatory, treatment, funding, legal), it is imperative to investigate whether diagnostic thresholds are reliable and defensible.

Finally, we consider a more basic question not necessarily tied to classification issues in the *DSM*: What are the important behavioral patterns of PD to track and target for intervention? Personality pathology is a dynamic phenomenon, generally reflecting processes that occur within and between levels of experience (e.g., motivational, cognitive, behavioral) over time, which result in maladaptive self-regulation and responses to environmental demands. The field's understanding of the actual dynamics of personality pathology relies heavily on clinical observation. This is the natural first step. However, there is little systematic knowledge of the frequency and the contingencies under which symptoms are expressed. Through a focus on dynamic processes in PD as opposed to diagnostic constructs, there is greater potential to understand the mechanisms of PD and move toward an idiographic science and practice that allows for flexibly applying diagnosis and treatment to individuals (van Os, Delespaul, Wigman, Myin-Germeys, & Wichers, 2013; for an alternative perspective on assessing dynamics, see Bornstein, 2011; see also Chapter 11, this volume).

In the remainder of the chapter, we discuss how contemporary statistical modeling can be brought to bear on these questions practitioners and researchers face when assessing PD. To answer the first three questions, we apply latent variable models to traditional diagnostic information (i.e., cross-sectional interview and self-report data). For the final question, we highlight new insights that have been gleaned from collecting and modeling intensively and repeatedly measured behavior (e.g., daily diary data; ecological momentary assessment).

LATENT VARIABLE MODELING: A BRIEF PRIMER

The first three questions we consider deal with traditional diagnostic information, the kind that emerges from diagnostic interviews and assessment inventories. This type of information, which includes symptoms and diagnoses, is generally treated as dispositional, or at least as characteristic of an individual at a particular time point. It is precisely this type of information that clinical assessors have been tasked to collect and organize during a standard diagnostic assessment. Although we have divided the issues associated with this type of data into three questions, in reality all deal with different facets of the underlying structure that gives rise to personality pathology. Accordingly, we discuss addressing these questions with different techniques that are all parts of a general suite of analytic approaches, *latent variable modeling*. Prior to exploring specific techniques as applied to the questions we pose, we provide a brief conceptual primer on latent variable modeling.

Latent variable modeling encompasses a range of techniques that have wide application in the behavioral and health sciences. The basic logic of latent variables is quite consistent with the current state of psychiatry and psychological science; namely, there are observable behaviors and symptoms that have unobserved and, in fact, directly unobservable underlying causes. For instance, a major depressive episode is not something that can be ascertained directly; rather, it is inferred when a patient presents complaining of anhedonia, depressed mood, decreased appetite, hypersomnia, psychomotor retardation, and thoughts of suicide. The *observed* or *manifest* signs and symptoms are presumed to be caused by an *unobserved* or *latent* entity that is hypothesized to exist, in this case depression. Similar to this, latent variable modeling presumes that manifest or observed variables (i.e., anything directly measurable, such as symptom ratings, answers to questionnaire items, levels of salivary cortisol, fMRI BOLD signals) arise from unobserved but hypothesized latent causes. In turn, the patterns of observations are used to estimate the latent structure that gives rise to the data.

Most readers will likely be familiar with at least one basic form of latent variable modeling, factor analysis. Readers will recall that factor analysis serves to estimate dimensions (i.e., factors) that represent patterns of covariation among items, questions, or tests. The goal of factor analysis is to reduce the complexity of the observed information such that a smaller number of dimensions explain the patterns of variance and covariance among the variables (e.g., symptoms, diagnoses). For instance, if each of five hypothetical symptoms covary (i.e., correlate with each other) within a sample of individuals, one interpretation is that a single latent dimension accounts for this pattern of co-occurrence. The top (Panel A) of Figure 5.1 provides a graphical depiction of this scenario. The oval represents the latent variable, in this case a factor or dimension, that gives rise to the individual symptoms, as represented by the arrows going from the latent variable to the observed symptoms. It is important to note here that although the latent variable is estimated using the pattern of covariation of observed variables in a sample, it is presumed to be causal, which is why the arrows emerge from it.[2] The arrows each represent the *factor loading*, or the proportion of variation in individual endorsement of each symptom accounted for by the latent dimension. The additional small

---

[2]Whether a latent variable is truly causal or merely descriptive is a topic with deep philosophical roots and important implications (Pearl, 2000). However, we do not consider this debate here.

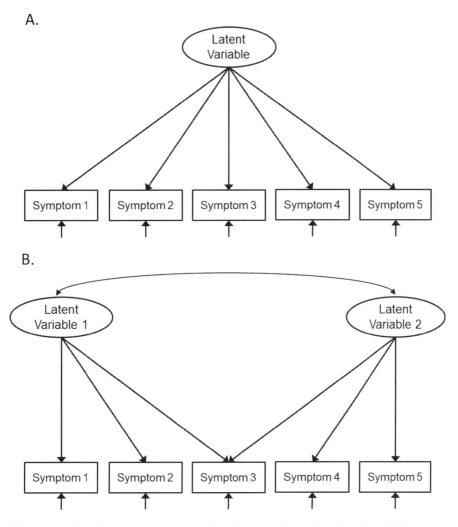

Figure 5.1. Graphical representation of a univariate (A) and multivariate (B) latent variable model.

arrows associated with each symptom represent unique variability, including measurement error, which contributes to their endorsement.

More complex models that include more than one latent variable can be estimated. Consider the lower panel (B) of Figure 5.1, which includes two latent factors that each explain two symptoms uniquely and share in the prediction of a third. An additional new feature in this second model is a curved arrow between the two latent variables. This represents the covariation among latent dimensions, which may or may not exist. If we take, for example, five symptoms, such as anhedonia, avolition, restless sleep, uncontrollable worry, and physiological arousal, the model in Panel B might be a reasonable hypothetical structure. Latent variable 1 might account for anhedonia, avolition, and restless sleep, whereas latent variable 2 might account for uncontrollable worry, physiological arousal, and restless sleep. Readers undoubtedly will recognize this as a simplified version of the *DSM*'s model for major depression and generalized anxiety disorders. The curved arrow in this case would be needed to account for the high rates of comorbidity among the two diagnoses.

Factor analysis is used here to provide an entrée to a general latent variable modeling framework. Many more complex and potentially illuminating models can be estimated, but the logic remains the same for each. For instance, *latent class analysis* (sometimes referred to as latent profile analysis) is a categorical latent variable modeling technique that accounts for patterns of covariation by estimating unobserved or latent groups that differ from each other in symptom endorsement or scale means. Other models can be estimated that have a hybrid latent structure, blending categories and dimensions to explain the observed data patterns. In general, models can be either *exploratory* (i.e., the investigator does not impose a hypothesized structure) or *confirmatory* (i.e., the investigator specifies a structure to test its fit to the data).

Additional attractive features of this analytic framework include the ability to test the fit of the model to the data, such that models can be retained or discarded on the basis of formal statistical rules. The same goes for comparing models to each other, allowing for sophisticated adjudication among models. Model testing is usually based on a *chi-square statistic*, which tests whether the estimated parameters of the model adequately reproduce the empirical data. A number of additional fit indices have been developed that are helpful in model selection. They balance different aspects influencing model fit, such as sample size, number of variables, and number of parameters, or compare fit relative to the null model (i.e., a model in which all relationships are fixed to zero). The most widely used and recommended fit indices in the current literature include the *root-mean-square error of approximation* (RMSEA), the *Tucker–Lewis index* (TLI), the *comparative fit index* (CFI), and the *standardized root-mean-square residual* (SRMR; Brown, 2006). Additionally, the *Akaike information criterion* (AIC) and the *Bayesian information criterion* (BIC) attempt to balance model fit and parsimony (see Vrieze, 2012). Many excellent comprehensive and technical treatments of latent variable models exist for the interested reader (e.g., Bollen, 1989; Brown, 2006; Collins & Lanza, 2010; McLachlan & Peel, 2000). However, our goal in this chapter is to limit the discussion of these models to the conceptual. In what follows we tether the clinical questions with statistical models, which we elaborate on in each section.

Why Do So Many Patients Meet the Criteria for Multiple PDs or PD-NOS?

There is probably no simple answer to the question of comorbidity (Krueger & Markon, 2006; Lilienfeld, Waldman, & Israel, 1994). Given that PD diagnoses are very common among patients, one possible explanation is that they "co-occur" simply due to chance, which would be the end of the issue. However, this explanation quickly becomes implausible when one acknowledges the fact that PD diagnoses (and, by implication, PD criteria of different PD categories) do not only simply co-occur but actually systematically covary (i.e., are correlated; see, e.g., Lenzenweger, Lane, Loranger, & Kessler, 2007; Trull, Vergés, Wood, & Sher, 2013; Zimmerman, Rothschild, & Chelminski, 2005). These patterns of covariation among PDs may arise for distinct reasons, including shared etiological pathways (e.g., some PDs may be affected by the same causal risk factor, such as childhood adversity), shared method variance (e.g., interviewers may be biased toward specific covariations of PDs), or shared underlying dimensions of personality pathology liability (e.g., PD criteria of different PDs may be indicators of the same latent dimension). The latter explanation might also account for the high prevalence of PD-NOS because persons with a high standing on a latent trait would display PD symptoms that cut across the categorical PD diagnoses.

Without doubt, latent variable modeling seems especially suited to shed light on these issues (Krueger & Markon, 2006). The technique that has received by far the most attention in this regard is factor analysis. As outlined above, factor analysis assumes that the patterns of covariation among PD diagnoses or criteria can be explained by a set of underlying latent dimensions. In the following section, we elaborate on some basic concepts necessary to understanding (exploratory) factor analysis and illustrate these concepts with selected studies on the covariation of PDs. In most of these studies, researchers collected cross-sectional data using a single assessment method (e.g., self-report). Such data obviously preclude inferences about the etiological status of the latent factors or the generalizability across different methods. However, we will close this section with an outlook on designs and extensions of factor-analytic methods that are able to address the question of comorbidity more comprehensively.

Exploratory Factor Analysis

The most prominent distinction in the family of factor-analytic methods is the distinction between *exploratory factor analysis* (EFA) and *confirmatory factor analysis* (CFA; see, e.g., Thompson, 2004). CFA is a theory-driven approach that aims for testing or comparing sets of assumptions about the relationships between indicators and factors. For example, the lower panel (B) of Figure 5.1 depicts a CFA that tests several assumptions about the covariation of five symptoms. Specifically, it is assumed that (a) latent factor 1 influences Symptoms 1 to 3 but is unrelated to Symptoms 4 and 5, (b) latent factor 2 influences Symptoms 3 to 5 but is unrelated to Symptoms 1 and 2, (c) the two latent factors are correlated, and (d) the unique variances of the five symptoms (including measurement error) are uncorrelated. Fit indices can be used to evaluate whether these assumptions fit the data reasonably well or whether they fit the data better than other assumptions (see Brown, 2006, for an excellent introduction to the technical aspects of CFA). In contrast, EFA is a data-driven approach that aims for identifying the appropriate number of latent factors and an optimal pattern of factor loadings. Although EFA requires fewer a priori specifications than does CFA, the researcher is also faced with a series of decisions (Fabrigar, Wegener, MacCallum, & Strahan, 1999). In particular, the researcher has to select procedures to estimate the latent variable model, to determine the appropriate number of factors, and to rotate the initial factor matrix to facilitate the interpretation of the factors (in the case of models with more than one factor). Commonly applied estimators are principal factors, maximum likelihood, and robust weighted least squares, all of which have their specific strengths and weaknesses (e.g., maximum likelihood provides descriptive fit indices and information criteria but requires continuous and normally distributed indicator variables). Note that principal component analysis (PCA) is often misclassified as an EFA estimation procedure. Although PCA may yield results similar to EFA under certain circumstances (e.g., when factors have many high-loading indicators), PCA does not differentiate between common and unique variance in observed indicators and thus is not in line with latent variable modeling (see Fabrigar et al., 1999, for details). This should be kept in mind when comparing results from exploratory studies on the factor structure of PDs, as several of these studies actually used PCA.

The decision on how many factors to extract should be guided by substantive considerations and statistical procedures. One of the most highly recommended procedures that has been extensively tested in simulation studies is *parallel analysis* (Horn, 1965; Timmerman & Lorenzo-Seva, 2011). Parallel analysis focuses on factors' *eigenvalues*, which represent the amount of variance in indicators explained by each factor. In short, the idea of parallel analysis is to extract all factors with eigenvalues that are greater than would be expected from "parallel" random data (i.e., data with the same number of indicators and participants). This procedure is demonstrably superior to the widespread *Kaiser criterion* (i.e., extracting all factors with an eigenvalue > 1), which is most often too liberal, or the *scree test* (i.e., visually searching for the last substantial decline in the magnitude of the eigenvalues and extracting all factors prior to that decline), which can be ambiguous and highly subjective. Other useful procedures for deciding on the number of factors include the *minimum average partial test* (Velicer, 1976) and *factor comparability coefficients* (Everett, 1983). When an estimation procedure provides a chi-square statistic (e.g., maximum likelihood), one can also inspect fit indices or information criteria to decide on the number of factors (Fabrigar et al., 1999; Lorenzo-Seva, Timmerman, & Kiers, 2011; Preacher, Zhang, Kim, & Mels, 2013). In practice, it is not uncommon for different procedures to recommend different numbers of factors. Although useful tools, the statistical procedures reviewed here are guides, and the researcher is ultimately responsible for choosing a substantively interpretable solution. We want to emphasize that the ultimate factor solution relies on the observed variables included in the model. Adding or removing variables to a model can substantially change a structure. For example, if only few markers of a given construct are included, it is unlikely to emerge as a separate factor.

After the appropriate number of factors has been determined, the final step in EFA is factor rotation. Because EFA models with more than one factor do not have a unique factor loading matrix, researchers must select one from an infinite number of equally fitting rotations (Fabrigar et al., 1999). Usually, researchers prefer rotation procedures that aim for simple structure, such that there is a factor loading matrix in which (a) each factor is defined by several indicators that have high loadings relative to the other indicators, and (b) each indicator has a high loading on one factor and close to zero loadings on the remaining factors. Simple structure can be achieved both with uncorrelated factors (i.e., orthogonal rotation such as *varimax*) and with correlated factors (i.e., oblique rotation such as *promax*). However, we note that simple structure might not always be the "best" solution from a conceptual point of view (see below).

The Dimensional Structure of DSM–IV *PDs*

A range of studies have investigated the latent structure of *DSM–IV* PDs with factor-analytic methods. These studies have used both CFA and EFA and have varied considerably in terms of the basic unit of analysis (e.g., individual PD criteria or dimensional PD scores), the assessment method (e.g., self- or clinician report), the sample type (e.g., community or clinical sample), and the statistical procedures (e.g., parallel analysis or scree test in EFA). A comprehensive summary of the findings is clearly beyond the scope of this chapter. However, several issues seem noteworthy here: First, studies focusing on PD diagnoses as the basic unit of analysis (i.e., either the presence or absence of diagnoses, or the number of criteria fulfilled) have failed to find strong support for the assumption that the pattern of covariation can be explained by three (correlated) latent dimensions representing the higher order clusters of odd-eccentric, dramatic-emotional, and anxious-fearful disturbances. In the majority of studies, CFA models showed unacceptable fit to the data (Bastiaansen, Rossi, Schotte, & de Fruyt, 2011; Chabrol, Rousseau, Callahan, & Hyler, 2007; Yang, Bagby, Costa, Ryder, & Herbst, 2002) or produced improper solutions (Trull et al., 2013), and EFA factors differed more often than not from the expected patterns (Fossati et al., 2000, 2006; Schotte, de Doncker, Vankerckhoven, Vertommen, & Cosyns, 1998). A latent structure that probably better accounts for diagnosis-level PD covariation requires more than three factors, which are likely to resemble major domains of general personality (Widiger & Trull, 2007). For example, O'Connor (2005) conducted a meta-analysis on PD data from 33 studies published between 1983 and 2000 and found evidence for a four-factor structure, with Dependent, Avoidant, Borderline, and Schizotypal PDs loading on high *Neuroticism*, Antisocial, Narcissistic, Histrionic, Paranoid, and Borderline PDs loading on low *Agreeableness*, Schizoid, Schizotypal, and Avoidant PD loading on low, and Histrionic PD loading on high *Extraversion*, and Obsessive-Compulsive PD loading on high *Conscientiousness*. With minor corrections and correlated latent factors, this model achieved a good CFA model fit in self-report data from 1,688 participants (Bastiaansen et al., 2011). However, a major limitation of focusing solely on covariation between PD diagnoses or scales is that they implicitly assume that PDs are unidimensional, coherent constructs.

Thus, we argue that factor-analytic studies based on individual PD criteria are likely to be more informative. Two studies based on clinician ratings and structured clinical interviews, respectively, tested the latent structure of *DSM–IV* PD criteria using CFA (Durrett & Westen, 2005; Huprich, Schmitt, Richard, Chelminski, & Zimmerman, 2010). They found only modest support for a model with 10 correlated factors that equal the 10 specific PDs, with fit indices around the lower bound of acceptability. The majority of studies explored the latent structure of *DSM–IV* PD criteria using EFA or PCA (Blackburn, Logan, Renwick, & Donnelly, 2005; Blais & Malone, 2013; Doering et al., 2007; Durrett & Westen, 2005; Howard, Huband, Duggan, & Mannion, 2008; Huprich et al., 2010; Nestadt et al., 2006; Schotte et al., 1998; Thomas, Turkheimer, & Oltmanns, 2003; Trull, Vergés, Wood, Jahng, & Sher, 2012).[3] The number of factors that were extracted differed considerably, ranging from five (Nestadt et al., 2006) to 11 factors (Schotte et al.,

---

[3] A detailed table of the samples, assessment methods, statistical procedures, and findings of these studies is not included due to space concerns but is available from the authors by request.

1998), with a median of nine factors. This difference might be in part due to differences in the sets of indicators, as two studies additionally included 15 conduct disorder symptoms (Blackburn et al., 2005; Howard et al., 2008) and two other studies additionally included the 14 criteria of depressive and passive-aggressive PD (Doering et al., 2007; Schotte et al., 1998). On the other hand, this difference might also be influenced by differences in decision rules, as only two studies consequently adhered to the results of parallel analysis, four studies employed the (inherently ambiguous) scree test, and four studies followed substantive considerations (e.g., consistence with prior literature, interpretability of factors). In any case, the findings of these studies might appear to run counter to the emerging consensus in PD research (Trull & Durrett, 2005; Widiger & Trull, 2007) by suggesting that more than four or five latent dimensions might be needed to comprehensively capture the covariation of *DSM–IV* PD criteria. However, we argue that a more parsimonious latent structure might still be valid at a higher level of abstraction (see below). Moreover, note that factor intercorrelations were predominantly positive but rather small: The five studies using oblique rotations found mean factor correlations ranging from .05 (Nestadt et al., 2006) to .23 (Trull et al., 2012), and in the remaining five studies, factor correlations were fixed to zero (i.e., by using orthogonal rotation), mostly because they were reported to be of trivial size.

When the content of the factors is reviewed, a complex picture emerges. We highlight two issues: First, only 16 out of the 86 factors (i.e., 18.6%) that were extracted in these studies had salient loadings of criteria that pertain to a single PD category, and more than half (i.e., 55.8%) of the factors had salient loadings of criteria from three or more PD categories. The only PDs that were replicated across studies as coherent, distinct latent dimensions were Obsessive-Compulsive PD (with a "clean" loading pattern in eight studies) and Schizotypal PD (with a "clean" loading pattern in four studies). This is not surprising, given that Obsessive-Compulsive PD and Schizotypal PD are more limited in their content related to constraint and oddity, respectively. In contrast, criteria of Avoidant, Paranoid, Schizoid, Histrionic, and Antisocial PD never appeared as the sole indicators of a latent dimension in any study. An obvious conclusion from this is that the criteria sets of most *DSM–IV* PD diagnoses do not sharply correspond to the underlying latent structure, making these distinctions look rather arbitrary. Second, criteria from Avoidant and Dependent PD, as well as Histrionic and Narcissistic PD, jointly indicated a latent dimension in nine and eight studies, respectively. This suggests that these PDs share, at least in part, a latent dimension. Moreover, it should be noted that across studies Borderline PD criteria were interrelated with criteria from nearly every other PD in indicating a variety of latent factors. This is in line with results from a multidimensional scaling analysis of PD criteria that indicates that borderline symptoms are at the core of personality pathology (i.e., rather than representing a specific content domain, they are common to the entire domain of PD; Turkheimer, Ford, & Oltmanns, 2008).

Current Developments

So, why do so many patients meet the criteria for multiple PDs or no specific PD? After one peruses the breadth of factor-analytic research, the answer appears to be because the current criteria sets do not "carve nature at its joints." In other words, they more often than not mix up indicators that mark different (correlated) latent dimensions. For sure, this is not the final word, because current developments in factor analysis will continue to refine our understanding of the optimal structure of personality pathology. Nevertheless, we want to call attention to the following: First, the search for simple structure (e.g., by means of varimax rotation) might miss the point in the domain of personality and personality pathology (e.g., Hopwood & Donnellan, 2010; Krueger, Derringer, Markon, Watson, & Skodol, 2012). Alternative strategies include *bifactor rotation*, which allows indicators to load on a general factor and encourages simple structure for the loadings on the remaining unique factors (Reise, Moore, & Haviland, 2010). Bifactor models seem promising for testing concepts such as generalized severity of PD (Hopwood et al., 2011; Jahng et al., 2011). Moreover, recent approaches such as *exploratory structural equation modeling* allow for a flexible integration of EFA and CFA and seem especially helpful when simple structure is unlikely to be present in the population (Marsh et al., 2010).

Second, there is an increasing interest in exploring the *hierarchical structure* of personality pathology, which involves estimating a series of factor models with an increasing number of factors and connecting these subsequent models using factor score correlations (Goldberg, 2006; Markon, Krueger, & Watson, 2005; Wright et al., 2012). One advantage of this strategy is that the question regarding the "true" number of factors becomes less important because solutions with fewer factors may come to light as plausible representations of the domain at a higher level of abstraction (cf. Leising & Zimmermann, 2011). This strategy might also be helpful for integrating other domains (e.g., clinical syndromes formerly represented on Axis I in *DSM*) into a general latent framework of psychopathology (Kotov et al., 2011; Markon, 2010; Røysamb et al., 2011). Indeed, as Markon (2010) demonstrated, many of the individual clinical syndromes and PD symptoms clustered together to form 20 specific factors that loaded on four more general factors.

Finally, factor analysis can be extended to handle more sophisticated designs and data structures. For example, multitrait-multimethod data allow for separating method from substantive factors (Blackburn, Donnelly, Logan,

& Renwick, 2004), and twin studies allow for disentangling genetic and environmental factors (Kendler et al., 2008). Both approaches pave the way for a deeper understanding of the comorbidity problem in PD research and practice.

Is Personality Pathology Dimensional, Categorical, or Some Hybrid of the Two?

Not surprisingly, this question has received the largest amount of intellectual attention and controversy over the years (Kendell, 1975; Livesley, Schroeder, Jackson, & Jang, 1994; Trull & Durrett, 2005), likely because it cuts to the very nature of the constructs in question and has large implications for practice, research, and policy. A number of methods with varying degrees of rigor exist for evaluating whether the data in a particular sample come from individuals whose pathology is organized along a dimension as opposed to emerging from distinct groups (Cleland, Rothschild, & Haslam, 2000). The latent variable modeling framework that we espouse here allows for a direct quantitative comparison and adjudication among models that assume dimensional, categorical, but also hybrid underlying structures.

One notable advantage of this approach is that it uses formal fit criteria that remove a great deal of subjectivity from model selection. Another benefit to this framework is that the hypothetical latent structures that can be estimated and compared are not limited to simplistic categorical versus dimensional dichotomies but rather encompass a *categorical–dimensional spectrum* (Masyn, Henderson, & Greenbaum, 2010). Thus, the modeled structures can range from the fully dimensional (i.e., factor analyses) to the fully categorical (i.e., latent class analysis), with variations that combine aspects of the two in between (see also Hallquist & Wright, 2014). Hybrid latent structures have traditionally been referred to as *factor mixture models*, but, as we show, factor analysis and latent class analysis are special cases of factor mixture models. Figure 5.2 provides graphical depictions of many, but not all, of the possible structures. Factor analysis (Panel A) represents one pole of the categorical–dimensional spectrum and assumes a fully dimensional latent structure, such that individuals vary continuously along a normally distributed latent trait (or traits). At the other end of the spectrum is latent class analysis (Panel F), which assumes a fully categorical latent structure, such that individuals differ discretely from each other exclusively in terms of a pattern of features shared among a homogenous subgroup. In terms of hybrid models, semiparametric factor analysis (Panel B) estimates a mixture of normally distributed groups along a common dimension to model a non-normal but continuous distribution. Thus, individuals vary along the same trait, but it allows for an extreme tail or other non-normal (e.g., bimodal) distributions. Alternatively, nonparametric factor analysis (also referred to as located latent class analysis;

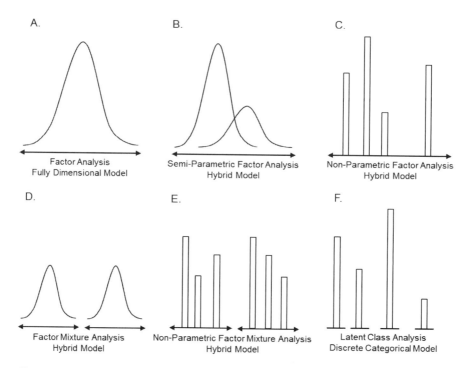

Figure 5.2. Graphical depiction of latent distributions associated with various factor mixture models. Lines at the base with arrows represent continuous dimensions. Columns represent groupings of individuals with no variance in latent scores.

Panel C) models discrete latent groups along a shared dimension. In this case, there are defined "gaps" between latent groups of individuals along the same latent trait. It is also possible to model factor structures that differ across groups (Panel D), which implies different latent dimensions or that the questions or symptoms have different meanings or function differently across groups. This can even be extended to include discrete disjunctions in those factors (Panel E). We do not provide an exhaustive catalogue or treatment of these models but rather a sampling to encourage researchers and practitioners to think in more nuanced ways about the possible latent structure of personality pathology. Of importance, these can all be estimated and compared with each other in real data to test theoretical assumptions about the actual latent structure of pathology.

Studies that directly compare a range of models including dimensional, categorical, and hybrid structures of PD remain rare but are starting to emerge. Conway, Hammen, and Brennan (2012) examined the latent structure of the DSM's nine Borderline Personality Disorder (BPD) criteria in a large community sample of young adults at risk for psychopathology. They compared dimensional, categorical, and hybrid models (nonparametric factor analyses) and found that a fully dimensional latent structure best fit the data (i.e., Figure 5.1, Panel A). Hallquist and Pilkonis (2012) also examined BPD symptoms but in a mixed clinical and nonclinical sample, finding that a hybrid model best fit the data. Their model suggested that there were largely symptomatic and asymptomatic classes that differed along a shared dimension of BPD severity (i.e., Figure 5.1, Panel C). Differences between the samples, assessment instruments, techniques, and the precise hybrid models tested prohibit strong conclusions about the nature of the latent structure of BPD based on these two studies alone. Confidence in the findings of these studies would be bolstered by independent replications. In this vein, Bornovalova, Levy, Gratz, and Lejuez (2010) estimated only a latent class model of BPD symptoms but implicitly found support for a dimensional model. This is because the four retained classes differed from each only in severity, not in the configuration of symptom endorsements (i.e., quantitative, not qualitative differences between classes). As in much of the PD literature, the focus has primarily been on BPD and the inclusion of other PD content is needed.

Expanding the lens somewhat further to include structural studies of broad domains of psychopathology (e.g., Internalizing, Externalizing, Psychosis), the finding has been consistent, with fit criteria favoring latent dimensional models over categorical or hybrid models (e.g., Eaton et al., 2013; Markon & Krueger, 2005; Walton, Ormel, & Krueger, 2011; Witkiewitz et al., 2013; Wright et al., 2013). These findings have direct bearing on structural questions in PDs because there is now accumulating evidence that PDs can be directly incorporated in to this framework (see above). However, a limitation of this growing body of work is that the studies have not been exhaustive in their tests of factor mixture models, instead restricting the explorations to a subset of common models (Hallquist & Pilkonis, 2012, is a notable exception).[4]

What Is a Reasonable Diagnostic Threshold for PD(s)?

Given the importance of diagnostic thresholds for scientific, clinical, and legal matters, it would stand to reason that the existing thresholds were developed with strong empirical support. They were not. In fact, most

---

[4]Readers familiar with traditional taxometric methods (e.g., MAMBAC, MAXCOV, and MAXEIG; see Ruscio, Haslam, & Ruscio, 2006, for a review) may wonder about the relationship between these methods and the analytic approach we suggest here. Although there are technical differences between these approaches, the key conceptual difference is that the traditional taxometric procedures are only able to compare a unidimensional to a "two-group" model, whereas factor mixture models are able to compare unidimensional, multidimensional, two-group, and multigroup categorical models, along with hybrids of all of the above. As such, the general latent variable framework is more flexible. We note, however, that for the majority of PD constructs—with the potential exception of schizotypal PD (see Lenzenweger, 2010)—taxometric evidence supports dimensional models (e.g., Arntz et al., 2009; Haslam, Holland, & Kuppens, 2012).

diagnostic thresholds were set arbitrarily without any formal investigation (Krueger, 2013); the exceptions being Borderline, Schizotypal (the criteria for which have since been changed; Spitzer, Endicott, & Gibbon, 1979), and Antisocial PDs (Widiger et al., 1996), which were each supported by only one study. The DSM model of PD is *polythetic*, such that to meet the threshold of for a particular disorder, a patient must exhibit a certain number of criteria from a larger set. From a quantitative modeling perspective, a polythetic model makes strong assumptions about the structure of PD. The obvious assumption about the categorical nature of PD can be set aside in this context, given that diagnostic thresholds will likely be necessary for practical reasons (e.g., study inclusion, reimbursement) with a dimensional system. Yet beyond this, a polythetic structure presumes that all symptoms are fungible and as such are equally good markers of the diagnostic construct (e.g., chronic emptiness is just as central to BPD as affective instability) and suggest equal degrees of severity in the pathology (e.g., inappropriate anger is just as severe as disassociation). It follows that all individuals with subthreshold symptom counts will be less severe than those "above the cut."

Item response theory (IRT) models (also called latent trait models; Embretson & Reise, 2000) can test these assumptions. IRT models can be understood as CFA models that use binary (i.e., 0/1 or present vs. absent) or ordinal (e.g., 0, 1, or 2; absent, present, severe) observed data. However, the model parameterization allows for drawing specific inferences about items. That is, IRT establishes the degree of information provided by each item (in this context an item is exhibiting a symptom) and where along the latent trait the item provides maximal information. The degree of information (referred to as the *alpha or "a"* parameter) can be understood as how well an item discriminates among individuals at different levels of the latent trait (conceptually, this is akin to a factor loading when using dimensional items in CFA). Where along the trait the item provides the most information is referred to as the difficulty (or *beta, "b"*) parameter, which is defined as the level of the trait an individual needs to possess to have a 50% chance of endorsing the item. Together these can be used to create an *item characteristic curve*, which describes the performance of the item relative to the latent trait.

To illustrate, let us consider a hypothetical example. For simplicity, we will use a fictional disorder with four criteria. If we were to run an IRT model, we might get results like those in Figure 5.3. A series of item characteristic curves are plotted in the top part of the figure. Note that the *x*-axis represents levels of a latent trait (e.g., PD severity), and the *y*-axis reflects the probability of endorsing a symptom. The table under the graph provides the parameter values associated with each symptom and curve. Note that Symptoms 3 and 4 are roughly equally discriminating (i.e., the curves are equally steep), but they are associated with markedly different levels of severity (i.e., difficulty

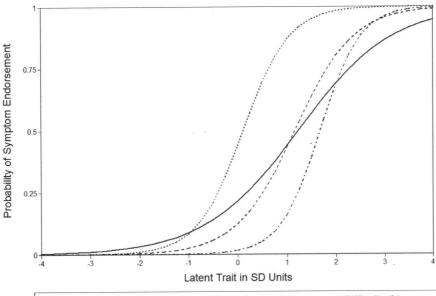

Item	Discrimination (a)	Difficulty (b)
Symptom 1 (Solid Line)	1.05	1.23
Symptom 2 (Dashed Line)	1.69	1.16
Symptom 3 (Dotted Line)	2.16	0.11
Symptom 4 (Dashed-Dotted Line)	2.46	1.68

Figure 5.3. Item characteristic curves and item response theory (IRT) model parameters for four hypothetical symptoms. SD = standard deviation.

parameters differ). Individuals at average levels of the trait ($SD = 0.11$) are likely to endorse Symptom 3, whereas relatively high levels of the trait are required before an individual is likely to endorse Symptom 4 ($SD = 1.68$). In contrast, Symptoms 1 and 2 are roughly the same in severity (i.e., similar difficulty parameters), but Symptom 2 is much more discriminating than Symptom 1. Note the gradual increase in probability of endorsement associated with Symptom 1 across levels of the latent trait.

IRT models have only recently been applied to PD research (e.g., Balsis, Gleason, Woods, & Oltmanns, 2007; Conway et al., 2012; Feske, Kirisci, Tarter, & Pilkonis, 2007), and results suggest that symptoms differ in both their severity and their relationship to the latent traits for which they are putative markers. Varying item parameters associated with symptoms has potentially large implications for diagnostic thresholds. These implications were examined in a series of recent studies that used an extension of IRT to determine the level of severity associated with a particular combination of symptoms (Balsis, Lowmaster, Cooper, & Benge, 2011; Cooper & Balsis,

2009; Cooper, Balsis, & Zimmerman, 2010). In the first two of these studies, the researchers demonstrated that for a given number of criteria, ranging from one through the maximum number for a PD, the level of the latent trait implied by the endorsed criteria varied dramatically depending on the combination. For example, the possible combinations of three criteria of BPD ranged from ~.6 SDs to ~1.1 SDs along the latent trait, suggesting a wide band of severity associated with three criteria. Alone, this may not warrant immediate cause for alarm, but we note that almost three quarters of possible response patterns overlapped in severity with a pattern at a different level of symptom endorsement (e.g., many four-criteria response patterns overlapped with many three-criteria and five-criteria response patterns). This means that many "subthreshold" patterns are actually more severe than the above-threshold patterns. The long-offered observation that individuals just shy of threshold are nonetheless impaired is not only true; at times, they can be more impaired than those who do meet the cutoff. Using the same technique, Balsis et al. (2011) examined whether similar levels of latent pathology (i.e., the latent trait) were needed to achieve diagnostic threshold (i.e., number of observed symptoms) across diagnoses. They found that diagnoses differed significantly in the level of latent trait needed. For example, only 1.54 SDs of latent schizoid pathology but a full 2.72 SDs of dependent pathology are required to meet threshold, suggesting that cutoffs were not consistent across disorders. The authors of these studies argue, and we agree, that cutting scores or diagnostic thresholds should be based on the level of the latent trait, not the number of criteria endorsed. In turn, this frees the practitioner from the task of criterion "bean counting" to a more nuanced and clinically relevant task of determining the level of severity in any given patient's pathology.

Additional attractive features of IRT models include the ability to test item parameters across relevant groups, such as age or gender (see, e.g., Balsis et al., 2007). Accordingly, different criteria could be developed or diagnostic rules could vary across groups of patients. For instance, as Balsis et al. (2007) have shown, the Schizoid PD criterion "lacks interest in sexual experiences" differs between younger and older adults, such that it represents elevated levels of the trait in young adults but not in older adults.

Which Are the Important Behavioral Patterns to Track and Target for Intervention?

Up to this point we have considered applying statistical models to traditional psychiatric assessment information (namely, symptoms and diagnoses). This type of information is often treated as dispositional or as a static feature of the individual. This is codified in the DSM through Criterion B of the general definition of a PD in Section II, which refers to a "pattern that is inflexible and pervasive across a broad range of personal and social situations" (American Psychiatric Association, 2013, pp. 646–647). At the same time, seasoned clinicians are aware that this is not strictly the case, recognizing that the symptomatic expression of PD varies not only between patients but also within a patient across time. Personality pathology reflects a dynamic interplay between the person and the environment through the behaviors emitted in response to stimuli (both external and internal), mental construal and interpretation of events, motivations and the manner in which they are pursued, and both how and how well self-regulation is enacted when motives and goals are frustrated. The key to clinical efficacy is to know which processes are central to and serve to maintain the pathology. Recent developments in assessment technology and statistical modeling allow for great insight on clinically rich information.

Assessing Dynamic Processes

To capture the type of information needed to understand the proximal processes of PD, we must move outside the consulting room to sample individuals in their everyday life (van Os et al., 2013). The goal is to capture individuals as they generally behave across a wide variety of situations in naturalistic settings. Referred to variously as *experience sampling methodology (ESM), ecological momentary assessment (EMA)*, and *ambulatory assessment (AA;* the moniker we use here), this approach samples an individual's behavior repeatedly in his or her natural environment (see Moskowitz, Russell, Sadikaj, & Sutton, 2009; Trull & Ebner-Priemer, 2013). In this framework, individuals are tasked with reporting on their behavior or experiences repeatedly and frequently as these are lived. For instance, a common protocol is to have individuals report on their behavior, emotions, and perception of the other person after every social interaction for 3 weeks. Figure 5.4 provides a graphical depiction of the appearance of a hypothetical individual's data stream over a 90-day assessment of symptoms (e.g., thoughts of self-harm), normative range behavior (e.g., basic emotions like anxiety), and key events (e.g., fights with significant other). The power of this approach to capture the dynamic interplay of people and their environments is impressive. An additional benefit is that they are robust to the well-known retrospective biases in self-reported functioning (Ebner-Priemer et al., 2006).

Designing an effective protocol requires consideration of numerous factors, chief among them (a) which variables to assess and (b) the temporal resolution of the sampling. We discuss these in tandem, as they are inextricably intertwined. Virtually any variable that an individual can self-report is amenable to experience sampling methods. Common targets include emotions, interpersonal behavior, stress, symptoms (e.g., self-injury),

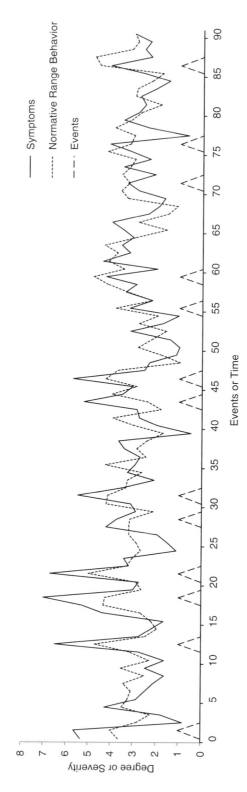

Figure 5.4. Hypothetical intensive repeated measurement data stream of symptoms, normal range behavior, and environmental events.

and substance use, to name a few. In addition, technology exists to sample additional behavior that the individual does not self-report, including physiological markers, such as heart rate and blood pressure, but also electronic audio recordings of ambient noise (Mehl, Pennebaker, Crow, Dabbs, & Price, 2001). The phenomenon of interest clearly dictates the types of variables being collected, but it also dictates the frequency of assessment. The temporal resolution must match the time scale on which the process in question occurs. For instance, mood fluctuations in BPD occur on the order of moments to hours, so daily sampling of mood would be insufficient for catching emotional lability in BPD. Alternatively, impulsive sex is likely to occur much less frequently. Asking people to report on their sexual behavior each hour would be excessive, but a daily question targeting this behavior is probably sufficient. Moreover, the sampling frame need not be tethered to time, as recordings can be event contingent as well (e.g., after each social interaction, following binges, when suicidal thoughts occur).

Modeling Dynamic Processes

The type of data that emerge from AA offers the ability to pose and answer new questions about PDs, and with this comes the need for different and even novel modeling approaches. Some of the most straightforward methods for AA involve calculating individual descriptive statistics that can then be used as outcomes or predictors. For example, an individual's mean, calculated as the average of all his (or her) assessments, is usually informative, but so too is his standard deviation, or the net amount of variability in his behavior over time (Fleeson, 2001). If we stick with traditional PD constructs for illustrative purposes, Borderline PD should be associated with higher individual standard deviations in affect, whereas Schizoid PD should be associated with lower individual standard deviations. Additional parameters can be derived from individual data streams, such as the mean square of successive differences, which captures instability over time (Ebner-Priemer, Eid, Kleindienst, Stabenow, & Trull, 2009). These methods offer a coarse view of dynamic processes.

A more detailed question is whether specific behaviors or features are linked within individuals across time and whether the within-person strength of that link is related to PD. For example, does perceived rejection elicit rage in BPD (Berenson, Downey, Rafaeli, Coifman, & Paquin, 2011), or do narcissists perceive assertiveness in others as hostility (Roche, Pincus, Hyde, Conroy, & Ram, 2013)? This type of question can be answered with *multilevel modeling* (MLM; also known as hierarchical linear modeling, random effects regression, or mixed modeling; see Hox, 2010, and Singer & Willett, 2003, for accessible texts). MLM is a form of regression that accounts for the fact that repeated measurements (Level 1) of target variables are nested within individuals (Level 2) in a sample. In MLM, the within-person association between the outcome and predictor is derived from the time-specific fluctuations on the variables, representing the temporal covariation of scores (e.g., are an individual's fluctuations in rejection perception at a given point in time associated with his or her rage at a given point in time?). Variability in these within-person effects is estimated as well. Thus, MLM provides an estimate of the average association strength (i.e., link) between a time-varying predictor and outcome (referred to as the fixed effect), as well as individual variability in association strength around that mean (referred to as the random effect). Additional features of the individual (e.g., gender, trait antagonism, PD diagnosis, childhood adversity) can be included at Level 2 to predict the strength of the link. MLM allows for the study of individual differences in within-person processes.

Finally, we draw the reader's attention to the potential for conducting idiographic or person-specific modeling with AA data. For example, the use of *P-technique factor analysis* (i.e., applying factor analysis to scores on multiple variables from one individual across multiple time points; Nesselroade & Ford, 1985) holds the potential to elucidate idiographic structure and change through time, especially when it is coupled with techniques such as *time-series analysis* (Hamaker, Dolan, & Molenaar, 2005). Novel hypotheses can be developed, such as that a person-specific factor model can provide insight in to psychological complexity (e.g., smaller numbers of factors suggest less differentiation across situations). Additionally, factor scores could be used to estimate the mental state an individual found himself in at a given point along the assessment stream (see, e.g., Figure 5.4). Space precludes a detailed discussion of these issues, but we mention them because rigorous statistical models applied to the individual hold incredible promise for personalized assessment and treatment. Methods can now be linked to theory and individual patients in ways that further the science and practice of assessing personality pathology, and the technology is rapidly becoming widespread and cheap.

Existing PD Research Using AA

Mirroring the research bias in the rest of the PD field, AA research has focused almost exclusively on BPD. The BPD construct is a natural first target, given the hallmark variability in emotions, self-esteem, and interpersonal behavior. Work has begun to show that structured patterns emerge that differentiate BPD from healthy and psychiatric controls. For example, individuals with BPD can be differentiated from nonclinical control participants based on higher levels of variability of interpersonal behavior over a 20-day period (Russell, Moskowitz, Zuroff, Sookman, & Paris, 2007). Ebner-Priemer et al. (2007) identified group-specific patterns of affective instability when comparing patients with BPD to healthy controls, with the former being distinguishable on the basis of rapid and dramatic declines from positive mood states in particular. Moreover, the sequence of experienced emotions (e.g., anxiety followed by anger) differed between these groups (Reisch, Ebner-Priemer, Tschacher, Bohus, & Linehan, 2008). Building on these results, Trull et al. (2008) used AA to investigate affective instability in BPD with a control group of individuals diagnosed with depressive disorder. It is noteworthy that these two groups did not differ on mean levels of positive or negative affect reported across time. In other words, they exhibited similar trait levels of affect. However, the variability in these scores differentiated the two groups, with BPD patients exhibiting greater variability. Moreover, BPD patients also exhibited more abrupt changes in hostility, fear, and sadness than did depressive controls. These results demonstrate that it is the temporal patterning and contingency of affective functioning that gives rise to the turbulent experience that clinicians recognize as BPD, even when compared to groups with similarity in overall negative affect. These techniques further differentiate individuals with diagnoses of BPD and PTSD from those with BPD alone and major depression with PTSD as well (Schneiderer, Wang, Tomko, Wood, & Trull, 2013).

Furthermore, MLM analyses have shown that individuals with BPD demonstrate stronger affective responses in response to less perceived warmth (Sadikaj, Russell, Moskowitz, & Paris, 2010) and rejection (Berenson et al., 2011) in interpersonal situations. They also show greater quarrelsomeness in response to others' quarrelsomeness (Sadikaj, Moskowitz, Russell, Zuroff, & Paris, 2013). Sadikaj, Moskowitz, Russell, and Zuroff (2010) compared patients with BPD to those carrying diagnoses of social phobia (SP), showing decreased perceptions of warmth in interpersonal situations are associated with higher negative affect for both groups. However, the association was strongest for anger in BPD and in embarrassment for SP. Furthermore, the two groups demonstrated specificity in the behavioral patterns associated with negative affect, with patients with BPD becoming more quarrelsome and patients with SP becoming more submissive. This type of result allows for highly articulated and precise description of symptoms and offers a look at the internal processes that gives rise to these symptoms. Finally, Coifman, Berenson, Rafaeli, and Downey (2012) showed that emotional and relational "polarity" (i.e., feeling all good or all bad) was higher in patients with BPD relative to controls, was strongest when the individual was under interpersonal stress, and was predictive of impulsive behaviors. This framework points to multiple possible sources of disturbed functioning (e.g., distortions in interpersonal perception and meaning-making processes; maladaptive, underdeveloped, or overvalued interpersonal goals, motives, expectancies, and competencies) that suggest more specific hypotheses for future research (Pincus, Lukowitsky, Wright, & Eichler, 2009).

SUMMARY, IMPLICATIONS, AND FURTHER QUESTIONS

At the start of this chapter we posed four clinical questions associated with the assessment and diagnosis of PD and then demonstrated how contemporary quantitative techniques are highly applicable to answering these questions. What answers did these models provide? In terms of the first question, we believe that the accumulation of factor-analytic research has convincingly shown that the *DSM*'s PD structure is erroneous. That is, not only do PD categories covary due to shared and correlated latent dimensions but at least most of them fall apart once symptoms are analyzed. We are far from the first to report what the science of PD has found with regard to the limitations of the current *DSM* structure. Nevertheless, we reiterate these points here because some believe this issue remains debatable.[5] As for the second question, we must be tentative given how little research has compared categorical, dimensional, and hybrid latent structures. The limited existing results suggest that the structure is likely to be either a fully dimensional one or a hybrid including a dimensional component, with categories being highly unlikely. The third question, related to the threshold issue, suggests there are alarming problems in the current polythetic approach to diagnosis and in its arbitrary assignment of most thresholds. This finding may matter more for research, given that clinicians generally choose to treat when there is impairment present, not based on the arbitrary criterion count. Finally, AA-based research is relatively new, but it has already demonstrated that it can model core features of existing constructs (e.g., BPD). There is incredible promise in this general approach to studying psychological and psychiatric phenomena in a more person-oriented and process-centered way.

Where should the field go from here? We believe there is much to be gained from continuing to apply the models we have discussed here to the PD domain. However, to what data they should be applied needs to be resolved. As others have noted before (Goldberg & Velicer, 2006) and as we mentioned above, the selection of variables in any statistical model will constrain the

---

[5]For example, some researchers have argued that prototypes resembling the *DSM* categories are advisable (Westen, Shedler, Bradley, & DeFife, 2012). However, results supporting this perspective have been based on a different data-analytic approach (i.e., *Q-factor analysis* of clinicians' ratings of patients; see Chapter 9, this volume) and thus cannot easily be compared with the results of conventional factor-analytic studies reviewed in this chapter. When using conventional PCA or EFA, Westen and colleagues did not find much support for the *DSM* categories emerging as distinct latent dimensions in their data sets (Shedler & Westen, 2004; Westen, Waller, Shedler, & Blagov, 2012).

outcome. This has both very specific and broad implications. For instance, because symptoms of most PD diagnoses tend to break apart (i.e., load on multiple factors) when additional content is added, testing the latent structure of a single diagnosis is not actually all that informative. Further studies on the latent structure of one specific PD are likely to be of limited value; instead, studies should include a broader representation of content in both theoretically related and distinct domains. We recommend that factor mixture models and especially AA are in need of expanding beyond the narrow focus on BPD. This is not to criticize existing work but rather to say there is real potential for new insights in examining the structure and dynamic processes of a broad range of personality pathology.

Furthermore, how the information is assessed and coded will matter a great deal for the ultimate conclusions. For example, consider coding the affective lability symptom for BPD from a traditional diagnostic interview. This highly complex process ordinarily gets transformed into a 0 or 1. Statistically speaking, this discards an incredible amount of information and introduces a lot of error into the data (i.e., all individuals with a 1 are treated as having the same mechanism present). Alternatively, consider using AA to actually collect the exact degree and patterning of someone's affective instability, which could then be extracted and used for more precise latent variable modeling. In much the same way an individual's physiological responses to interpersonal challenge tasks in the laboratory, reaction times to performance-based tasks, BOLD recordings from fMRI scans of amygdala activity, or plasma or salivary levels of hormones could all be used as observed variables in the estimation of (potentially novel) latent constructs. These are but a few examples to suggest that these models need not be wedded to psychiatric criteria as assessed only by traditional interviews and self-report scales. Novel data collection procedures may achieve greater fidelity in capturing the important features of PD.

More broadly, the composition and coverage of the *DSM* criteria set themselves are debatable. For example, roughly one fifth of the individual criteria tap behavioral tendencies that are specific to a particular class of situations, whereas the remaining ones refer to dispositions that generalize across situations (Leising & Zimmermann, 2011). This amount of situational specificity may be judged as too high or too low, depending on the underlying theory of personality or personality pathology (Eaton, South, & Krueger, 2009). Moreover, the *DSM* criteria set predominantly captures impairments in interpersonal and cognitive functioning and places less weight on impairments in affectivity and impulse control (Bornstein, Bianucci, Fishman, & Biars, 2014). Adopting more critical views, others have argued that the *DSM* criteria set lacks important content coverage (Westen & Arkowitz-Westen, 1998; Widiger & Trull, 2007) or that individual PD criteria are ill conceived, as they mix up "symptoms, traits, functions, and consequences" (Morey &

Skodol, 2013, p. 192). This view raises conceptual questions about the basic unit or definition of PD that probably cannot be fully answered with quantitative methods (Leising & Zimmermann, 2011; Zachar & Kendler, 2010). However, it also suggests that researchers may do well to go beyond the DSM criteria set when investigating the latent structure or dynamic interplay of personality pathology (Clark, Livesley, Schroeder, & Irish, 1996; Shedler & Westen, 2004).

These issues are timely, as we currently find ourselves (and it is unclear for how long) in the unprecedented position of having a DSM with two full PD models (Krueger, 2013; Skodol, 2012). The Section III model in DSM–5 has adopted a very different structure, which warrants evaluation using the types of modeling we have discussed here. Although the model appears very promising and provides an impressive step toward both clinical theory and scientific results, there are challenges to modeling the hypothesized structure. Among the most interesting but difficult to resolve will be how Criterion A (general PD functioning dimension) differs from and interfaces with Criterion B (hierarchical pathological trait model) conceptually and in practice. Criterion A uses process-based language to describe its content, suggesting that perhaps it will require the application of methods that can capture this type of information (e.g., AA). Further, the DSM–5 retains a series of categorical PD diagnoses that should be amenable for investigation with various latent variable modeling approaches.

At the same time, despite our enthusiasm for these advanced methods, we would not want to leave readers with the impression that more established methods, such as correlation, multiple regression, and analysis of variance, are no longer valuable. Quite to the contrary, the techniques described here are meant to augment, but not replace, the statistical armamentarium of the psychopathologist. What remains most important is that the right method be paired with a sophisticated and clinically interesting research question in a way that it can clearly communicate new information. Advanced statistics cannot stand in for this whole equation. There are some questions for which the methods we have described here are ideal, and as such we encourage researchers to learn them and pursue them. We look forward to seeing the emerging research and hope our review of methods will inspire other investigators to use them.

CONCLUSION

We have tried to demonstrate that questions that emerge directly from clinical assessment can be translated into statistical models and investigated with powerful quantitative tools. In the process, we have reviewed a large and growing body of research on the application of these models to the domain of PD. Regrettably, we had to be selective in our review of the literature, and many interesting lines of work that run parallel or even directly relevant to what we discussed here were not covered. Nevertheless, we hope we were convincing in arguing that basic clinical questions and modern quantitative methods do not contradict each other but actually have the potential to stimulate each other. The clinical questions we examined here, and the tentative answers suggested by applying the statistical models to PD data, cut to the very heart of the psychiatric nosology's validity. Due to the privileged position the *DSM* enjoys in modern mental health practice, nosological failures become magnified when they are used as the basis for the allocation of scarce public resources (e.g., the type of research that gets funded), which in turn dictates the likelihood of successfully identifying etiological and maintenance mechanisms (e.g., which patients are chosen for inclusion in laboratory studies) and ultimately whether or not treatments are developed (e.g., who qualifies for treatment studies). These issues are not esoteric: They directly impede clinical care by complicating communication, both between practitioners and between practitioners and patients, and by providing limited prognostic value and prescriptive information for treatment selection. Patients deserve better.

REFERENCES

American Psychiatric Association. (1994). *Diagnostic and statistical manual of mental disorders* (4th ed.). Washington, DC: Author.

American Psychiatric Association. (2013). *Diagnostic and statistical manual of mental disorders* (5th ed.). Arlington, VA: Author.

Arntz, A., Bernstein, D., Gielen, D., van Nieuwenhuyzen, M., Penders, K., Haslam, N., & Ruscio, J. (2009). Taxometric evidence for the dimensional structure of Cluster-C, paranoid, and borderline personality disorders. *Journal of Personality Disorders, 23,* 606–628. doi:10.1521/pedi.2009.23.6.606

Balsis, S., Gleason, M. E. J., Woods, C. M., & Oltmanns, T. F. (2007). An item response theory analysis of *DSM–IV* personality disorder criteria across younger and older age groups. *Psychology and Aging, 22,* 171–185. doi:10.1037/0882-7974.22.1.171

Balsis, S., Lowmaster, S., Cooper, L. D., & Benge, J. F. (2011). Personality disorder diagnostic thresholds correspond to different levels of latent pathology. *Journal of Personality Disorders, 25,* 115–127. doi:10.1521/pedi.2011.25.1.115

Bastiaansen, L., Rossi, G., Schotte, C., & de Fruyt, F. (2011). The structure of personality disorders: Comparing the *DSM–IV–TR* Axis II classification with the five-factor model framework using structural equation modeling. *Journal of Personality Disorders, 25,* 378–396. doi:10.1521/pedi.2011.25.3.378

Berenson, K. R., Downey, G., Rafaeli, E., Coifman, K. G., & Paquin, N. L. (2011). The rejection–rage contingency in borderline personality disorder. *Journal of Abnormal Psychology, 120,* 681–690. doi:10.1037/a0023335

Blackburn, R., Donnelly, J. P., Logan, C., & Renwick, S. J. D. (2004). Convergent and discriminative validity of interview and questionnaire measures of personality disorder in mentally disordered offenders: A multitrait-multimethod analysis using confirmatory factor analysis. *Journal of Personality Disorders, 18,* 129–150. doi:10.1521/pedi.18.2.129.32779

Blackburn, R., Logan, C., Renwick, S. J. D., & Donnelly, J. P. (2005). Higher-order dimensions of personality disorder: Hierarchical structure and relationships with the five-factor model, the Interpersonal Circle, and psychopathy. *Journal of Personality Disorders, 19,* 597–623. doi:10.1521/pedi.2005.19.6.597

Blagov, P. S., Bradley, R., & Westen, D. (2007). Under the Axis II radar. *Journal of Nervous and Mental Disease, 195,* 477–483. doi:10.1097/NMD.0b013e318064e824

Blais, M. A., & Malone, J. C. (2013). Structure of the *DSM–IV* personality disorders as revealed in clinician ratings. *Comprehensive Psychiatry, 54,* 326–333. doi:10.1016/j.comppsych.2012.10.014

Bollen, K. A. (1989). *Structural equations with latent variables.* New York, NY: Wiley.

Bornovalova, M. A., Levy, R., Gratz, K. L., & Lejuez, C. W. (2010). Understanding the heterogeneity of BPD symptoms through latent class analysis: Initial results and clinical correlates among inner-city substance users. *Psychological Assessment, 22,* 233–245. doi:10.1037/a0018493

Bornstein, R. F. (2011). Toward a process-focused model of test score validity: Improving psychological assessment in science and practice. *Psychological Assessment, 23,* 532–544. doi:10.1037/a0022402

Bornstein, R. F., Bianucci, V., Fishman, D. P., & Biars, J. W. (2014). Toward a firmer foundation for *DSM–5.1*: Domains of impairment in *DSM–IV/DSM–5* personality disorders. *Journal of Personality Disorders, 28,* 212–224. doi:10.1521/pedi_2013_27_116

Brown, T. A. (2006). *Confirmatory factor analysis for applied research.* New York, NY: Guilford Press.

Chabrol, H., Rousseau, A., Callahan, S., & Hyler, S. E. (2007). Frequency and structure of *DSM–IV* personality disorder traits in college students. *Personality and Individual Differences, 43,* 1767–1776. doi:10.1016/j.paid.2007.05.015

Clark, L. A., Livesley, W. J., Schroeder, M. L., & Irish, S. L. (1996). Convergence of two systems for assessing specific traits of personality disorder. *Psychological Assessment, 8,* 294–303. doi:10.1037/1040-3590.8.3.294

Clarkin, J. F., Yeomans, F., & Kernberg, O. F. (2006). *Psychotherapy of borderline personality: Focusing on object relations.* Washington, DC: American Psychiatric Publishing.

Cleland, C. M., Rothschild, L., & Haslam, N. (2000). Detecting latent taxa: Monte Carlo comparison of taxometric, mixture model, and clustering procedures. *Psychological Reports, 87,* 37–47. doi:10.2466/pr0.2000.87.1.37

Coifman, K. G., Berenson, K. R., Rafaeli, E., & Downey, G. (2012). From negative to positive and back again: Polarized affective and relational experience in borderline personality disorder. *Journal of Abnormal Psychology, 121,* 668–679. doi:10.1037/a0028502

Collins, L. M., & Lanza, S. T. (2010). *Latent class and latent transition analysis: With applications in the social behavioral, and health sciences.* Hoboken, NJ: Wiley.

Conway, C., Hammen, C., & Brennan, P. (2012). A comparison of latent class, latent trait, and factor mixture models of *DSM–IV* borderline personality disorder criteria in a community setting: Implications for *DSM–5. Journal of Personality Disorders, 26,* 793–803. doi:10.1521/pedi.2012.26.5.793

Cooper, L. D., & Balsis, S. (2009). When less is more: How fewer diagnostic criteria can indicate greater severity. *Psychological Assessment, 21,* 285–293. doi:10.1037/a0016698

Cooper, L. D., Balsis, S., & Zimmerman, M. (2010). Challenges associated with a polythetic diagnostic system: Criteria combinations in the personality disorders. *Journal of Abnormal Psychology, 119,* 886–895. doi:10.1037/a0021078

Doering, S., Renn, D., Höfer, S., Rumpold, G., Smrekar, U., Janecke, N., . . . Schüssler, G. (2007). Validierung der deutschen Version des Fragebogens zur Erfassung von *DSM–IV* Persönlichkeitsstörungen (*ADP–IV*) [Validation of the German version of the Assessment of *DSM–IV* Personality Disorders (*ADP–IV*) Questionnaire]. *Zeitschrift für Psychosomatische Medizin und Psychotherapie, 53,* 111–128. doi:10.13109/zptm.2007.53.2.111

Durrett, C., & Westen, D. (2005). The structure of Axis II disorders in adolescents: A cluster- and factor-analytic investigation of *DSM–IV* categories and criteria. *Journal of Personality Disorders, 19,* 440–461. doi:10.1521/pedi.2005.19.4.440

Eaton, N. R., Krueger, R. F., Markon, K. E., Keyes, K. M., Skodol, A. E., Wall, M., . . . Grant, B. F. (2013). The structure and predictive validity of the internalizing disorders. *Journal of Abnormal Psychology, 122,* 86–92. doi:10.1037/a0029598

Eaton, N. R., South, S. C., & Krueger, R. F. (2009). The Cognitive–Affective Processing System (CAPS) approach to personality and the concept of personality disorder: Integrating clinical and social-cognitive research. *Journal of Research in Personality, 43,* 208–217. doi:10.1016/j.jrp.2009.01.016

Ebner-Priemer, U. W., Eid, M., Kleindienst, N., Stabenow, S., & Trull, T. J. (2009). Analytic strategies for understanding affective (in)stability and other dynamic processes in psychopathology. *Journal of Abnormal Psychology, 118,* 195–202. doi:10.1037/a0014868

Ebner-Priemer, U. W., Kuo, J., Kleindienst, N., Welch, S. S., Reisch, T., Reinhard, I., . . . Bohus, M. (2007). State affective instability in borderline personality disorder assessed by ambulatory monitoring. *Psychological Medicine, 37,* 961–970. doi:10.1017/S0033291706009706

Ebner-Priemer, U. W., Kuo, J., Welch, S. S., Thielgen, T., Witte, S., Bohus, M., & Linehan, M. M. (2006). A valence-dependent group-specific recall bias of retrospective self-reports: A study of borderline personality disorder in everyday life. *Journal of Nervous and Mental Disease, 194,* 774–779. doi:10.1097/01.nmd.0000239900.46595.72

Embretson, S. E., & Reise, S. (2000). *Psychometric methods: Item response theory for psychologists.* Mahwah, NJ: Erlbaum.

Everett, J. (1983). Factor comparability as a means of determining the number of factors and their rotation. *Multivariate Behavioral Research, 18,* 197–218. doi:10.1207/s15327906mbr1802_5

Fabrigar, L. R., Wegener, D. T., MacCallum, R. C., & Strahan, E. J. (1999). Evaluating the use of exploratory factor analysis in psychological research. *Psychological Methods, 4,* 272–299. doi:10.1037/1082-989X.4.3.272

Feske, U., Kirisci, L., Tarter, R. E., & Pilkonis, P. A. (2007). An application of item response theory to the *DSM–III–R* criteria for borderline personality disorder. *Journal of Personality Disorders, 21,* 418–433. doi:10.1521/pedi.2007.21.4.418

Fleeson, W. (2001). Toward a structure- and process-integrated view of personality: Traits as density distributions of states. *Journal of Personality and Social Psychology, 80,* 1011–1027. doi:10.1037/0022-3514.80.6.1011

Fossati, A., Beauchaine, T. P., Grazioli, F., Borroni, S., Carretta, I., de Vecchi, C., . . . Maffei, C. (2006). Confirmatory factor analyses of *DSM–IV* Cluster C personality disorder criteria. *Journal of Personality Disorders, 20,* 186–203. doi:10.1521/pedi.2006.20.2.186

Fossati, A., Maffei, C., Bagnato, M., Battaglia, M., Donati, D., Donini, M., . . . Prolo, F. (2000). Patterns of covariation of *DSM–IV* personality disorders in a mixed psychiatric sample. *Comprehensive Psychiatry, 41,* 206–215. doi:10.1016/S0010-440X(00)90049-X

Goldberg, L. R. (2006). Doing it all bass-ackwards: The development of hierarchical factor structures from the top down. *Journal of Research in Personality, 40,* 347–358. doi:10.1016/j.jrp.2006.01.001

Goldberg, L. R., & Velicer, W. F. (2006). Principles of exploratory factor analysis. In S. Strack (Ed.), *Differentiating normal and abnormal personality* (2nd ed., pp. 209–237). New York, NY: Springer.

Hallquist, M. N., & Pilkonis, P. A. (2012). Refining the phenotype of borderline personality disorder: Diagnostic criteria and beyond. *Personality Disorders: Theory, Research, and Treatment, 3,* 228–246. doi:10.1037/a0027953

Hallquist, M. N., & Wright, A. G. C. (2014). Mixture modeling methods for the assessment of normal and abnormal personality, Part I: Cross-sectional models. *Journal of Personality Assessment, 96,* 256–268. doi:10.1080/00223891.2013.845201

Hamaker, E. L., Dolan, C. V., & Molenaar, P. C. M. (2005). Statistical modeling of the individual: Rationale and application of multivariate stationary time series analysis. *Multivariate Behavioral Research, 40,* 207–233.

Haslam, N., Holland, E., & Kuppens, P. (2012). Categories versus dimensions in personality and psychopathology: A quantitative review of taxometric research. *Psychological Medicine, 42,* 903–920. doi:10.1017/S0033291711001966

Hopwood, C. J., & Donnellan, M. B. (2010). How should the internal structure of personality inventories be evaluated? *Personality and Social Psychology Review, 14,* 332–346. doi:10.1177/1088868310361240

Hopwood, C. J., Malone, J. C., Ansell, E. B., Sanislow, C. A., Grilo, C. M., McGlashan, T. H., . . . Morey, L. C. (2011). Personality assessment in *DSM–5:* Empirical support for rating severity, style, and traits. *Journal of Personality Disorders, 25,* 305–320. doi:10.1521/pedi.2011.25.3.305

Horn, J. L. (1965). A rationale and test for the number of factors in factor analysis. *Psychometrika, 30,* 179–185. doi:10.1007/BF02289447

Howard, R. C., Huband, N., Duggan, C., & Mannion, A. (2008). Exploring the link between personality disorder and criminality in a community sample. *Journal of Personality Disorders, 22,* 589–603. doi:10.1521/pedi.2008.22.6.589

Hox, J. J. (2010). *Multilevel analysis: Techniques and applications* (2nd ed.). New York, NY: Routledge.

Huprich, S. K., Schmitt, T. A., Richard, D. C. S., Chelminski, I., & Zimmerman, M. A. (2010). Comparing factor analytic models of the *DSM–IV* personality disorders. *Personality Disorders: Theory, Research, and Treatment, 1,* 22–37. doi:10.1037/a0018245

Jahng, S., Trull, T. J., Wood, P. K., Tragesser, S. L., Tomko, R., Grant, J. D., . . . Sher, K. J. (2011). Distinguishing general and specific personality disorder features and implications for substance dependence comorbidity. *Journal of Abnormal Psychology, 120,* 656–669. doi:10.1037/a0023539

Kendell, R. C. (1975). *The role of diagnosis in psychiatry.* Oxford, England: Blackwell Scientific.

Kendler, K. S., Aggen, S. H., Czajkowski, N., Røysamb, E., Tambs, K., Torgersen, S., . . . Reichborn-Kjennerud, T. (2008). The structure of genetic and environmental risk factors for *DSM–IV* personality disorders: A multivariate twin study. *Archives of General Psychiatry, 65,* 1438–1446. doi:10.1001/archpsyc.65.12.1438

Kotov, R., Ruggero, C. J., Krueger, R. F., Watson, D., Yuan, Q., & Zimmerman, M. A. (2011). New dimensions in the quantitative classification of mental illness. *Archives of General Psychiatry, 68,* 1003–1011. doi:10.1001/archgenpsychiatry.2011.107

Krueger, R. F. (2013). Personality disorders are the vanguard of the post-*DSM–5.0* era. *Personality Disorders: Theory, Research, and Treatment, 4,* 355–362. doi:10.1037/per0000028

Krueger, R. F., Derringer, J., Markon, K. E., Watson, D., & Skodol, A. E. (2012). Initial construction of a maladaptive personality trait model and inventory for *DSM–5*. *Psychological Medicine, 42,* 1879–1890. doi:10.1017/S0033291711002674

Krueger, R. F., & Markon, K. E. (2006). Reinterpreting comorbidity: A model-based approach to understanding and classifying psychopathology. *Annual Review of Clinical Psychology, 2,* 111–133. doi:10.1146/annurev.clinpsy.2.022305.095213

Leising, D., & Zimmermann, J. (2011). An integrative conceptual framework for assessing personality and personality pathology. *Review of General Psychology, 15,* 317–330. doi:10.1037/a0025070

Lenzenweger, M. F. (2010). *Schizotypy and schizophrenia: The view from experimental psychopathology.* New York, NY: Guilford Press.

Lenzenweger, M. F., Lane, M. C., Loranger, A. W., & Kessler, R. C. (2007). *DSM–IV* personality disorders in the National Comorbidity Survey Replication. *Biological Psychiatry, 62,* 553–564. doi:10.1016/j.biopsych.2006.09.019

Lilienfeld, S. O., Waldman, I. D., & Israel, A. C. (1994). A critical examination of the use of the term and concept of comorbidity in psychopathology research. *Clinical Psychology: Science and Practice, 1,* 71–83. doi:10.1111/j.1468-2850.1994.tb00007.x

Livesley, W. J., Schroeder, M. L., Jackson, D. N., & Jang, K. L. (1994). Categorical distinctions in the study of personality disorder: Implications for classification. *Journal of Abnormal Psychology, 103,* 6–17. doi:10.1037/0021-843X.103.1.6

Lorenzo-Seva, U., Timmerman, M. E., & Kiers, H. A. L. (2011). The Hull method for selecting the number of common factors. *Multivariate Behavioral Research, 46,* 340–364. doi:10.1080/00273171.2011.564527

Markon, K. E. (2010). Modeling psychopathology structure: A symptom-level analysis of Axis I and II disorders. *Psychological Medicine, 40,* 273–288. doi:10.1017/S0033291709990183

Markon, K. E., & Krueger, R. F. (2005). Categorical and continuous models of liability to externalizing disorders: A direct comparison in NESARC. *Archives of General Psychiatry, 62,* 1352–1359. doi:10.1001/archpsyc.62.12.1352

Markon, K. E., Krueger, R. F., & Watson, D. (2005). Delineating the structure of normal and abnormal personality: An integrative hierarchical approach. *Journal of Personality and Social Psychology, 88,* 139–157. doi:10.1037/0022-3514.88.1.139

Marsh, H. W., Lüdtke, O., Muthén, B., Asparouhov, T., Morin, A. J. S., Trautwein, U., & Nagengast, B. (2010). A new look at the Big Five factor structure through exploratory structural equation modeling. *Psychological Assessment, 22,* 471–491. doi:10.1037/a0019227

Masyn, K. E., Henderson, C. E., & Greenbaum, P. E. (2010). Exploring the latent structures of psychological constructs in social development using the dimensional–categorical spectrum. *Social Development, 19,* 470–493. doi:10.1111/j.1467-9507.2009.00573.x

McLachlan, G. J., & Peel, D. (2000). *Finite mixture models*. New York, NY: Wiley.

Mehl, M. R., Pennebaker, J. W., Crow, D. M., Dabbs, J., & Price, J. H. (2001). The Electronically Activated Recorder (EAR): A device for sampling naturalistic daily activities and conversations. *Behavior Research Methods, Instruments, & Computers, 33*, 517–523. doi:10.3758/BF03195410

Morey, L. C., & Skodol, A. E. (2013). Convergence between *DSM–IV–TR* and *DSM–5* diagnostic models for personality disorder: Evaluation of strategies for establishing diagnostic thresholds. *Journal of Psychiatric Practice, 19*, 179–193. doi:10.1097/01.pra.0000430502.78833.06

Moskowitz, D. S., Russell, J. J., Sadikaj, G., & Sutton, R. (2009). Measuring people intensively. *Canadian Psychology/Psychologie canadienne, 50*, 131–140.

Nesselroade, J. R., & Ford, D. H. (1985). P-technique comes of age. Multivariate, replicated, single-subject designs for research on older adults. *Research on Aging, 7*, 46–80. doi:10.1177/0164027585007001003

Nestadt, G., Hsu, F.-C., Samuels, J., Bienvenu, O. J., Reti, I., Costa, P. T., & Eaton, W. W. (2006). Latent structure of the *Diagnostic and Statistical Manual of Mental Disorders, Fourth Edition* personality disorder criteria. *Comprehensive Psychiatry, 47*, 54–62.

O'Connor, B. P. (2005). A search for consensus on the dimensional structure of personality disorders. *Journal of Clinical Psychology, 61*, 323–345. doi:10.1002/jclp.20017

Pearl, J. (2000). *Causality: Models, reasoning, and inference*. Cambridge, England: Cambridge University Press.

Pincus, A. L., Lukowitsky, M. R., Wright, A. G., & Eichler, W. C. (2009). The interpersonal nexus of persons, situations, and psychopathology. *Journal of Research in Personality, 43*, 264–265. doi:10.1016/j.jrp.2008.12.029

Preacher, K. J., Zhang, G., Kim, C., & Mels, G. (2013). Choosing the optimal number of factors in exploratory factor analysis: A model selection perspective. *Multivariate Behavioral Research, 48*, 28–56. doi:10.1080/00273171.2012.710386

Reisch, T., Ebner-Priemer, U. W., Tschacher, W., Bohus, M., & Linehan, M. M. (2008). Sequences of emotions in patients with borderline personality disorder. *Acta Psychiatrica Scandinavica, 118*, 42–48. doi:10.1111/j.1600-0447.2008.01222.x

Reise, S. P., Moore, T. M., & Haviland, M. G. (2010). Bifactor models and rotations: Exploring the extent to which multidimensional data yield univocal scale scores. *Journal of Personality Assessment, 92*, 544–559. doi:10.1080/00223891.2010.496477

Roche, M. J., Pincus, A. L., Hyde, A. L., Conroy, D. E., & Ram, N. (2013). Within-person covariation of agentic and communal perceptions: Implications for interpersonal theory and assessment. *Journal of Research in Personality, 47*, 445–452. doi:10.1016/j.jrp.2013.01.007

Røysamb, E., Kendler, K. S., Tambs, K., Ørstavik, R. E., Neale, M. C., Aggen, S. H., . . . Reichborn-Kjennerud, T. (2011). The joint structure of *DSM–IV*

Axis I and Axis II disorders. *Journal of Abnormal Psychology, 120,* 198–209. doi:10.1037/a0021660

Ruscio, J., Haslam, N., & Ruscio, A. M. (2006). *Introduction to the taxometric method: A practical guide.* Mahwah, NJ: Erlbaum.

Russell, J. J., Moskowitz, D. S., Zuroff, D. C., Sookman, D., & Paris, J. (2007). Stability and variability of affective experience and interpersonal behavior in borderline personality disorder. *Journal of Abnormal Psychology, 116,* 578–588. doi:10.1037/0021-843X.116.3.578

Sadikaj, G., Moskowitz, D. S., Russell, J. J., & Zuroff, D. C. (2010, June). *On the dynamic association between interpersonal perception, interpersonal behavior, and affect: Effects of social anxiety and borderline personality disorder.* Paper presented at the meeting of the Society for Interpersonal Theory and Research, Philadelphia, PA.

Sadikaj, G., Moskowitz, D. S., Russell, J. J., Zuroff, D. C., & Paris, J. (2013). Quarrelsome behavior in borderline personality disorder: Influence of behavioral and affective reactivity to perceptions of others. *Journal of Abnormal Psychology, 122,* 195–207. doi:10.1037/a0030871

Sadikaj, G., Russell, J. J., Moskowitz, D. S., & Paris, J. (2010). Affect dysregulation in individuals with borderline personality disorder: Persistence and interpersonal triggers. *Journal of Personality Assessment, 92,* 490–500. doi:10.1080/00223891.2010.513287

Schneiderer, E. M., Wang, T., Tomko, R., Wood, P. K., & Trull, T. J. (2013). *Negative affect instability among individuals with comorbid borderline personality disorder and posttraumatic stress disorder.* Manuscript submitted for publication.

Schotte, C. K., de Doncker, D., Vankerckhoven, C., Vertommen, H., & Cosyns, P. (1998). Self-report assessment of the *DSM–IV* personality disorders. Measurement of trait and distress characteristics: The ADP-IV. *Psychological Medicine, 28,* 1179–1188. doi:10.1017/S0033291798007041

Shedler, J., & Westen, D. (2004). Dimensions of personality pathology: An alternative to the five-factor model. *The American Journal of Psychiatry, 161,* 1743–1754. doi:10.1176/appi.ajp.161.10.1743

Singer, J. D., & Willett, J. B. (2003). *Applied longitudinal data analysis: Modeling change and event occurrence.* Oxford, England: Oxford University Press.

Skodol, A. E. (2012). Personality disorders in *DSM–5. Annual Review of Clinical Psychology, 8,* 317–344. doi:10.1146/annurev-clinpsy-032511-143131

Spitzer, R. L., Endicott, J., & Gibbon, M. (1979). Crossing the border into borderline personality and borderline schizophrenia. The development of criteria. *Archives of General Psychiatry, 36,* 17–24. doi:10.1001/archpsyc.1979.01780010023001

Thomas, C., Turkheimer, E., & Oltmanns, T. F. (2003). Factorial structure of pathological personality as evaluated by peers. *Journal of Abnormal Psychology, 112,* 81–91. doi:10.1037/0021-843X.112.1.81

Thompson, B. (2004). *Exploratory and confirmatory factor analysis: Understanding concepts and applications.* Washington, DC: American Psychological Association.

Timmerman, M. E., & Lorenzo-Seva, U. (2011). Dimensionality assessment of ordered polytomous items with parallel analysis. *Psychological Methods, 16,* 209–220. doi:10.1037/a0023353

Trull, T. J., & Durrett, C. A. (2005). Categorical and dimensional models of personality disorder. *Annual Review of Clinical Psychology, 1,* 355–380. doi:10.1146/annurev.clinpsy.1.102803.144009

Trull, T. J., & Ebner-Priemer, U. (2013). Ambulatory assessment. *Annual Review of Clinical Psychology, 9,* 151–176. doi:10.1146/annurev-clinpsy-050212-185510

Trull, T. J., Solhan, M. B., Tragesser, S. L., Jahng, S., Wood, P. K., Piasecki, T. M., & Watson, D. (2008). Affective instability: Measuring a core feature of borderline personality disorder with ecological momentary assessment. *Journal of Abnormal Psychology, 117,* 647–661. doi:10.1037/a0012532

Trull, T. J., Vergés, A., Wood, P. K., Jahng, S., & Sher, K. J. (2012). The structure of *Diagnostic and Statistical Manual of Mental Disorders* (4th edition, text revision) personality disorder symptoms in a large national sample. *Personality Disorders: Theory, Research, and Treatment, 3,* 355–369. doi:10.1037/a0027766

Trull, T. J., Vergés, A., Wood, P. K., & Sher, K. J. (2013). The structure of *DSM–IV–TR* personality disorder diagnoses in NESARC: A reanalysis. *Journal of Personality Disorders, 27,* 727–734. doi:10.1521/pedi_2013_27_107

Turkheimer, E., Ford, D. C., & Oltmanns, T. F. (2008). Regional analysis of self-reported personality disorder criteria. *Journal of Personality, 76,* 1587–1622. doi:10.1111/j.1467-6494.2008.00532.x

van Os, J., Delespaul, P., Wigman, J., Myin-Germeys, I., & Wichers, M. (2013). Beyond *DSM* and *ICD*: Introducing "precision diagnosis" for psychiatry using momentary assessment technology. *World Psychiatry, 12,* 113–117. doi:10.1002/wps.20046

Velicer, W. F. (1976). Determining the number of components from the matrix of partial correlations. *Psychometrika, 41,* 321–327. doi:10.1007/BF02293557

Verheul, R., & Widiger, T. A. (2004). A meta-analysis of the prevalence and usage of the Personality Disorder Not Otherwise Specified (PDNOS) diagnosis. *Journal of Personality Disorders, 18,* 309–319. doi:10.1521/pedi.2004.18.4.309

Vrieze, S. I. (2012). Model selection and psychological theory: A discussion of the differences between the Akaike information criterion (AIC) and the Bayesian information criterion (BIC). *Psychological Methods, 17,* 228–243. doi:10.1037/a0027127

Walton, K. E., Ormel, J., & Krueger, R. F. (2011). The dimensional nature of externalizing behaviors in adolescence: Evidence from a direct comparison of categorical, dimensional, and hybrid models. *Journal of Abnormal Child Psychology, 39,* 553–561. doi:10.1007/s10802-010-9478-y

Westen, D., & Arkowitz-Westen, L. (1998). Limitations of Axis II in diagnosing personality pathology in clinical practice. *The American Journal of Psychiatry, 155,* 1767–1771.

Westen, D., Shedler, J., Bradley, B., & DeFife, J. A. (2012). An empirically derived taxonomy for personality diagnosis: Bridging science and practice in conceptualizing personality. *The American Journal of Psychiatry, 169*, 273–284. doi:10.1176/appi.ajp.2011.11020274

Westen, D., Waller, N. G., Shedler, J., & Blagov, P. S. (2012). Dimensions of personality and personality pathology: Factor structure of the Shedler–Westen Assessment Procedure-II (SWAP-II). *Journal of Personality Disorders, 28*, 281–318. doi:10.1521/pedi_2012_26_059

Widiger, T. A., Cadoret, R., Hare, R., Robins, L., Rutherford, M., Zanarini, M., . . . Allen, F. (1996). *DSM–IV* antisocial personality disorder field trial. *Journal of Abnormal Psychology, 105*, 3–16. doi:10.1037/0021-843X.105.1.3

Widiger, T. A., & Rogers, J. H. (1989). Prevalence and comorbidity of personality disorders. *Psychiatric Annals, 19*, 132–136. doi:10.3928/0048-5713-19890301-07

Widiger, T. A., & Trull, T. J. (2007). Plate tectonics in the classification of personality disorder: Shifting to a dimensional model. *American Psychologist, 62*, 71–83. doi:10.1037/0003-066X.62.2.71

Witkiewitz, K., King, K., McMahon, R. J., Wu, J., Luk, J., Bierman, K. L., . . . Pinderhughes, E. E. (2013). Evidence for a multi-dimensional latent structural model of externalizing disorders. *Journal of Abnormal Child Psychology, 41*, 223–237. doi:10.1007/s10802-012-9674-z

Wright, A. G. C., Krueger, R. F., Hobbs, M. J., Markon, K. E., Eaton, N. R., & Slade, T. (2013). The structure of psychopathology: Toward an expanded quantitative empirical model. *Journal of Abnormal Psychology, 122*, 281–294. doi:10.1037/a0030133

Wright, A. G. C., Thomas, K. M., Hopwood, C. J., Markon, K. E., Pincus, A. L., & Krueger, R. F. (2012). The hierarchical structure of *DSM–5* pathological personality traits. *Journal of Abnormal Psychology, 121*, 951–957. doi:10.1037/a0027669

Yang, J., Bagby, R. M., Costa, P. T., Ryder, A. G., & Herbst, J. H. (2002). Assessing the *DSM–IV* structure of personality disorder with a sample of Chinese psychiatric patients. *Journal of Personality Disorders, 16*, 317–331. doi:10.1521/pedi.16.4.317.24127

Zachar, P., & Kendler, K. S. (2010). Philosophical issues in the classification of psychopathology. In T. Millon, R. F. Krueger, & E. Simonsen (Eds.), *Contemporary directions in psychopathology: Scientific foundations of the* DSM–5 and ICD–11 (pp. 127–148). New York, NY: Guilford Press.

Zimmerman, M., Rothschild, L., & Chelminski, I. (2005). The prevalence of *DSM–IV* personality disorders in psychiatric outpatients. *The American Journal of Psychiatry, 162*, 1911–1918. doi:10.1176/appi.ajp.162.10.1911

6

LESSONS LEARNED FROM LONGITUDINAL STUDIES OF PERSONALITY DISORDERS

ALEX S. KEUROGHLIAN AND MARY C. ZANARINI

The *Diagnostic and Statistical Manual of Mental Disorders* (DSM) has consistently defined *personality disorders* (PDs) as inherently stable over time, from the first edition (American Psychiatric Association, 1952) to the fourth edition, text revision (*DSM–IV–TR*; American Psychiatric Association, 2000). This conceptualization has been in contrast to that of Axis I disorders, which have been viewed as more episodic (Grilo, McGlashan, Quinlan, et al., 1998). Since the classification of PDs on an independent diagnostic axis in the *DSM–III* (American Psychiatric Association, 1980), a proliferation of new research has challenged the notion that these disorders are entirely stable constructs over time (Morey & Meyer, 2012). The use of more standardized and structured instruments for diagnosing PDs (Zimmerman, 1994) brought increased rigor to this research, yielding findings that further called into question the notion of stability over time (Grilo & McGlashan, 1999; Grilo, McGlashan, &

http://dx.doi.org/10.1037/14549-007
Personality Disorders: Toward Theoretical and Empirical Integration in Diagnosis and Assessment,
S. K. Huprich (Editor)

Oldham, 1998; Mattanah, Becker, Levy, Edell, & McGlashan, 1995; McDavid & Pilkonis, 1996; Paris, 2003; Zimmerman, 1994).

Furthermore, the notion that PDs endure throughout the entire life span is at odds with the empirical findings that PDs in adulthood are linked to adverse childhood experience (Cohen, Crawford, Johnson, & Kasen, 2005). For example, there is a strong relationship between childhood trauma and PDs in adulthood (Cohen, Brown, & Smailes, 2001). Additionally, there is some evidence that antisocial PD and borderline personality disorder (BPD) become less severe in older adults (Paris & Zweig-Frank, 2001; Stevenson, Meares, & Comerford, 2003), in contrast to the increase in severity of Cluster A and Cluster C PDs that can occur with age (Seivewright, Tyrer, & Johnson, 2002).

Thus far, questions about the stability of PDs over time have best been addressed methodologically by researchers who have studied them in a prospective and longitudinal manner (Morey & Meyer, 2012). Long-term prospective follow-up studies allow empirical assessment of how these disorders endure and evolve throughout the life span. These studies leverage the use of reliable and valid assessment tools for diagnosing PDs at several follow-up intervals throughout the duration of these studies and the life spans of their participants.

In recent years, four principal longitudinal prospective follow-up studies of PDs have emerged in the United States: the Children in the Community Study (CIC; Cohen et al., 2005); the ongoing Longitudinal Study of Personality Disorders (LSPD; Lenzenweger, 1999); the McLean Study of Adult Development (MSAD; Zanarini, Frankenburg, Hennen, Reich, & Silk, 2005), which also continues to collect data; and the Collaborative Longitudinal Personality Disorders Study (CLPS; Skodol et al., 2005). It should also be noted that Daniel Klein at SUNY Stony Brook is studying the longitudinal interactions of early temperament, emotional style, personality, and mood and anxiety disorders in a community sample of young children (Bufferd, Dougherty, Carlson, Rose, & Klein, 2012).

In this chapter, we focus on BPD as an exemplar of what can be learned from the longitudinal study of PDs. We discuss findings from the MSAD and CLPS, which have applied rigorous research methodologies to the prospective study of BPD and have generated extensive findings about the long-term stability and chronicity of this disorder. We provide an overview of findings regarding BPD-related remissions, recurrences, and recovery, as well as comorbidities over time and the relationship of BPD to physical health in a longitudinal context. In addition, we discuss the implications of these longitudinal studies of BPD with regard to the utility of categorical versus dimensional models of PDs. We conclude by proposing much-needed future directions for longitudinal research on BPD.

CHILDREN IN THE COMMUNITY STUDY

The CIC has focused on early emergence and development of PDs (Cohen et al., 2005). The researchers recruited a sample of 800 children from the community in two residential counties of New York, starting in 1975. The study rapidly evolved from a needs assessment for services benefiting children into an investigation with a primary goal of empirically assessing the development of personality and associated psychopathology in children as they grew into adults (Cohen et al., 2005). Participants were as young as 9 years at index admission and were evaluated with a combination of reports by their mothers and self-report. PDs were assessed in early adolescence (mean age of 14), mid-adolescence (mean age of 16), early adulthood (mean age of 22), and adulthood (mean age of 33).

During mid-adolescence, PDs were most prevalent among 12-year-old boys and 13-year-old girls, with particularly high rates of obsessive-compulsive, narcissistic, and schizotypal PDs (Bernstein et al., 1993). These findings pointed to the emergence of PDs early in life (Morey & Meyer, 2012), showing that the average number of symptoms of PD decreases overall from early adolescence onward and is generally lowest in adults, with stabilization in the mean level of PD symptomatology by the late 20s (Johnson et al., 2000). Moreover, those PD symptoms found in adolescence appeared to become more severe in adulthood.

Within Cluster A, paranoid symptoms were the most stable throughout the study period, and Cluster A disorders were more likely to endure into adulthood when these were comorbid in early life with a disruptive disorder (Cohen et al., 2005). Among Cluster B disorders, the greatest decrease in symptomatology during the transition into adulthood was observed in narcissistic PD (Cohen et al., 2005). Cluster B disorder stability was highly influenced by school life as well as relationships with parents and peers (Cohen et al., 2005). For Cluster C disorders, the presence of a comorbid anxiety disorder quadrupled the probability of the PD persisting into adulthood.

The CIC has provided an opportunity to assess the effect of PDs in early life on the quality of life in adults (Chen et al., 2006; Skodol, Johnson, Cohen, Sneed, & Crawford, 2007; Winograd, Cohen, & Chen, 2008) and on adult behaviors, such as maladaptive parenting (Johnson, Cohen, Kasen, Ehrensaft, & Crawford, 2006). The estimated rate of PDs in the CIC based on point prevalence ranged from 12.7% to 14.6%, whereas the cumulative lifetime rate across all follow-up assessments was 28.2%, indicating variability in the presence of PD symptoms over time (Morey & Meyer, 2012).

THE LONGITUDINAL STUDY OF PERSONALITY DISORDERS

The LSPD was designed to empirically examine the longitudinal course of PDs (Lenzenweger, 1999). It recruited 250 undergraduate students, as opposed to patients pursuing treatment, who were screened and selected to provide a representative sample of various PD symptoms (Morey & Meyer, 2012). The investigators divided the sample into a possible PD group (129 participants at risk of having at least one PD) and a no PD group (121 participants with fewer than 10 PD symptoms; Lenzenweger, Loranger, Korfine, & Neff, 1997).

Participant assessments occurred three times throughout the 4-year study period, and the mean level of PD symptomatology declined throughout this period in both study groups, despite significant stability over time within PD Cluster A, Cluster B, and Cluster C (Lenzenweger, 1999). More recent assessment of the study's data using individual growth curve analysis, as opposed to the method of repeated measures, found that PD features decreased steadily with time, at a rate of approximately 1.4 features annually (Lenzenweger, Johnson, & Willett, 2004). Thus, the study demonstrated both stability and improvement in PDs over time. Its limitations included the exclusive use of college student participants, resulting in relative homogeneity of socioeconomic status and age, as well as use of the Millon Clinical Multiaxial Inventory II (Millon, 1987), which is limited in its utility for assessing DSM PDs (Morey & Meyer, 2012; Widiger, Williams, Spitzer, & Frances, 1985).

THE McLEAN STUDY OF ADULT DEVELOPMENT

The MSAD has undertaken a longitudinal examination of BPD compared with other PDs (Zanarini et al., 2005; Zanarini, Frankenburg, Hennen, & Silk, 2003), thus yielding extensive results about a full range of PD symptomatology. Unlike the community or college samples recruited for the CIC or LSPD, the MSAD study sample of 290 men and women between 18 and 35 years of age was originally recruited from an inpatient psychiatric setting and thus focused on patients with more severe initial psychiatric illness. The MSAD continues to follow patients with BPD longitudinally for over 20 years (Zanarini et al., 2005), with follow-up interviews conducted every 2 years to assess changes in psychosocial functioning, psychiatric treatment, and psychopathology in DSM–IV–TR Axes I and II.

The MSAD has provided evidence that PDs, even when severe, are less enduring than their characterization in the DSM suggests (Morey & Meyer, 2012), with most patients experiencing remission of BPD by 6-year follow-up (Zanarini et al., 2003), and over 90% achieving remission by 10-year follow-up (Zanarini, Frankenburg, Reich, & Fitzmaurice, 2010a; Zanarini et al., 2007). Moreover, BPD relapses were found to be rare, indicating long-term stability of symptomatic improvement. Another key finding of the MSAD is that certain borderline symptoms were more likely to change over time than others: Rates of self-harm behaviors and suicidal ideation decreased from 81% at baseline to 25% at 6-year follow-up (Zanarini et al., 2003), whereas affective and interpersonal features were more enduring over time (Zanarini et al., 2007). The MSAD also showed that recovery from BPD, defined as symptomatic remission combined with good occupational and social functioning, is substantially more difficult to attain than mere remission and occurs in only 50% of participants by 10-year follow-up, with subsequent loss of this level of psychosocial functioning in a third of participants (Zanarini, Frankenburg, Reich, & Fitzmaurice, 2010b).

THE COLLABORATIVE LONGITUDINAL PERSONALITY DISORDERS STUDY

The CLPS was a longitudinal multisite study that examined the long-term course of personality psychopathology and associated phenomena (Morey & Meyer, 2012). It followed recently treated or treatment-seeking patients between 18 and 45 years of age with borderline, avoidant, and obsessive-compulsive PDs, as well as a group of comparison patients with major depressive disorder (MDD) and no PD, throughout a 10-year period (Skodol et al., 2005). Although the CLPS did initially include a schizotypal PD study group, these participants were not included in the final 10-year report due to difficulty collecting data from in vivo observations about this group, as assessments later in the study were increasingly being performed by telephone (Gunderson et al., 2011). Of note, MDD was chosen as a comparison group, given its well-established episodic course, high rates in the general population, and extensive empiric characterization (Morey & Meyer, 2012).

The CLPS has revealed lower stability of categorical PDs than implied in *DSM–IV–TR* (American Psychiatric Association, 2000) definitions, substantial stability in the dimensional degree of PD features observed, more persistent impairment in psychosocial functioning over time, and higher stability of personality traits than of *DSM–IV–TR* symptoms over time.

IN-DEPTH ANALYSIS OF BORDERLINE PERSONALITY DISORDER

Background

From 1985 to 1995, four large retrospective studies of the longitudinal course of borderline PD (BPD) were completed (McGlashan, 1986; Paris, Brown, & Nowlis, 1987; Plakun, Burkhardt, & Muller, 1985; Stone, 1990).

These studies found that patients with BPD tended to improve clinically over time. A mean of 14 to 16 years after initial admission to the hospital, patients with BPD in these studies achieved fairly good functional outcomes on the Health–Sickness Rating Scale (Luborsky, 1962) or the Global Assessment Scale (Endicott, Spitzer, Fleiss, & Cohen, 1976), which was subsequently replaced by the Global Assessment of Functioning (GAF) Scale. These findings challenged the widely held view of BPD as a chronic illness that is refractory to treatment and has poor long-term outcomes with regard to social and occupational functioning. Given the methodological limitations of these follow-back studies, however, this work instilled only limited optimism among mental health clinicians and researchers about the long-term potential for recovery among patients with BPD (Gunderson et al., 2011). The suboptimal design of these studies also contributed to doubts about the diagnostic validity of BPD as a distinct psychiatric illness, based on validation standards outlined by Robins and Guze (1970).

To understand the long-term course of BPD with more rigorously designed methodologies, the National Institute of Mental Health approved grants in the 1990s for two prospective studies.

Design of These Studies

In the MSAD, all participants were initially hospitalized on inpatient units at McLean Hospital. Inclusion criteria consisted of age between 18 and 35; IQ of at least 71; no past or present symptoms of schizophrenia, schizoaffective disorder, bipolar I disorder, or organic brain conditions that could cause psychiatric symptoms; and fluency in English. At baseline, each participant met with a highly skilled interviewer blind to the patient's clinical diagnoses for a comprehensive psychosocial and treatment history as well as a diagnostic assessment. These 2-year follow-up interviews consist of four semistructured interviews: the Revised Borderline Follow-Up Interview (Zanarini, Sickel, Yong, & Glazer, 1994), the Structured Clinical Interview for DSM–III–R Axis I Disorders (Spitzer, Williams, Gibbon, & First, 1992), the Revised Diagnostic Interview for Borderlines (Zanarini, Gunderson, Frankenburg, & Chauncey, 1989), and the Diagnostic Interview for DSM–III–R Personality Disorders (Zanarini, Frankenburg, Chauncey, & Gunderson, 1987). Every 24 months, at each of the 10 follow-up interviews, similar interview methods were used to assess changes in psychosocial functioning, psychiatric treatment, and psychopathology in Axes I and II.

The CLPS was a multisite, naturalistic study that recruited patients from Brown, Columbia, Harvard, and Yale universities, at a total of 19 subsites. Outpatient mental health clinics were the most common source of the study's participant sample (43%), and 12% of participants were recruited from psychiatric inpatient units. Participants at baseline ranged from 18 to 45 years of age, with exclusion criteria similar to those in the MSAD. PDs were diagnosed with the Diagnostic Interview for *DSM–IV* PDs (Zanarini, Frankenburg, Sickel, & Yong, 1996) at baseline, at 6- and 12-month follow-up, and at 2-, 4-, 6-, 8-, and 10-year follow-up, by study staff blind to the participants' diagnoses. The PDs were also assessed over time with a follow-along version of the Diagnostic Interview for *DSM–IV* Personality Disorders (Zanarini & Shea, 1996) by interviewers who were not blind to the participants' diagnoses. The severity of MDD and other Axis I disorders was quantified with weekly psychiatric status ratings (PSRs): PSR = 1, *no symptoms*; PSR = 2, *moderate symptoms but participant does not meet full diagnostic criteria*; PSR = 3, *participant meets full diagnostic criteria*.

Study Samples

In the MSAD, 290 participants met rigorous diagnostic criteria for BPD at baseline, and 72 participants met criteria for at least one nonborderline Axis II disorder but not BPD (Zanarini, Frankenburg, Reich, & Fitzmaurice, 2012). Over 16 years of follow-up, 87.5% of patients with BPD who remained alive continued to participate in the study (Zanarini et al., 2012); among Axis II comparison subjects, 82.9% of surviving participants (*n* = 58/70) were reinterviewed for each of the eight follow-up intervals.

In the CLPS, 63% of participants with BPD at the study's baseline continued to participate for the entire 10-year follow-up period, as did 62% of those with avoidant PD, 74% of those with obsessive-compulsive PD, and 64% of those with MDD (Gunderson et al., 2011; McGlashan et al., 2000).

Remission, Recurrence, and Recovery Over Time

BPD Remission

The MSAD findings at 16-year follow-up shed light on the longitudinal course of BPD (Zanarini et al., 2012). Remission in the study was defined as no longer meeting criteria for BPD based on both the Revised Diagnostic Interview for Borderlines and the *DSM–III–R*, or for any other PD based on the *Diagnostic and Statistical Manual of Mental Disorders* (3rd ed., rev.; *DSM–III–R*; American Psychiatric Association, 1987) for at least 2 years. Over 16 years, high rates of remission were found among both borderline and Axis II comparison subjects. Specifically, remissions lasting 8 years were observed among 78% of participants with BPD and 97% of participants with other PDs. Remissions lasting at least two years were observed among 99% of participants with BPD and 99% of participants with other PDs.

Of note, patients with BPD in the MSAD achieved remission more slowly than those with other PDs: Remission at the first possible 2- or 8-year time interval was achieved by 30% of participants with BPD, whereas 85% of those with other PDs achieved either 2-year or 8-year remissions as soon as possible. This slower remission among participants with BPD may be reflective of more severe psychopathology than that observed among Axis II comparison subjects.

In the CLPS 10-year final report, remission of BPD in comparison to other PDs was defined as meeting two or fewer *DSM–IV–TR* criteria for 12 months. Ninety-one percent of participants with BPD achieved remission over 10 years based on the 2-month criteria, and 85% achieved remission with the 12-month criteria. These remissions did not necessarily require the presence of ongoing therapies focused on BPD (Gunderson et al., 2011). Time to remission was slower for BPD than it was both for MDD and for a combined avoidant and obsessive-compulsive PD comparison group.

One 10-year report from the MSAD examined subsyndromal phenomenology of BPD, focusing specifically on the longitudinal course and time to remission of 24 borderline symptoms (Zanarini et al., 2007). Twelve of these symptoms decreased precipitously over 10 years of follow-up and were endorsed at the end of this period by less than 15% of patients with BPD who initially reported them. These more rapidly remitting symptoms included features of impulsivity, such as self-injury and suicide attempts, as well as efforts to actively resolve interpersonal problems, such as difficulties with demandingness or entitlement and treatment regressions. Features pertaining to dysphoric affect, such as anger and loneliness or emptiness, as well as interpersonal problems related to feeling abandoned or being dependent, such as aloneness intolerance and being counterdependent, remitted more slowly. Thus there emerges a distinction between more acutely manifested components of BPD versus those dimensions of the disorder that are more persistent and temperamental in nature.

In the CLPS, there was a significant decrease in the average number of *DSM–IV* criteria for BPD met by participants with BPD, from 6.7 at baseline to 4.3 at the end of the first year, with a subsequent 0.29 annual rate of decline in the number of criteria, down to a mean of 1.7 criteria per participant in the 10th year of follow-up. At 10-year follow-up, only 9% of patients with BPD continued to meet five or more *DSM–IV* criteria for BPD. The number of BPD criteria present at each follow-up interval was inversely predictive of the following year's GAF score, though GAF scores were not predictive of the BPD criterion count in the following year. All nine borderline diagnostic criteria decreased by approximately 50% over 10 years. Affective instability remained the most prevalent *DSM–IV* criterion throughout the 10-year follow-up period, whereas the criterion of self-injury/suicide attempts was least prevalent. Affective, behavioral, or interpersonal phenotypic symptom clusters were not individually stable over time but rather seemed to decrease together as one construct at a consistent rate.

BPD Recurrence and Relapse

Over 16 years in the MSAD, the rate of symptomatic recurrence for BPD after a 2-year remission was 36%, whereas 10% of patients with BPD who had a remission lasting 8 years subsequently experienced a recurrence (Zanarini et al., 2012). Recurrences after remissions lasting 2 to 6 years occurred significantly sooner among patients with BPD than those with other PDs, which again may be attributable to more severe psychopathology among patients with BPD. Nevertheless, the relatively high remission and low recurrence rates for BPD over 16 years provide a more optimistic long-term prognosis for BPD than do the remission and recurrence rates for MDD (Mueller et al., 1999; Solomon et al., 1997) and bipolar I disorder (Judd et al., 2002, 2008).

The definition of BPD relapse in the CLPS was a return to at least five *DSM–IV* criteria, the *DSM–IV* threshold for BPD, for at least 2 months following a remission. The rate of relapse over 10 years among participants with BPD was 11% based on the 12-month remission definition, compared with a 25% relapse rate over 10 years among participants with other baseline PDs. This difference with the 16-year findings from the MSAD, in which higher recurrence rates were observed among patients with BPD than those with other PDs, may be due to higher participant retention rates in the MSAD, as well as the fact that 13% of participants with Obsessive Compulsive PD in the CLPS also had a baseline diagnosis of BPD (Zanarini et al., 2012). The BPD relapse rate was 21% based on the 2-month remission criteria, compared with a 67% relapse rate over 10 years in the MDD group. Most BPD relapses were observed during the first 4 years of follow-up. This relatively low rate of relapse may be due to increased resiliency, adaptiveness, or social supports gained during the remission phase (Gunderson et al., 2011). Relapses of BPD over 10 years occurred less frequently than for MDD, bipolar disorder, panic disorder, or social phobia (Bruce et al., 2005; Gunderson et al., 2011; Keller, Lavori, Coryell, Endicott, & Mueller, 1993; Mueller et al., 1999; Winokur et al., 1994).

Psychosocial Functioning and Recovery in Patients With BPD

Findings from the MSAD have shed light on the long-term course of psychosocial functioning in patients with BPD. At 6-year MSAD follow-up, patients with BPD demonstrated improved psychosocial functioning: 26% reported good overall psychosocial functioning at baseline compared with 56% at 6 years (Zanarini et al., 2005). Patients with BPD nevertheless had significantly lower psychosocial functioning over 6 years than did participants with other PDs. Symptomatic remission over this period was related to improved social functioning with a good friend or spouse and one parent, as well as good performance at school or work, maintenance over time of school or work activities, and a GAF score ≥ 61. The rate of participants with BPD with a GAF score ≥ 61 was 0% at baseline and increased among remitted patients with BPD to 43% at 6-year follow-up. Thus, the 6-year MSAD report revealed a high rate of enhanced psychosocial functioning among patients with BPD and demonstrated that these improvements more frequently occur in cases of symptomatic remission from BPD. A subsequent MSAD study at 10-year follow-up found that a consistent vocational record, with sustained history of work or school activities, is a strong predictor of faster time to remission from BPD, underscoring the importance of good psychosocial functioning for improvement in borderline symptoms (Zanarini, Frankenburg, Hennen, Reich, & Silk, 2006).

Another 10-year MSAD report found the prevalence of Social Security Disability Insurance (SSDI) receipt among patients with BPD was 3 times greater than the rate among patients with other PDs (Zanarini, Jacoby, Frankenburg, Reich, & Fitzmaurice, 2009). Approximately 40% of patients with BPD were able to stop receiving payments at some point, though 43% of those who had discontinued SSDI later started receiving federal benefits again. Moreover, 39% of patients with BPD first received SSDI benefits during the 10-year follow-up period; moreover, 55% of them had attended work or school during 50% or more of the prior 2-year interval, approximately 70% reporting having at least one supportive friend, and over 50% endorsed having a good romantic relationship.

An additional report from the MSAD at 10-year follow-up was more sobering (Zanarini et al., 2010b). Patients with BPD reported difficulty attaining good psychosocial functioning at baseline, difficulty retaining this level of functioning over 10 years, and difficulty regaining it. Poor occupational functioning rather than social impairment was the basis of poor psychosocial functioning in over 90% of cases.

Improved psychosocial functioning including full-time work or school is closely embedded in the concept of recovery from illness. In the MSAD, *recovery* was operationally defined based on the following requirements: GAF ≥ 61; remission from the primary PD; having one or more emotionally sustaining relationships with a spouse, life partner, or close friend; and working or going to school full-time and in a reliable manner (Zanarini et al., 2012). Over 16 years, 60% of patients with BPD achieved a 2-year recovery and 40% achieved an 8-year recovery. Time to recovery was significantly longer among patients with BPD than among those with other PDs. Only 10% of participants with BPD recovered within the earliest 2- or 8-year period possible. Impaired occupational functioning is most associated with a failure to recover from BPD, despite improved interpersonal functioning and no longer meeting diagnostic criteria for BPD (Zanarini et al., 2009, 2010a, 2010b). These results are consistent with earlier MSAD reports that patients with BPD have poorer occupational functioning (Zanarini, Frankenburg, Reich, & Fitzmaurice, 2010a) and are more likely than participants with other PDs to have disability benefits as their primary income source (Zanarini et al., 2009).

The rate of loss of BPD recovery in the MSAD over 16 years was 44% for 2-year recoveries and 20% for 8-year recoveries. At 2-year CLPS follow-up, borderline and schizotypal patients were significantly more impaired with regard to employment, social relationships, and recreation than patients with either obsessive-compulsive PD or MDD (Skodol et al., 2002). There were small but statistically significant improvements in mean GAF scores in the CLPS over 10 years among participants with BPD (53–57). Hierarchical linear modeling showed that the mean GAF score for participants with BPD was significantly lower than for those with other PDs, though this difference between BPD and each of the other two study groups decreased over time. Twenty-one percent of patients with BPD achieved a GAF score greater than 70 over 10 years of follow-up, which was significantly lower than the rate of achievement of this psychosocial functioning level by participants with obsessive-compulsive PD (48%) or those with MDD (61%). Participants with BPD were significantly less likely to achieve full-time employment over 10 years than were those with other PDs or with MDD.

Implications and Future Directions

Thus, a clear theme emerges from both the MSAD and the CLPS: Sustained remission of BPD over time occurs at a dramatic rate, with infrequent long-term recurrences, in contrast to the slower and more modest recovery of social and occupational functioning among these patients. Some patients with BPD showed chronic psychosocial impairment, particularly in their ability to maintain full-time competent work or school performance, in both the MSAD and CLPS. This characteristic longitudinal course of BPD is distinct from the course of common mood and anxiety disorders (Coryell et al., 1993; Judd et al., 2008; Stout, Dolan, Dyck, Eisen, & Keller, 2001) and provides a compelling argument for the diagnostic validity of the BPD construct. Future studies could focus on refining diagnostic criteria for BPD to reflect its distinctive persistent social and vocational impairment over time. Investigators ought to also characterize the extent to which borderline-specific treatment modalities improve psychosocial functioning, as well as pioneering novel treatments geared toward social and vocational rehabilitation (Gunderson et al., 2011; Zanarini et al., 2010a, 2012).

CONCLUSION

The MSAD and the CLPS have shed a great deal of light on the long-term course of BPD, including (a) remission, recurrence, psychosocial functioning, and recovery; and (b) interactions over time with mood disorders, anxiety disorders, substance use disorders, and eating disorders. Future longitudinal research will help elucidate the course of BPD through older age. When coupled with emerging neurobiological research approaches, longitudinal studies will help uncover the biological and temperamental basis of BPD as it evolves throughout the life span.

REFERENCES

American Psychiatric Association. (1952). *Diagnostic and statistical manual of mental disorders*. Washington, DC: Author.

American Psychiatric Association. (1980). *Diagnostic and statistical manual of mental disorders* (3rd ed.). Washington, DC: Author.

American Psychiatric Association. (1987). *Diagnostic and statistical manual of mental disorders* (3rd ed., rev.). Washington, DC: Author.

American Psychiatric Association. (2000). *Diagnostic and statistical manual of mental disorders* (4th ed., text rev.). Washington, DC: Author.

Bernstein, D. P., Cohen, P., Velez, C. N., Schwab-Stone, M., Siever, L. J., & Shinsato, L. (1993). Prevalence and stability of the *DSM–III* personality disorders in a community-based survey of adolescents. *The American Journal of Psychiatry, 150,* 1237–1243.

Bruce, S. E., Yonkers, K. A., Otto, M. W., Eisen, J. L., Weisberg, R. B., Pagano, M., . . . Keller, M. B. (2005). Influence of psychiatric comorbidity on recovery and recurrence in generalized anxiety disorder, social phobia, and panic disorder: A 12-year prospective study. *The American Journal of Psychiatry, 162,* 1179–1187. doi:10.1176/appi.ajp.162.6.1179

Bufferd, S. J., Dougherty, L. R., Carlson, G. A., Rose, S., & Klein, D. N. (2012). Psychiatric disorders in preschoolers: Continuity from ages 3 to 6. *The American Journal of Psychiatry, 169,* 1157–1164. doi:10.1176/appi.ajp.2012.12020268

Chen, H., Cohen, P., Crawford, T. N., Kasen, S., Johnson, J. G., & Berenson, K. (2006). Relative impact of young adult personality disorders on subsequent quality of life: Findings of a community-based longitudinal study. *Journal of Personality Disorders, 20,* 510–523. doi:10.1521/pedi.2006.20.5.510

Cohen, P., Brown, J., & Smailes, E. (2001). Child abuse and neglect and the development of personality disorders in the general population. *Development and Psychopathology, 13,* 981–999.

Cohen, P., Crawford, T. N., Johnson, J. G., & Kasen, S. (2005). The Children in the Community study of developmental course of personality disorder. *Journal of Personality Disorders, 19*, 466–486. doi:10.1521/pedi.2005.19.5.466

Coryell, W., Scheftner, W., Keller, M., Endicott, J., Maser, J., & Klerman, G. L. (1993). The enduring psychosocial consequences of mania and depression. *The American Journal of Psychiatry, 150*, 720–727.

Endicott, J., Spitzer, R. L., Fleiss, J. L., & Cohen, J. (1976). The Global Assessment Scale: A procedure for measuring overall severity of psychiatric disturbance. *Archives of General Psychiatry, 33*, 766–771. doi:10.1001/archpsyc.1976.01770060086012

Grilo, C. M., & McGlashan, T. H. (1999). Stability and course of personality disorders. *Current Opinion in Psychiatry, 12*, 157–162. doi:10.1097/00001504-199903000-00003

Grilo, C. M., McGlashan, T. H., & Oldham, J. M. (1998). Course and stability of personality disorders. *Journal of Practical Psychiatry and Behavioral Health, 4*, 61–75.

Grilo, C. M., McGlashan, T. H., Quinlan, D. M., Walker, M. L., Greenfeld, D., & Edell, W. S. (1998). Frequency of personality disorders in two age cohorts of psychiatric inpatients. *The American Journal of Psychiatry, 155*, 140–142.

Gunderson, J. G., Stout, R. L., McGlashan, T. H., Shea, M. T., Morey, L. C., Grilo, C. M., . . . Skodol, A. E. (2011). Ten-year course of borderline personality disorder: Psychopathology and function from the Collaborative Longitudinal Personality Disorders study. *Archives of General Psychiatry, 68*, 827–837. doi:10.1001/archgenpsychiatry.2011.37

Johnson, J. G., Cohen, P., Kasen, S., Ehrensaft, M. K., & Crawford, T. N. (2006). Associations of parental personality disorders and Axis I disorders with child-rearing behavior. *Psychiatry: Interpersonal and Biological Processes, 69*, 336–350. doi:10.1521/psyc.2006.69.4.336

Johnson, J. G., Cohen, P., Kasen, S., Skodol, A. E., Hamagami, F., & Brook, J. S. (2000). Age-related change in personality disorder trait levels between early adolescence and adulthood: A community-based longitudinal investigation. *Acta Psychiatrica Scandinavica, 102*, 265–275. doi:10.1034/j.1600-0447.2000.102004265.x

Judd, L. L., Akiskal, H. S., Schettler, P. J., Endicott, J., Maser, J., Solomon, D. A., . . . Keller, M. B. (2002). The long-term natural history of the weekly symptomatic status of bipolar I disorder. *Archives of General Psychiatry, 59*, 530–537. doi:10.1001/archpsyc.59.6.530

Judd, L. L., Schettler, P. J., Solomon, D. A., Maser, J. D., Coryell, W., Endicott, J., & Akiskal, H. S. (2008). Psychosocial disability and work role function compared across the long-term course of bipolar I, bipolar II and unipolar major depressive disorders. *Journal of Affective Disorders, 108*, 49–58. doi:10.1016/j.jad.2007.06.014

Keller, M. B., Lavori, P. W., Coryell, W., Endicott, J., & Mueller, T. I. (1993). Bipolar I: A five-year prospective follow-up. *Journal of Nervous and Mental Disease, 181*, 238–245. doi:10.1097/00005053-199304000-00005

Lenzenweger, M. F. (1999). Stability and change in personality disorder features: The Longitudinal Study of Personality Disorders. *Archives of General Psychiatry, 56*, 1009–1015. doi:10.1001/archpsyc.56.11.1009

Lenzenweger, M. F., Johnson, M. D., & Willett, J. B. (2004). Individual growth curve analysis illuminates stability and change in personality disorder features: The Longitudinal Study of Personality Disorders. *Archives of General Psychiatry, 61*, 1015–1024. doi:10.1001/archpsyc.61.10.1015

Lenzenweger, M. F., Loranger, A. W., Korfine, L., & Neff, C. (1997). Detecting personality disorders in a nonclinical population: Application of a 2-stage procedure for case identification. *Archives of General Psychiatry, 54*, 345–351. doi:10.1001/archpsyc.1997.01830160073010

Luborsky, L. (1962). Clinician's judgments of mental health. *Archives of General Psychiatry, 7*, 407–417. doi:10.1001/archpsyc.1962.01720060019002

Mattanah, J. J., Becker, D. F., Levy, K. N., Edell, W. S., & McGlashan, T. H. (1995). Diagnostic stability in adolescents followed up 2 years after hospitalization. *The American Journal of Psychiatry, 152*, 889–894.

McDavid, J. D., & Pilkonis, P. A. (1996). The stability of personality disorder diagnosis. *Journal of Personality Disorders, 10*, 1–15. doi:10.1521/pedi.1996.10.1.1

McGlashan, T. H. (1986). The Chestnut Lodge follow-up study: III. Long-term outcome of borderline personalities. *Archives of General Psychiatry, 43*, 20–30. doi:10.1001/archpsyc.1986.01800010022003

McGlashan, T. H., Grilo, C. M., Skodol, A. E., Gunderson, J. G., Shea, M. T., Morey, L. C., . . . Stout, R. L. (2000). The Collaborative Longitudinal Personality Disorders Study: Baseline Axis I/II and II/II diagnostic co-occurrence. *Acta Psychiatrica Scandinavica, 102*, 256–264. doi:10.1034/j.1600-0447.2000.102004256.x

Millon, T. (1987). *Manual for the Millon Clinical Multiaxial Inventory II (MCMI-II)*. Minneapolis, MN: National Computer Systems.

Morey, L. C., & Meyer, J. K. (2012). Course of personality disorders. In T. A. Widiger (Ed.), *The Oxford handbook of personality disorders* (pp. 275–298). New York, NY: Oxford University Press.

Mueller, T. I., Leon, A. C., Keller, M. B., Solomon, D. A., Endicott, J., Coryell, W., . . . Maser, J. D. (1999). Recurrence after recovery from major depressive disorder during 15 years of observational follow-up. *The American Journal of Psychiatry, 156*, 1000–1006.

Paris, J. (2003). Personality disorders over time: Precursors, course and outcome. *Journal of Personality Disorders, 17*, 479–488. doi:10.1521/pedi.17.6.479.25360

Paris, J., Brown, R., & Nowlis, D. (1987). Long-term follow-up of borderline patients in a general hospital. *Comprehensive Psychiatry, 28*, 530–535. doi:10.1016/0010-440X(87)90019-8

Paris, J., & Zweig-Frank, H. (2001). A 27-year follow-up of patients with borderline personality disorder. *Comprehensive Psychiatry, 42*, 482–487. doi:10.1053/comp.2001.26271

Plakun, E. M., Burkhardt, P. E., & Muller, J. P. (1985). Fourteen-year follow-up of borderline and schizotypal personality disorders. *Comprehensive Psychiatry, 26,* 448–455. doi:10.1016/0010-440X(85)90081-1

Robins, E., & Guze, S. B. (1970). Establishment of diagnostic validity in psychiatric illness: Its application to schizophrenia. *The American Journal of Psychiatry, 126,* 983–987.

Seivewright, H., Tyrer, P., & Johnson, T. (2002). Change in personality status in neurotic disorders. *The Lancet, 359,* 2253–2254. doi:10.1016/S0140-6736(02)09266-8

Skodol, A. E., Gunderson, J. G., McGlashan, T. H., Dyck, I. R., Stout, R. L., Bender, D. S., . . . Oldham, J. M. (2002). Functional impairment in patients with schizotypal, borderline, avoidant, or obsessive-compulsive personality disorder. *The American Journal of Psychiatry, 159,* 276–283. doi:10.1176/appi.ajp.159.2.276

Skodol, A. E., Gunderson, J. G., Shea, M. T., McGlashan, T. H., Morey, L. C., Sanislow, C. A., . . . Stout, R. L. (2005). The Collaborative Longitudinal Personality Disorders Study (CLPS): Overview and implications. *Journal of Personality Disorders, 19,* 487–504. doi:10.1521/pedi.2005.19.5.487

Skodol, A. E., Johnson, J. G., Cohen, P., Sneed, J. R., & Crawford, T. N. (2007). Personality disorder and impaired functioning from adolescence to adulthood. *British Journal of Psychiatry, 190,* 415–420. doi:10.1192/bjp.bp.105.019364

Solomon, D. A., Keller, M. B., Leon, A. C., Mueller, T. I., Shea, M. T., Warshaw, M., . . . Endicott, J. (1997). Recovery from major depression: A 10-year prospective follow-up across multiple episodes. *Archives of General Psychiatry, 54,* 1001–1006. doi:10.1001/archpsyc.1997.01830230033005

Spitzer, R. L., Williams, J. B., Gibbon, M., & First, M. B. (1992). The Structured Clinical Interview for DSM–III–R (SCID). I: History, rationale, and description. *Archives of General Psychiatry, 49,* 624–629. doi:10.1001/archpsyc.1992.01820080032005

Stevenson, J., Meares, R., & Comerford, A. (2003). Diminished impulsivity in older patients with borderline personality disorder. *The American Journal of Psychiatry, 160,* 165–166. doi:10.1176/appi.ajp.160.1.165

Stone, M. H. (1990). *The fate of borderline patients: Successful outcome and psychiatric practice.* New York, NY: Guilford Press.

Stout, R. L., Dolan, R., Dyck, I., Eisen, J., & Keller, M. B. (2001). Course of social functioning after remission from panic disorder. *Comprehensive Psychiatry, 42,* 441–447. doi:10.1053/comp.2001.27894

Widiger, T. A., Williams, J. B., Spitzer, R. L., & Frances, A. (1985). The MCMI as a measure of DSM–III. *Journal of Personality Assessment, 49,* 366–378. doi:10.1207/s15327752jpa4904_4

Winograd, G., Cohen, P., & Chen, H. (2008). Adolescent borderline symptoms in the community: Prognosis for functioning over 20 years. *Journal of Child Psychology and Psychiatry, 49,* 933–941. doi:10.1111/j.1469-7610.2008.01930.x

Winokur, G., Coryell, W., Akiskal, H. S., Endicott, J., Keller, M., & Mueller, T. (1994). Manic-depressive (bipolar) disorder: The course in light of a prospective 10-year follow-up of 131 patients. *Acta Psychiatrica Scandinavica, 89*, 102–110. doi:10.1111/j.1600-0447.1994.tb01495.x

Zanarini, M. C., Frankenburg, F. R., Chauncey, D. L., & Gunderson, J. G. (1987). The Diagnostic Interview for Personality Disorders: Interrater and test–retest reliability. *Comprehensive Psychiatry, 28*, 467–480. doi:10.1016/0010-440X(87)90012-5

Zanarini, M. C., Frankenburg, F. R., Hennen, J., Reich, D. B., & Silk, K. R. (2005). Psychosocial functioning of borderline patients and Axis II comparison subjects followed prospectively for six years. *Journal of Personality Disorders, 19*, 19–29. doi:10.1521/pedi.19.1.19.62178

Zanarini, M. C., Frankenburg, F. R., Hennen, J., Reich, D. B., & Silk, K. R. (2006). Prediction of the 10-year course of borderline personality disorder. *The American Journal of Psychiatry, 163*, 827–832. doi:10.1176/appi.ajp.163.5.827

Zanarini, M. C., Frankenburg, F. R., Hennen, J., & Silk, K. R. (2003). The longitudinal course of borderline psychopathology: 6-year prospective follow-up of the phenomenology of borderline personality disorder. *The American Journal of Psychiatry, 160*, 274–283. doi:10.1176/appi.ajp.160.2.274

Zanarini, M. C., Frankenburg, F. R., Reich, D. B., & Fitzmaurice, G. (2010a). The 10-year course of psychosocial functioning among patients with borderline personality disorder and Axis II comparison subjects. *Acta Psychiatrica Scandinavica, 122*, 103–109. doi:10.1111/j.1600-0447.2010.01543.x

Zanarini, M. C., Frankenburg, F. R., Reich, D. B., & Fitzmaurice, G. (2010b). Time to attainment of recovery from borderline personality disorder and stability of recovery: A 10-year prospective follow-up study. *The American Journal of Psychiatry, 167*, 663–667. doi:10.1176/appi.ajp.2009.09081130

Zanarini, M. C., Frankenburg, F. R., Reich, D. B., & Fitzmaurice, G. (2012). Attainment and stability of sustained symptomatic remission and recovery among patients with borderline personality disorder and Axis II comparison subjects: A 16-year prospective follow-up study. *The American Journal of Psychiatry, 169*, 476–483. doi:10.1176/appi.ajp.2011.11101550

Zanarini, M. C., Frankenburg, F. R., Reich, D. B., Silk, K. R., Hudson, J. I., & McSweeney, L. B. (2007). The subsyndromal phenomenology of borderline personality disorder: A 10-year follow-up study. *The American Journal of Psychiatry, 164*, 929–935. doi:10.1176/appi.ajp.164.6.929

Zanarini, M. C., Frankenburg, F. R., Sickel, A. E., & Yong, L. (1996). *The Diagnostic Interview for DSM–IV Personality Disorders (DIPD-IV)*. Belmont, MA: McLean Hospital.

Zanarini, M. C., Gunderson, J. G., Frankenburg, F. R., & Chauncey, D. L. (1989). The Revised Diagnostic Interview for Borderlines: Discriminating BPD from other axis II disorders. *Journal of Personality Disorders, 3*, 10–18. doi:10.1521/pedi.1989.3.1.10

Zanarini, M. C., Jacoby, R. J., Frankenburg, F. R., Reich, D. B., & Fitzmaurice, G. (2009). The 10-year course of Social Security disability income reported by patients with borderline personality disorder and Axis II comparison subjects. *Journal of Personality Disorders, 23,* 346–356. doi:10.1521/pedi.2009.23.4.346

Zanarini, M. C., & Shea, M. T. (1996). *The Diagnostic Interview for DSM–IV Personality Disorders–Follow-Along Version (DIPD-FA).* Belmont, MA: McLean Hospital.

Zanarini, M. C., Sickel, A. E., Yong, L., & Glazer, L. J. (1994). *Revised Borderline Follow-up Interview.* Belmont, MA: McLean Hospital.

Zimmerman, M. (1994). Diagnosing personality disorders: A review of issues and research methods. *Archives of General Psychiatry, 51,* 225–245. doi:10.1001/archpsyc.1994.03950030061006

7

BIOLOGICAL BASES OF PERSONALITY DISORDERS

SUSAN C. SOUTH

The goal in this chapter is to review the state of current knowledge with regard to behavior and molecular genetics of personality disorders (PDs). Behavior genetics focuses on quantitative modeling of genetic and environmental influences on individual differences (e.g., personality), while molecular genetics aims to determine the actual sequences of DNA that can explain variations in thinking, feeling, and behaving. Building on previous recent reviews of this area (Livesley & Jang, 2008; South & DeYoung, 2013; South, Reichborn-Kjennerud, Eaton, & Krueger, 2012), I review the methodologies and techniques of both behavior and molecular genetics before turning to major findings in both areas. Throughout this chapter, an effort is made to integrate findings with the most recent edition of the *Diagnostic and Statistical Manual of Mental Disorders* (DSM–5; American Psychiatric Association, 2013), and consideration is given to how this work will move forward based

http://dx.doi.org/10.1037/14549-008
Personality Disorders: Toward Theoretical and Empirical Integration in Diagnosis and Assessment,
S. K. Huprich (Editor)

on retention of the PD diagnoses from the fourth edition text revision of the *DSM* (*DSM–IV–TR*; American Psychiatric Association, 2000) to *DSM–5*.

BEHAVIOR GENETICS OF PERSONALITY DISORDERS

The term *behavior genetics* encompasses a host of methodologies that all aim to accomplish the same goal: to estimate the genetic and environmental influences on a phenotype, or observed variable. Before the advent of molecular genetic techniques made it possible to sequence DNA and examine the associations between measured genes and personality traits, behavior genetic techniques were used to determine the relative magnitude of genetic and environmental etiological influences. It is axiomatic today to state that every personality trait and almost every psychologically meaningful variable that differs between individuals in the population, including PDs, are due to a combination of nature and nurture. Findings from the field of behavior genetics were instrumental in showing that genetic differences between people contributed to differences in observed characteristics, including personality. Further, these techniques were important in showing that the unique aspects of the environment also impacted development.

Behavior genetic techniques make certain assumptions about the phenotype under study. Arguably, the most important assumption is that of a multifactorial, polygenic model of inheritance, in which there is a continuum of liability underlying the variable of interest; this continuum is roughly normally distributed in the population and results from multiple genetic and environmental influences (Falconer, 1965; Gottesman & Shields, 1967). This model of influence fits well with a dimensional-spectrum conceptualization of psychopathology, particularly PDs; in fact, most behavior genetic modeling of PDs utilizes symptom count variables, as opposed to categorical diagnoses per se. Although it is possible to directly test the assumption of a continuum of liability, research with other psychopathology variables (e.g., attention-deficit/hyperactivity disorder; Levy, Hay, McStephen, Wood, & Waldman, 1997) generally disregards discrete cutoffs in favor of continuums of liability. This has never been done with PD symptoms, although it is likely that similar findings would emerge if applied to PD data (e.g., Eaton, Krueger, South, Simms, & Clark, 2011). This is clearly an avenue for future research.

In this section, I review the major family of behavior genetic research designs that have been used to examine the genetic and environmental influences on normal and pathological personality, including PDs. First, I review the basic univariate twin design, before moving on to extensions of this twin design that can handle multiple personality traits, longitudinal data, and even gene–environment interplay. The methods and assumptions of adoption, family, and extended family designs are also covered.

Twin and Family Methods

The Basic Twin Design

The basic univariate twin design takes advantage of the fact that twins raised together in the same family are a fascinating form of natural experiment: Monozygotic (MZ) or identical twins share 100% of their DNA, but dizygotic (DZ) or fraternal twins are no more alike than any two non-twin siblings, sharing approximately 50% of their segregating DNA. The two types of twins share the same family experience. It is possible to compare the agreement between MZ twins and the agreement between DZ twins on a measured variable, such as a PD, and arrive at an estimate of genetic and environmental influences on that disorder. A rough estimate of the well-known heritability statistic $h2$ (the proportion of variance in a phenotype that is due to genetic differences between people) can be computed by subtracting the correlation between DZ twins from the correlation between MZ twins and multiplying the result by 2; that is, $2*(rMZ\text{-}rDZ)$.

More formal statistical modeling with structural equation modeling software (Neale, Boker, Xie, & Maes, 2003) can be used to decompose the variance in the personality phenotype of interest. The phenotype can be a dimensional personality trait, a total PD symptom count, or even a categorical yes/no variable for whether a PD is present or not (with some modifications to the model to account for categorical variables). For example, Figure 7.1 presents a path diagram of the basic univariate twin design. The total variance in the observed personality phenotype, represented by the box in the figure, is decomposed into three latent sources of variance that are unobserved but estimated from the model, represented by circles in the diagram: (a) *additive genetic influences*, abbreviated A, that represent the combined, or summed, influence of many genes that "add up" to the total genetic influence; (b) *shared, or common, family environment*, abbreviated C, that represents the shared family experiences that make twins more similar to each other (e.g., having the same parents, neighborhood, and socioeconomic status); and (c) *unique, nonshared environment*, abbreviated E, which represents environmental influences that make two people growing up in the same family less similar to each other (e.g., things like having different peer groups or traumatic experiences). Following from the abbreviations of the latent sources of variance, the univariate twin model is often referred to as the ACE model.

As applied to the study of PDs, the basic univariate twin model is useful for determining the relative magnitude of genetic and environmental influences on PDs. Although it may seem obvious that any individual difference

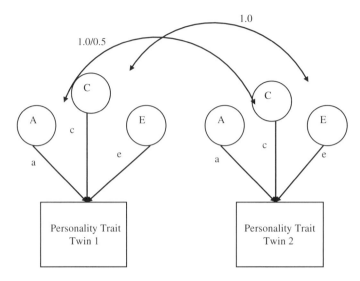

Figure 7.1. ACE path diagram for the univariate twin model. Three sources of variance are represented as latent variables: A = additive genetic influences; C = common environmental influences shared between family members; E = nonshared environmental influences. The correlations between genetic factors and common environmental factors are set to 1.0/0.5 (MZ twins/DZ twins) and 1.0/1.0 (MZ/DZ). The total variance in the phenotype (P) is calculated by summing the squared paths leading to it: $P = a^2 + c^2 + e^2$. MZ = monozygotic; DZ = dyzygotic.

characteristic would have at least some genetic component (e.g., Turkheimer, 2000), it is still important to document this in regard to PDs. PDs are among the most controversial disorders in the *DSM*, as evidenced by recent debates throughout the *DSM–5* process (e.g., Skodol et al., 2011; South & DeYoung, 2013; Widiger, 2011). Establishing genetic influences on the PDs substantiates them as valid disorders, as family and genetic factors have long been considered a critical indicator of construct validity (Robins & Guze, 1970). An important area for future research will be to examine the genetic and environmental influences on the trait system included in Section III of the *DSM–5;* if the heritability estimates for the higher order domains included in this trait system were larger and/or more consistent than heritability estimates for the *DSM–5* Section II categorical PDs, that would be one line of support in favor of the trait system over the categorical diagnoses, which could be bolstered by evidence from other lines of inquiry (e.g., clinical utility studies).

There are several important caveats about the univariate twin model. First, any source of error is included in the estimate of E. Second, many variables that are putatively included in the C estimate may in fact be better thought of as estimates of E. For instance, two siblings can grow up with the same parents (theoretically included under C) but have vastly different relationships with those parents (which would more appropriately be considered E). Third, the univariate ACE model, as well as multivariate extensions of this twin model, attempts to explain the *variance* in a phenotype. The ACE estimates do not describe how much, or which, genetic or environmental influences affect a specific person's personality. People within the population will vary on a personality trait (hence the term *individual differences*), and the goal of the twin design is to estimate the influence of differences in genes and environment on the reason that people's personalities differ. Fourth, and related to the last point, the estimates obtained from the twin model are specific to that sample and the population of interest. Thus, as with any descriptive statistic, these estimates may change depending on the uniqueness of the specific sample. There may also be important differences within each sample. For example, there may be differences between men and women on magnitude of the ACE estimates. More recently, an extension of the univariate twin model was developed (see more on gene × environment models below) that made it possible to determine if genetic and environmental estimates on a phenotype differed for different segments within the population (e.g., ACE estimates for antisocial behavior at different levels of socioeconomic status; see Tuvblad, Grann, & Lichtenstein, 2006). Finally, it is also possible to run an ADE model (D for dominant) that includes both additive and nonadditive genetic effects. The D is somewhat of a misnomer, as nonadditive genetic effects include both dominant effects (interactions of genes at the same locus) and epistatic effects (interactions of genes at different loci). The limitations of the model preclude the estimation of all four sources of variance at once (i.e., ADCE models are not possible).

Multivariate Twin Designs

The basic univariate twin design has also been extended to handle multiple phenotypes at once. This is particularly appropriate for normal and pathological personality traits, where multiple phenotypes (or traits) are necessary to capture the totality of personality "space." These multivariate designs have the advantage of being able to estimate genetic and environmental influences on individual personality traits (as in the univariate case) as well as the amount of overlap between influences on multiple traits. With regard to PDs, these models have several purposes. First, they can determine whether the comorbidity between PDs can be explained by overlapping genetic or environmental influences. They can also be used to examine whether the etiological structure of PDs parallels the phenotypic structure. For instance, researchers can determine whether there is validity to the *DSM* three-cluster organization system at the genetic and environmental level. Further, these multivariate models can be applied to examine the overlap between PDs and other, related clinical disorders (e.g., substance use disorders, mood disorders). Finally, multivariate models can be used to examine the etiological overlap between PDs and normal personality.

The first type of multivariate twin model is the *triangular (Cholesky) decomposition* model. This model includes multiple measured phenotypes (e.g., two or more PDs), and it is possible to decompose the variance in each phenotype as well as the covariance between the multiple phenotypes. The Cholesky model is able to provide estimates of genetic and environmental influences on each variable, but, more important, it is able to provide genetic and environmental correlations between variables. A genetic correlation (rA) estimates the amount of overlap between the genetic influences on two variables. Similar correlations are produced for shared (rC) and nonshared (rE) environment. These types of correlations are particularly applicable when examining the etiological influences on personality traits, as it is then possible to determine whether different personality traits share genetic or environmental influences. The second type of multivariate model is an *independent pathways (IP) model*. This model is more structured than a Cholesky model, as it includes a set of latent A, C, and E factors that directly influence the phenotypes (here, PDs). In addition, there are residual ACE effects for each individual variable. Thus, it is possible for each phenotype in the model to share genetic and environmental influences with other phenotypes as well as have residual influences not shared with the other variables. The final type of multivariate model is a *common pathway (CP) model*. This model is the biometric modeling equivalent to a regular factor analysis but with the estimate of ACE variance components added. As with a phenotypic factor, the common latent variable is assumed to explain the covariance among the lower order variables (e.g., multiple personality traits); the variance of this latent factor is decomposed into genetic and environmental influences.

These three models—Cholesky, IP, and CP—can be directly compared within the same data set because they are nested within each other. This direct comparison then allows for statistical tests of model fit between different conceptualizations of the shared etiological influences among different personality traits. For instance, a researcher with twin data on all 10 *DSM* PDs could compare a Cholesky model including the 10 PDs with (a) an IP model including, perhaps, three latent factors to correspond to the three-cluster organization of the *DSM* and (b) a CP model that formally models three latent factors, again corresponding to the three clusters.

Longitudinal Twin Designs

Some multivariate biometric models allow for examination of etiological influences on personality over time. One option is to use a Cholesky model, but with personality variables measured over time as opposed to cross-sectionally; this design would be appropriate for examining the origins of differential stability or the amount of consistency in the rank order of individuals over time (Roberts & DelVecchio, 2000). Depending on the time points measured, these types of models are appropriate for understanding whether genetic or environmental influences contribute to stability of personality over time. PDs by definition are chronic, long-standing patterns of behavior present by adolescence (American Psychiatric Association, 2013) that follow a long and debilitating course; indeed, PDs have long been thought resistant to treatment for this reason. Researchers, however, have questioned this assumption, suggesting that PDs fluctuate to a similar degree as major clinical disorders (e.g., Clark, 2005; Krueger, 2005). Longitudinal biometric models may help to answer this question by determining whether new genetic or environmental influences come "online" for PDs over the course of the life span.

Another option is to use a biometric model extension of a latent growth curve model. Phenotypic latent growth curve models estimate latent intercept and slope growth factors that represent the average at first time point and change over time, respectively. Growth curve models are appropriate for examining absolute stability, or mean level changes in personality over time; they also have the advantage of providing variance around the mean-level trend by including a random effect term. The biometric extension of this model decomposes the variance of the growth factors into genetic and environmental influences. When applied to PDs, this model could be used to examine the genetic and environmental origins of individual differences in changes in PD symptoms over time.

Adoption, Family and Extended-Family Designs

In addition to using twins, researchers can take advantage of other types of family units to examine the genetic and environmental basis of PDs. For instance, family studies can examine first-degree relatives of probands with the PD diagnosis of interest to determine whether the disorder tends to aggregate within families (e.g., Zanarini, Barison, Frankenburg, Reich, & Hudson, 2009). Adoption studies are a strong complement to twin studies for examining the importance of genetic influences on a phenotype like personality. In the basic adoption design, assessments are collected from the biological parent(s), adopted parent(s), and adopted offspring. If there has been no contact between the adopted child and the biological parent, any resemblance between the two would be due to genetic influences alone. More recently, researchers have utilized a variety of extended-family designs that use biological full- and half-siblings as well as adopted offspring to examine etiological influences. Consider the case of nonbiologically related adopted siblings raised in the same household, who provide a direct test of the shared environment.

Findings From Twin and Family Studies

Over the past several decades the field of behavior genetics has comprehensively demonstrated that almost every psychologically meaningful individual difference between people in the population—including intelligence, psychopathology, and personality—has a measurable genetic component (Turkheimer, 2000). There are strong associations between normal and pathological personality traits (Markon, Krueger, & Watson, 2005), to the point where PDs can be modeled as combinations of extreme normal personality traits like the five-factor model (FFM; Widiger & Costa, 2002). Researchers have argued that the problems with the *DSM* PD diagnoses, including arbitrary boundaries, heterogeneity within disorders, and comorbidity across disorders, could be ameliorated by using a dimensional conceptualization of PDs (e.g., Widiger & Simonsen, 2005). Thus, in this section I first briefly review what is known about the biometric modeling of genetic and environmental influences on normal personality traits. There is less research into PDs per se, and much of this has been done with pathological personality inventories as opposed to *DSM* PD symptoms or disorders. Both types of work are reviewed below.

Normal Personality Traits

Given the dominance of trait theory in personality research over the last several decades (e.g., John, Naumann, & Soto, 2008), it is not surprising that most biometric modeling of normal personality has focused on using inventories of trait models. Three of the most common personality inventories used in biometric modeling of normal personality are the NEO Personality Inventory—Revised (NEO-PI–R) and its variants, the most popular assessment measure for the FFM (Costa & McCrae, 1992); the Multidimensional Personality Questionnaire (MPQ), an inventory to assess Tellegen's Big Three (Tellegen & Waller, in press); and the Eysenck Personality Questionnaire (EPQ), a measure to assess Eysenck's three-factor model (Eysenck, 1991; Eysenck & Eysenck, 1975). Of importance, there is considerable overlap between the traits included in these three models, and these different scales all tend to load together in factor models (e.g., Markon et al., 2005). Across different samples and assessment instruments, most of the variance in the FFM trait domains of extraversion, conscientiousness, neuroticism, openness, and agreeableness can be split between genetic and nonshared environmental influences, with heritability around .40–.50 for the broad domains (Bouchard & Loehlin, 2001). For instance, one study of the NEO-PI–R reported broad heritabilities (including both additive and dominant genetic influences, known as *broad-sense* heritability) of 44% (conscientiousness), 41% (agreeableness), 41% (neuroticism), 53% (extraversion), and 61% (openness;

Jang, Livesley, & Vernon, 1996). Similarly, the variance in the EPQ domains (Bouchard & Loehlin, 2001) and in the MPQ higher order traits (Finkel & McGue, 1997; Tellegen et al., 1988) can be roughly split between genetic and nonshared environmental influences.

Of course, normal personality trait domains are hierarchically organized, and it is possible to decompose the variance in lower-order traits as well as the higher order domains. Lower order traits generally seem to have moderate genetic influences, with again little evidence of the shared environment (Jang, McCrae, Angleitner, Riemann, & Livesley, 1998; Yamagata et al., 2006). For instance, additive genetic influences on the lower order facets of the NEO-PI–R in one study ranged from .26 (Anxiety, N domain) to .52 (Gregariousness, E domain; Jang, Livesley, & Vernon, 1996). There is also some evidence of gender differences in the estimates of genetic and environmental influences on the facets and domains. Bergeman et al. (1993) reported greater genetic influence on conscientiousness in men than in women (41% vs. 11%), and Finkel and McGue (1997) also found higher heritability for men on the MPQ control subscale; in contrast, Blonigen, Carlson, Hicks, Krueger, and Iacono (2008) found that parameters for genetic influences on MPQ scales could be set equal across gender with no significant reduction in fit.

Adoption studies are generally commensurate with twin studies in finding moderate genetic influences, no or minimal shared family influences, and sizable nonshared environmental influences (e.g., Bouchard & Loehlin, 2001; Plomin, Corley, Caspi, Fulker, & DeFries, 1998). One important difference is that adoption studies will report somewhat lower heritability estimates than will twin studies (e.g., Plomin et al., 1998). One reason for this discrepancy can be explained by the presence of nonadditive genetic effects. In twin studies, nonadditive genetic effects can have the effect of increasing heritability because MZ twins share 100% of their genes (including any nonadditive genetic effects), but DZ twins share 50% of their additive genes, on average, and thus the similarity between DZ twins will be less affected by nonadditive effects. There is some evidence from twin studies for nonadditive genetic effects on normal personality traits (e.g., Bergeman et al., 1993; Jang, Livesley, & Vernon, 1996), but there are two important limitations; as noted above, nonadditive genetic effects cannot be modeled along with both shared and nonshared environmental effects, and large samples are necessary to estimate these models (Martin, Eaves, Kearsey, & Davies, 1978). Adoption studies and extended family designs that use twins, siblings, and unrelated (adopted) offspring have found evidence of nonadditive genetic effects on personality (e.g., Keller, Coventry, Heath, & Martin, 2005).

Findings from multivariate models of normal personality have also added to understanding of the etiology of the joint multivariate space of normal personality traits. Studies have now utilized the multivariate biometric models described above (Cholesky, IP, and CP) to examine the structure of normal personality traits. Most major trait theories of personality posit a hierarchical structure, with lower-order trait facets (e.g., gregariousness, warmth) underlying higher order domains (e.g., Extraversion). Behavior genetic studies have tested whether genetic and environmental influences parallel the phenotypic structure of major trait theories, finding mixed results regarding the correspondence between phenotypic and genotypic data (Jang, Livesley, Angleitner, Riemann, & Vernon, 2002; Yamagata et al., 2006). For instance, Johnson and Krueger (2004) modeled trait adjectives representing the Big Five domains. They found that some domains (Neuroticism, Extraversion) were best represented by unitary latent factors (CP model fit best) while others (Conscientiousness, Openness) had a "looser" organizational structure (IP model fit best). However, Jang et al. (2002) reported good congruence between the phenotypic and genetic structure of the NEO-PI–R, based on factor analysis of the genetic covariance structure.

Multivariate biometric modeling has also been used to examine the genetic and environmental contributions to personality over time. Studies using a variation of the Cholesky decomposition to look at the origins of differential stability generally find genetic contributions to stability and nonshared environmental influences on change (Blonigen et al., 2008; McGue, Bacon, & Lykken, 1993). Note that these studies used only two time points assessed during adolescence to early adulthood. More recent biometric modeling of longitudinal growth curves found genetic influences on both stability (the intercept growth factor) and change (the slope growth factor), depending on the personality trait studied (Bleidorn, Kandler, Riemann, Angleitner, & Spinath, 2009; Hopwood et al., 2011). Hopwood et al. (2011) reported that the slope factor for MPQ constraint was due to significant genetic (.504) and nonshared environmental (.496) influences; the slope factor for MPQ negative emotionality was due largely to nonshared environmental influences (.792), with only minimal impact of genetic effects (.122).

In summary, findings from twin studies and adoption and extended family designs confirm substantial genetic influences on most major normal personality traits. There is still work to be done to determine the relative influence of nonadditive versus additive genetic effects, and it could have important implications for finding measured genes that are associated with personality traits. Research on the etiological influences on personality trait structure and development suggest somewhat mixed findings. These results have implications for PD research. Some argue for a conceptualization of PDs as maladaptive variants of normal personality (e.g., Widiger & Mullins-Sweatt, 2009). Thus, understanding the etiological structure of normal personality traits, for instance, will inform how PDs are described in terms of normal personality traits.

Pathological Personality Traits

For some time, there has been a push for a dimensional conceptualization of personality pathology (for a review, see Widiger & Simonsen, 2005). This follows from numerous problems plaguing the current categorical system, including heterogeneity within diagnosis, poor thresholds for diagnostic cutoffs, unreliability of diagnostic assessment, and comorbidity among PDs (see Widiger & Trull, 2007). It also follows from a broader move toward dimensionalization of psychopathology in general (Widiger & Samuel, 2005). Many have argued that a dimensional model of PDs would alleviate the problems inherent in the current *DSM* definitions, and a growing amount of empirical research also seems to support dimensions over categories (e.g., Eaton et al., 2011). There is strong and growing evidence that PDs can be captured by using extreme variants of normal personality already included in most major trait models. For instance, a large body of evidence now exists that describes the *DSM* PD constructs using the domains and facets of the FFM of normal personality (see Samuel & Widiger, 2008). As of this writing, there are no known biometric studies that examine the etiological influences on five-factor model profiles of PD constructs. This is clearly an interesting area for future research; finding genetic influences on the FFM PD profiles would be strong evidence in support of this type of conceptualization.

There are, however, numerous studies that examine the genetic and environmental influences on trait inventories of pathological personality traits. Most of these studies have centered on the Dimensional Assessment of Personality Pathology (DAPP; Livesley & Jackson, 2001), a 290-item trait measure of pathological personality that includes 18 lower-order dimensions (e.g., submissiveness, identify problems, affective lability) that are subsumed by four higher order domains of dissocial behavior, inhibitedness, compulsivity, and emotional dysregulation (Jang et al., 1998). Biometric modeling with the DAPP has found heritability estimates of 38% for compulsivity, 50% for dissocial behavior, 52% for inhibitedness, and 53% for emotional dysregulation (Jang, Livesley, Vernon, & Jackson, 1996), with little evidence of the shared environment; thus, etiological influences on these domains of pathological personality are commensurate with influences on higher order domains of normal personality.

There are many parallels between biometric modeling of the DAPP traits and modeling of normal personality traits (e.g., with versions of the NEO). Similar to modeling of normal personality trait domains and facets, the lower order scales of the DAPP generally had moderate genetic influences (although one study estimated heritability of DAPP conduct disorder at 0%; Livesley, Jang, Jackson, & Vernon, 1993). Also similar to normal personality traits, there was evidence of nonadditive genetic effects; these nonadditive effects were found for affective lability (48%), identity problems

(19%), intimacy problems (38%), narcissism (64%), self-harm (15%), social avoidance (10%), and oppositionality (3%). There was little effect of the shared environment, with only two lower order DAPP scales demonstrating substantial influences: conduct problems (53%) and submissiveness (28%). Finally, many of the DAPP lower order traits demonstrated significant residual heritability after accounting for the higher order domains on which they load (Jang et al., 1998). Similarly, the NEO-PI–R lower order facets show substantial heritability after partialing out the higher order domains (Jang et al., 1998). Phenotypic research suggests a great deal of overlap between pathological personality trait inventories like the DAPP and normal personality trait inventories like the NEO-PI–R and its variants (e.g., Markon et al., 2005). Jang and Livesley (1999) investigated the source of this overlap by conducting multivariate biometric modeling with the DAPP and the NEO Five-Factor Inventory (NEO-FFI) in a volunteer community twin sample. There was a great deal of variability in the genetic and environmental correlations between DAPP and NEO scales; in general, DAPP scales had the greatest number of correlations with the NEO Neuroticism domain (from .05 for DAPP stimulus seeking to .81 for DAPP anxiousness). Of the five NEO domains, openness showed the fewest genetic or environmental correlations with any of the DAPP scales. Genetic correlations were generally greater than nonshared environmental correlations, and the genetic correlations were often larger than the phenotypic correlations. Jang and Livesley concluded that their findings supported the use of normal personality trait inventories, like the NEO-FFI, for the assessment of pathological personality problems. It is important to note that studies described in this section have comprised volunteer (nonclinical) twin samples, and research with samples including more extreme levels of personality variation may result in different findings.

DSM Personality Disorders

There are several family studies of PDs that were the first to provide evidence of familial aggregation of PD, particularly schizotypal and borderline personality disorders (e.g., Loranger, Oldham, & Tulis, 1982). Adoption studies with patients who have PDs have also been conducted, often with a focus on antisocial behavior and related constructs. For instance, work by Cadoret, Yates, Troughton, Woodworth, and Stewart (1995) with adopted offspring who had a positive biological family history of antisocial behavior demonstrated the importance of genetic and environmental effects on aggressive and antisocial behavior.

Biometric modeling of twin data on PD constructs is relatively sparse compared with studies of normal personality and pathological personality traits (e.g., using the DAPP) and is limited to a few disorders. For instance, one study (Distel et al., 2010) found that a latent factor representing a borderline personality disorder (BPD) construct (measured with the Personality Assessment Inventory, Borderline Features scale [Morey, 1991]) was explained by genetics (51%) and unique environment (49%). A meta-analysis of behavior genetic studies found that variance in antisocial behavior could be attributed to additive genetic influences (32%), nonadditive genetic influences (9%), shared environment (16%) and nonshared environment (43%), although the operationalization of diagnosis had a significant moderating effect; when limited to studies where the phenotype was antisocial personality disorder (ASPD), shared environment was lower (10%) and nonshared environment was higher (54%; Rhee & Waldman, 2002).

Only a handful of studies have conducted biometric modeling of all *DSM*-defined PDs. In a sample of 112 child twin pairs, Coolidge, Thede, and Jang (2001) asked parents to report on PD symptoms; univariate twin modeling of this data revealed that heritability estimates ranged from 50% (paranoid) to 81% (dependent, schizotypal). There was no appreciable influence of the shared environment on any of the PDs. A later study in a sample of Norwegian adult twins partially recruited from psychiatric facilities conducted structured diagnostic interviews for *DSM–III–R* PDs and reported heritability estimates from 28% (paranoid, avoidant) to 77% (narcissistic, obsessive-compulsive; Torgersen et al., 2000). Estimates were not computed for ASPD due to the low number of cases in the sample. The most recent biometric modeling of PDs used data from structured interviews (Structured Interview for *DSM–IV* Personality; Pfohl, Blum, & Zimmerman, 1997) of *DSM–IV* PD symptoms collected from twins in the Norwegian Institute of Public Health Twin Panel (NIPHTP). Estimates from this study were among the lowest of the three, ranging from 21% (paranoid) to 38% (antisocial; Kendler et al., 2006; Reichborn-Kjennerud, Czajkowski, Neale, et al., 2007; Torgersen et al., 2008).

It is not surprising that specific heritability estimates for the individual PDs differed across these three studies, given the differences in population, age of the samples, and method of assessment. The last is particularly important, as research has shown that the way PD is conceptualized and assessed can impact estimates of genetic influences. For instance, meta-analysis put the heritability of "antisocial behavior" around 40% (Ferguson, 2010; Miles & Carey, 1997; Rhee & Waldman, 2002), but using only *DSM*-defined ASPD results in higher estimates of the unique environment and lower estimates of heritability (Ferguson, 2010). In other work, Kendler et al. found that using latent factors comprising both self-report questionnaires and structured interview resulted in higher heritability estimates in Cluster A PDs than did a structured interview alone, partly explaining the lower estimates of heritability found in the NIPHTP sample (Kendler, Myers, Torgersen, Neale,

& Reichborn-Kjennerud, 2007). Further, they directly compared self-report questionnaires with structured interviews and found that there were residual genetic effects specific only to the self-report questionnaires; this suggests that structured interviews had greater specificity with regard to genetic risk underlying the latent domain of Cluster A pathology.

Perhaps more illuminating than univariate twin studies that establish genetic and environmental influences on PDs are multivariate twin studies that can begin to answer questions about why PDs tend to be correlated and whether they are truly etiologically distinct constructs. Researchers conducted a series of analyses using the NIPHTP twin data to examine the PDs separately by cluster. Kendler et al. (2006) fit an IP model to the Cluster A PDs and found that although heritability was modest for all three disorders, schizotypal PD had the highest loading on the general factor of genetic influences, suggesting it was the PD that most closely reflect latent genetic liability for Cluster A type pathology. A similar analysis among Cluster B personality disorders found a latent genetic factor that influenced all four personality disorders, a genetic factor that influenced only ASPD and BPD, and residual genetic influences on ASPD and narcissistic PD (Torgersen et al., 2008). Finally, modeling of the Cluster C PDs indicated one set of genetic and environmental factors influencing all three disorders; however, the common genetic factor explained only 11% of the variance in obsessive–compulsive personality disorder (OCPD), suggesting it was etiologically distinct from the other two PDs in that cluster. Of note, none of the models for any of the clusters revealed significant shared environmental influences.

To date, only one multivariate twin studied has been conducted that included all 10 of the *DSM* PDs. Again using the NIPHTP twin data set, Kendler et al. (2008) ran a series of models to examine the genetic and environmental structure underlying the 10 PDs. A CP model did not fit the data well; the best fitting model was an IP model that included three genetic factors and three nonshared environmental factors but no shared environmental factors. The first genetic factor has substantial loadings (explaining more than 8% of the phenotypic variance) on paranoid, histrionic, borderline, narcissistic, dependent, and obsessive–compulsive PDs; the second genetic factor had substantial loadings on ASPD and BPD, and the third genetic factor had substantial loadings on schizoid and avoidant PDs. Kendler et al. interpreted these findings as reflecting general tendencies toward personality pathology/negative emotionality, aggressive/impulsive behavior, and pathological introversion, respectively. In contrast, the nonshared environmental influences better reflected the three-cluster system found in *DSM–IV*. Finally, there were specific genetic effects on several of the PDs, particularly OCPD.

In addition to clarifying the etiological influences on the comorbidity of PDs, biometric modeling can begin to examine the relationships between

PDs and other clinical disorders in the *DSM*. As reviewed elsewhere, there is a great deal of comorbidity between PDs and the *DSM–IV* Axis I disorders (Dolan-Sewell, Krueger, & Shea, 2001). Multivariate phenotypic modeling of symptoms of clinical disorders suggests that major common forms of mental disorders group into internalizing syndromes—mood, anxiety, and eating disorders (e.g., Krueger & Markon, 2006)—and externalizing syndromes of substance dependence, conduct disorder, and antisocial behavior (Krueger, Skodol, Livesley, Shrout, & Huang, 2007). More recently, these models have been begun to include PDs. For instance, Kotov et al. (2011), using structured interview data for Axis I and Axis II of *DSM–IV*, found that Cluster C PDs (dependent, obsessive–compulsive) fell under an internalizing factor. The Cluster A PDs were best grouped into a thought disorder domain with mania and psychosis; ASPD cross-loaded on an externalizing factor and an antagonism factor; and borderline, histrionic, and narcissistic were subsumed under the antagonism domain (borderline also cross-loaded on internalizing).

Family and adoption studies have long suggested a shared familial risk for certain PDs and clinical disorders, including schizotypal PD and schizophrenia (e.g., Asarnow et al., 2001) and BPD and major depression (e.g., Riso, Klein, Anderson, & Ouimette, 2000). These findings are bolstered by work from twin studies. One study demonstrated that the covariance between borderline, avoidant, and paranoid personality disorders and major depression could be accounted for by one genetic factor (Reichborn-Kjennerud et al., 2010). Another study found identical genetic risk underlying social phobia and avoidant PD but uncorrelated environmental factors, suggesting that whether one develops avoidant PD or social phobia is largely a result of unique environmental risk factors (Reichborn-Kjennerud, Czajkowki, Torgersen, et al., 2007). Other work has shown that symptoms of ASPD fit well within a highly heritable externalizing spectrum (Krueger et al., 2002) that also includes conduct disorder, alcohol dependence, drug dependence, and the personality trait of constraint (reversed); this externalizing factor is also transmitted from parents to offspring (Hicks, Krueger, Iacono, McGue, & Patrick, 2004).

There has been only one biometric modeling study to include PDs and other major forms of clinical disorders. Using the NIPHTP data set, Kendler et al. (2011) modeled the joint structure of all 10 *DSM–IV* PDs as well as 12 *DSM–IV* Axis I disorders: major depression (MD), dysthymia (DYS), specific phobia (SP), social phobia (SoP), panic disorder (PD), agoraphobia (AG), generalized anxiety disorder (GAD), somatoform disorder (SD), eating disorders (ED), alcohol abuse/dependence (AD), illicit drug abuse/dependence (DD), and conduct disorder (CD). They conducted an exploratory factor analysis of the genetic and environmental correlations between the 22 disorders. Results revealed four genetic factors: an Axis I internalizing factor (PD, MD, AG, SD, SP, ED, GAD), an Axis II internalizing factor (SD, DYS, SZ, STP, AVD, DEP, SoP, PD), an Axis I externalizing factor (ASPD, DD, CD, AD, BOR), and an Axis II externalizing factor (ED, DEP, HIS, NARC, OC, PAR, BOR). Of note, four disorders had substantial cross loadings (ED, DEP, SD, PD, BD). In contrast, the environmental influences on the 22 disorders were structured quite differently, with one environmental factor for all personality disorders, one for all Axis I internalizing disorders, and one that distinguished anxiety disorders from externalizing disorders. Kendler et al. (2011) concluded that these results generally supported keeping a distinction between PDs and clinical disorders, or between disorders that are more chronic versus more transient in nature, respectively.

Gene × Environment Interplay

Behavior genetic studies have historically been invaluable in establishing genetic influences on personality and PDs. The limitation of this work, of course, is that it does not say anything about which genes or which environments are included in those estimates of the A, C, and E variance components. They are simply estimates of what contributes to the fact that PDs vary in the population. Further, heritability and environmental estimates average across the sample-specific population, just as means are an average that may hide important within-sample differences. More recent biometric models, however, have been developed that examine within-sample differences in ACE estimates and start to identify the interplay between environmental and genetic influences on PDs and related traits.

These *biometric moderation models* (Purcell, 2002) are so named because they allow for the possibility that certain environments may "moderate" genetic and environmental influences on a phenotype. That is, instead of obtaining ACE estimates that are the same for everyone in the sample, it is possible to obtain ACE estimates that differ for people at very high, average, and very low levels of an environmental "moderator" variable (or anywhere in between). Figure 7.2 displays an example from a study by Krueger, South, Johnson, and Iacono (2008). In this example, the biometric moderation model was applied to the phenotype of the personality trait of negative emotionality (NEM) from the MPQ (Tellegen & Waller, in press), scored in the direction of lower NEM, obtained from a sample of adolescent twins in the Minnesota Twin Family Study. Instead of producing one set of ACE estimates, in Figure 7.2 different ACE estimates are plotted at different levels of the moderator variable, which in this case is the amount of regard in the adolescent's relationship with his or her parent. Estimates of the shared and nonshared environment remain the same at every level of regard; genetic

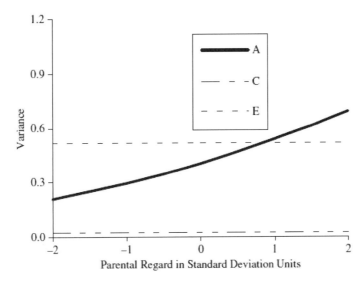

Figure 7.2. Example of a biometric moderation model demonstrating gene ×
environment interaction for the personality trait of negative emotionality. This
graph illustrates variance in negative emotionality as a function of parental regard
at age 17. A = additive genetic variance. C = shared environmental variance.
E = nonshared environmental variance. From "The Heritability of Personality Is
Not Always 50%: Gene–Environment Interactions and Correlations Between
Personality and Parenting," by R. F. Krueger, S. C. South, W. Johnson, and W.
Iacono, 2008, *Journal of Personality, 76,* p. 1507. Copyright 2008 by the authors.
Reprinted with permission.

variance, however, increases from low to high levels of regard. Thus, high
levels of regard in the parent–adolescent relationship allow for the expression
of genetic influences on low NEM.

These moderation models have several potential uses. First, they may
help in molecular gene-hunting efforts, which to date have been plagued
by difficulties with replication (see below). Second, they may aid in understanding the etiological models of PDs by providing support for different
theories of PD development. These models have been shown to support
diathesis-stress models of psychopathology (e.g., South & Krueger, 2008),
in which genetic influences on a phenotype are higher in the more maladaptive end of the environmental moderator. Alternatively, these models
may also support a social push model of psychopathology, in which greater
genetic influences are found in the more adaptive, advantaged end of the
environment. In one of the few studies that have applied this biometric
model to a PD phenotype, Tuvblad et al. (2006) found support for grater

genetic influences on antisocial behavior among individuals from higher socioeconomic status. Finally, if genetic influences were higher at both the adaptive and maladaptive ends of the environment, this might suggest that biological sensitivity to context would be operating on PD traits (e.g., South & Krueger, 2013).

Conclusions From Behavior Genetics: DSM–5 and the Future

At this point, it is possible to conclude that major domains of normal personality and pathological personality as well as *DSM* PD symptom clusters have significant and generally moderate genetic influences, with little evidence of the shared environment. It is reasonable to ask how behavior genetic studies of pathological personality and *DSM* PDs move forward from this point. After a widely debated series of suggested changes to the *DSM–5* section (Skodol, 2011; Skodol et al., 2011; Widiger, 2011), the final proposal for a dimensional trait system was rejected and the *DSM–IV* classification of PDs was retained for *DSM–5*. As noted in a previous review, it was also not clear how findings from twin and family studies played into the PD work groups' proposed (and ultimately rejected) changes (South & DeYoung, 2013).

Going forward, is it useful to continue to conduct univariate biometric modeling of *DSM*-based PDs? Replication is certainly key to scientific inquiry, so continuing to establish the genetic and environmental basis of individual differences in PD pathology is important, given how few studies have been conducted. It would also be important to replicate the work of Kendler et al. (2011), who found separate, genetically influenced factors for clinical disorders and PDs. These findings were important support for retaining a separate PD chapter in the *DSM*; at times during the *DSM–5* proposal process, there was concern that the PD chapter would be removed completely in favor of moving the PDs to other chapters within the *DSM* (e.g., BPD to mood disorders; see South & DeYoung, 2013). It would be particularly important to replicate this work longitudinally.

Potentially more useful, however, are multivariate forms of biometric modeling that can begin to tackle unanswered questions. Phenotypic research using data from the Collaborative Longitudinal Personality Disorders Study showed that normal personality traits prospectively predicted change in *DSM* PDs, but PDs did not predict personality change longitudinally (Warner et al., 2004). It would be particularly informative to extend that type of work to biometric modeling. Indeed, given the push toward a dimensional model of PDs (a provisional model for "further study" is included in the *DSM–5*), perhaps the most critical work that could be done in the future is to understand the overlap between etiological influences on normal and pathological personality traits. If normal and pathological personality traits had genetic and environmental influences in common but still retained their own specific genetic and environmental influences, this would suggest that extreme personality traits, not included in normal personality trait measures like the NEO, are needed to capture the totality of multivariate personality space. The *DSM–5* contains a trait inventory, the PID (Krueger, Derringer, Markon, Watson, & Skodol, 2012), to assess the provisional trait model; as of this writing, no biometric modeling has been conducted with this instrument. Understanding the genetic and environmental influences on the PID domains and on the covariances between the PID, normal personality traits, and other clinical disorders, would be an important next step.

MOLECULAR GENETICS OF PERSONALITY DISORDERS

Work from the field of behavior genetics has firmly established that PDs, like normal personality traits, psychopathology, intelligence, and other important individual differences, are all at least moderately heritable. Following from advances in DNA sequencing technology, researchers began turning in earnest in the 1990s to finding the measured genes for personality (and, more recently, PDs). Molecular genetics researchers examining the genes for personality follow a polygenic model of inheritance, looking for many genes of small effect size. Even though PDs are defined as categorical in the *DSM*, for purposes of molecular genetic analysis they are generally treated as dimensional entitles. This not only fits with theoretical and empirical conceptualizations of normal and abnormal personality (e.g., Eaton et al., 2011) but also confers certain statistical advantages. For instance, the search for quantitative trait loci (QTL) that affect a dimensional personality trait, as opposed to susceptibility genes for a categorical disorder, requires smaller sample sizes. Finding replicable associations between *any* measured genes and *any* personality traits, normal or abnormal, has been a daunting task, leading many to question what has happened to the "missing heritability" (Manolio et al., 2009). In this section, I first review different techniques for finding measured genes for personality and PDs, before turning to the major findings to date. I finish with thoughts on the future and how emerging methods may finally move this field forward.

Molecular Genetic Methods

Below, I briefly review the most commonly used techniques to data; this review is not meant to be comprehensive, and interested readers are referred to more in-depth reviews and descriptions of these techniques (e.g., Sham & McGuffin, 2002). It is fairly well accepted at this point that there are many genes "responsible" for personality and PDs, each of small effect size. Thus, molecular genetics researchers interested in personality do not look for dominant, Mendelian-influenced traits (although see above regarding nonadditive genetic findings) but instead try to identify the many small genes that together influence personality (also known as quantitative trait loci, or QTL). Common gene variants that are found widely in the population (greater than 1%) are called *polymorphisms*. There are various types of polymorphisms, including *variable number tandem repeats* (VNTRs), in which certain sequences of base pairs are replicated a variable number of times, and *single nucleotide polymorphisms* (SNPs), a switch in one of the four bases that make up DNA. To date, molecular genetic studies of personality and PDs are focused on identifying polymorphisms that may be linked to personality traits assessed with various self-report questionnaires.

The most theoretically driven analysis of the molecular genetics of personality and PDs relies on *candidate gene analysis*. These candidate genes are selected on the basis of what is known about their mechanisms of action. For instance, many genes examined in psychiatric genetics are known to affect neurotransmitters that have significant relationships with psychopathology (e.g., serotonin genes and internalizing disorders of mood and anxiety). Similarly, candidate genes examined for personality are mostly genes known to code for or affect neurotransmission in the brain.

Less theoretically driven than the candidate gene approach is the technique of linkage analysis. Linkage analysis takes advantage of the fact that during DNA recombination, segments of DNA from the mother and father are combined in unique ways on the new chromosomes of the developing offspring. Thus, a child's chromosome is not simply a direct copy of that of the mother or father but a unique combination of both. Genes that are close together on the chromosome are "linked" and more likely to be transmitted together onto the new chromosome. Linkage analysis uses samples of related individuals (i.e., biological families) and analyzes how close or distant two areas of a chromosome are to arrive at hypotheses about genes that may be involved in the phenotype of interest. The drawback of linkage analysis is that it is best suited to find genes of large effect size, and it is widely agreed that the genetic model of inheritance for personality and PDs is one of many genes of very small effect.

The latest tool in molecular genetics of personality is *genome-wide association studies* (GWAS). GWAS extends basic association analysis by scanning genetic markers across the genome (hundreds of thousands and up to one million in the latest platforms) to detect an association between the presence of a marker and the presence of the phenotype. This method relies on the idea that there are millions of SNPs or one-base-pair substitutions on the human genome, and these SNPs either may be directly responsible for associated phenotypic differences or may indicate the presence of other genes that are related to the phenotype.

Findings From Molecular Genetics

Cluster A

Given the close links found between schizophrenia and the schizophrenia-spectrum disorders, particularly with family studies (e.g., Kendler et al., 1993), it is not surprising that many of the studies looking for the genetic basis of Cluster A disorders have focused on risk genes for schizophrenia. Indeed, in one interesting study, the authors conducted a genome-wide linkage analysis of schizotypy in the nonpsychotic relatives of high-risk schizophrenia families (Fanous et al., 2007). The findings provided support for a genetic correlation between schizotypy and schizophrenia, as a subset of susceptibility genes for schizophrenia also appeared to affect schizotypy; however, no significant markers for schizotypy were found.

In the last several years, a growing number of studies have examined whether risk alleles for schizophrenia might also be associated with schizotypal personality traits. For instance, Ohi et al. (2012) investigated the association between the risk allele of the *p250GAP* gene and schizotypal personality traits. Using a Japanese sample assessed with a translated version of the Schizotypal Personality Questionnaire (SPQ; Raine, 1991), they found a significant association between the risk A/A genotype and the SPQ interpersonal factor scale score. The *p250GAP* gene is involved in N-methyl-d-aspartate (NMDA) receptor glutamate transmission or signaling, suggesting a role for NMDA in the pathogenesis of schizophrenia and schizotypal personality traits. Other genes implicated in schizotypal PD include catechol-O-methyltransferase (*COMT*), particularly the val to met substitution at codon 158 (Avramopoulos et al., 2002; Schürhoff et al., 2007; Stefanis et al., 2004), neuregulin 1 (*NRG1*; Lin et al., 2005), dystrobrevin-binding protein 1 (*DTNBP1*; Kircher et al., 2009), and the Zinc Finger Protein 804A (*ZNF804A*; Yasuda et al., 2011). In one of the few studies to extend beyond the schizotypal phenotype, Rosmond et al. (2001) examined genetic associations with men assessed for nine of the *DSM–IV* PDs (all but antisocial) and found that a polymorphism in exon 6 of the dopamine 2 receptor gene (*DRD2*) was significantly associated with Cluster A PDs.

Cluster B

The majority of research on the Cluster B PDs has focused on ASPD and BPD. Studies examining all Cluster B PDs are more rare. One research group compared healthy controls and a PD patient group diagnosed with structured interviews and found that Cluster B PDs were related to a *TPH2* polymorphism (Gutknecht et al., 2007) and *MAOA* (Jacob et al., 2005).

There is a deep and growing research literature on the genetics of antisocial, aggressive, violent, and psychopathic behavior, broadly defined (Gunter, Vaughn, & Philibert, 2010). There are large differences in the specific phenotype examined among these studies, but in general it appears that polymorphisms related to *MAOA* and *5-HTTLPR* are most important for antisocial spectrum disorders (Gunter et al., 2010). Far fewer studies have examined ASPD specifically as the phenotype. In one exception, the serotonin-transporter-linked polymorphic region and the serotonin transporter *VNTR* (Garcia, Aluja, Fibla, Cuevas, & Garcia, 2010) were associated with ASPD. Instead, much of this work seems to focus on antisocial behavior in the context of comorbid substance dependence. For example, Li et al. (2012) found in a sample of individuals with substance dependence that ASPD was associated with a SNP in the collagen XXV alpha 1 gene (*COL25A1*), which codes for the collagen-like Alzheimer amyloid plaque component precursor.

One large GWAS of adult antisocial behavior was conducted with data from 4,816 individuals who completed either a self-report questionnaire or a diagnostic assessment (Tielbeek et al., 2012). Results demonstrated no significant associations between any polymorphisms and antisocial behavior; the top 50 SNP markers explained only 1% of the variance in antisocial behavior. Further, there were no significant associations with traditional candidate genes previously found to be associated with antisocial phenotypes (e.g., *5-HTTLPR, COMT, MAOA*), although it is possible that heterogeneity of the samples used or assessment method variance may have contributed to the null findings.

Many serotonin-related genes have been studied in relation to BPD, including tryptophan hydroxylase 1 (*TPH1*; Wilson et al., 2009), *5-HTTLPR* (Lyons-Ruth et al., 2007; Maurex, Zaboli, Ohhman, Asberg, & Leopardi, 2010), and several polymorphisms within the serotonin transporter gene (including *5-HTTLPR* and the *VNTR* in intron 2; Ni, Chan, et al., 2006). Almost all have shown significant associations with BPD, but several studies have reported null findings (Tadic et al., 2008, 2009). One study also failed to replicate the findings of Ni et al. (Pascual et al., 2008). In a later study, Ni, Chan, Chan, McMain, and Kennedy (2009) genotyped 27 SNPs across seven serotonin genes (*5-HT1A, 5-HT1B, 5-HT1D, 5-HT2C, 5-HT3A, TPH1, TPH2*), finding significant associations between BPD and two of the genes (*5-HT2C, TPH2*) as well as significant interactions between genes (e.g., between *5-HT2C* and *TPH2*). In another study, the same research group found no significant association between the serotonin 2A receptor gene (*HTR2A*) and BPD, although certain normal personality traits (e.g., extraversion) did demonstrate significant associations with genetic markers for the gene (Ni, Bismil, et al., 2006). Other studies have found significant associations between BPD and MAOA (Ni et al., 2007) and the dopamine transporter gene *DAT1* (Joyce et al., 2006). A later study failed to replicate an association with *DAT1* but did find significant associations with *DRD2* and *DRD4* polymorphisms (Nemoda et al., 2010).

Cluster C

One study examined the association between the serotonin transporter gene and all *DSM–IV* PDs in a community sample (Blom et al., 2011). The short allele of the *5-HTTLPR* polymorphism, which is known to be associated with more maladaptive outcomes, was significantly associated with avoidant PD. Interesting gender differences emerged with regard to OCPD, with the risk allele decreasing susceptibility in men and increasing susceptibility in women. In a sample of depressed patients, researchers found that polymorphisms of the *DRD4* receptor were associated with avoidant PD and OCPD and a *DRD3* polymorphism was significantly associated with OCPD; of note, there were no significant associations were personality traits from the Temperament and Character Inventory (Joyce et al., 2003). A later study with two independent samples failed to support the association of *DRD3* with OCPD, but a meta-analysis (using all three samples) concluded that individuals with the risk genotype were 2.4 times more likely to meet diagnosis of OCPD (Light et al., 2006). Light et al. (2006) acknowledged that the mechanism of action of this gene on OCPD behavior is unknown, but, on the basis of animal studies, they suggested a role for the receptor on locomotor inhibition.

Summary

Research on the molecular genetics of PDs is growing, but this work is certainly still in its infancy. Most studies to date have relied on candidate gene analysis, and GWAS has rarely been used (e.g., antisocial). This is likely due to the fact that GWAS requires very large sample sizes, and few studies of large samples have included PD assessment. Further, there is relatively little research on certain disorders (e.g., schizoid, paranoid, narcissistic). Studies conducted to date have other limitations. They are often restricted to small samples, male samples (e.g., Lin et al., 2005), Caucasian samples (e.g., Blom et al., 2011), or patient samples (e.g., Joyce et al., 2003). Future work in this area may wish to focus on expanding the number of PDs studied, collecting larger and more diverse samples, and using multiple informant sources for PD assessment.

Normal Personality

The modern era of personality molecular genetics began in 1996 with the publication of two articles simultaneously in *Nature Genetics:* one (Ebstein et al., 1996) showing an association between the dopamine receptor gene *DRD4* variable number tandem repeat and the personality trait of novelty seeking (from Cloninger's Tridimensional Personality Questionnaire; Cloninger, Svrakic, & Przybeck, 1993) and one (Benjamin et al., 1996) showing an association between the same polymorphism and novelty seeking estimated from scores on the NEO-PI–R (Costa & McCrae, 1992). Shortly thereafter, a third study reported an association between the *VNTR* polymorphism in the serotonin transporter promoter region and NEO-PI–R neuroticism (Lesch et al., 1996).

Since then, the story has been a generally gloomy and pessimistic one, with many failures to find any significant associations and replication attempts for those that are found generally unsuccessful. To date, the best evidence for significant relationships between a gene and a measured personality trait exists for (a) serotonin-related genes (e.g., the serotonin transporter polymorphism) and neuroticism, and (b) dopamine genes (e.g., *DRD4*) and novelty seeking (see Ebstein & Israel, 2009).The largely null results found for normal personality traits have implications for PDs. As noted above, there is a large push among PD researchers to conceptualize pathological personality as extreme variants of normal personality traits (e.g., the FFM domains; Widiger & Mullins-Sweatt, 2009). The failure to find replicable, significant genetic effects for normal personality would suggest that defining PDs by using normal personality trait domains will not make gene hunting for PDs any easier.

Two recent genome-wide searches of the FFM domains illustrate the complexity of finding genes for personality. In one study, the authors conducted an extensive and comprehensive GWAS of the FFM domains (de Moor et al., 2012). The researchers used data on approximately 2.4 million SNPs from 17,375 adults for the discovery samples and 3,294 adults for the replication studies. All adults were of European ancestry and had completed the NEO-FFI. Results indicated that Openness was associated with two SNPs on chromosome *5q14.3*, implicating the *RASA1* gene which is involved in cellular proliferation and differentiation and intracellular signaling; further, Conscientiousness was associated with a SNP on chromosome *18q21.1* in the intron region of the *KATNAL2* gene, which may play a role in neurodevelopment. These associations were not significant in the replication samples. de Moor et al. (2012) concluded that the SNPs that contribute to variation in human personality may be even smaller than the ones found here, which explained about .2% of personality variation.

In the second study, Amin et al. (2012) conducted a genome-wide linkage analysis in a family-based study. All participants completed the NEO-FFI, which was used to create cases (> 90th percentile of the distribution for each quantitative trait) and controls. Amin et al. found numerous significant associations between FFM personality traits and genetic markers, unlike in the FFM GWAS described above. They concluded, in contrast to studies that assume many genes of small effect size, that there may be rare genes that have large effects on normal personality.

Gene × Environment Interaction, Epigenetics, and Endophenotypes

One of the most exciting developments in molecular psychiatry occurred just over a decade ago, when Caspi and colleagues published a series of papers examining gene × environment interaction, or the idea that certain environments moderate the expression of "risky" genes on the phenotype of interest (Caspi et al., 2002, 2003, 2005). Most relevant to personality pathology, they examined the likelihood of antisocial behavior as a function of childhood maltreatment before age 12 and presence of the "low activity" risk allele for the MAOA gene (Caspi et al., 2002). There was no main effect of MAOA on the composite index of antisocial behavior; however, men with the high-activity MAOA allele who had experienced maltreatment were much less likely to display aggressive and antisocial behavior as adults than were individuals with the low activity MAOA gene. Since this original publication, there have been numerous unsuccessful attempts at replication (see Haberstick et al., 2014, for a recent example), although two meta-analyses have supported the original finding (Kim-Cohen et al., 2006; Taylor & Kim-Cohen, 2007).

Research into the molecular genetics of PDs and pathological personality traits is at a relatively young stage, and certainly gene–environment interplay between measured genes and risky environmental contexts should play a part in future research. Most work to date has again focused on only a small set of disorders and risk factors, particularly antisocial or aggressive behavior. Douglas et al. (2011) tested for an interaction between adverse childhood experiences and the serotonin transporter polymorphism on risk for ASPD. They found tentative evidence of an interaction between the 5-HTTLPR risk allele and child maltreatment but only for African-American women, and the sample size for this group was small. Collecting a large enough sample to have the power to detect effects is only one concern for measured gene × environment studies; other areas for concern with future work include collecting diverse samples, thoroughly assessing the phenotype of interest, and ensuring a wide variety of environmental contexts measured at both extremes (see Dick, 2011).

Another possible mechanism that researchers have only begun to examine is the role of *epistatic* processes. In contrast to dominance, which refers to the interaction between alleles at the same locus, epistasis refers to the interaction between genes at different loci. Thus, the expression of one gene on a phenotype will depend on the presence of one or more other genes that modify its expression. Evidence is tentative at best but is beginning to accumulate. For instance, Tadić et al. (2009) found no main effects of the *HTR1B* or the *BDNF* genes on BPD, but they did report preliminary evidence that an interaction between these two genes may increase the risk for BPD. In another study, Cuartas Arias et al. (2011) examined the genetic association and interaction between 10 candidate genes related to serotonin located at 11 different loci in relation to ASPD. Data were obtained from prison inmates assessed for ASPD with a structured interview. Findings demonstrated an interaction between *COMT*, *5-HTR2A*, and tryptophan hydroxylase. Although this work is again preliminary, it suggests that understanding the interactions between different genes may help inform the biological networks underlying personality pathology.

A final issue to consider in understanding the molecular basis of PDs is the possible utility of *endophenotypes*. As detailed elsewhere (Gottesman & Gould, 2003; Walters & Owen, 2007), endophenotypes are constructs that exist at a more basic level than the phenotype of interest. They are biochemical, neuropsychological, cognitive, affective, and neuroanatomical processes that that lie closer on the pathway to disease than the phenotype. By existing at a lower level to the genotype, it is assumed, endophenotypes will aid not only in classifying and conceptualizing of pathology but also in understanding the genetic basis for a disorder. Endophenotypes are also assumed to be heritable, to occur more frequently in affected individuals and family members of probands, and to be present in an individual regardless of whether she or he is demonstrating signs of the disorder.

Endophenotypes are discussed quite often in regard to psychiatric disorders. Indeed, endophenotypes play a prominent role in the National Institute of Mental Health's new Research Domain Criteria (RDoC) initiative (Sanislow et al., 2010). Some have suggested that PDs may serve as endophenotypes (e.g., depressive PD; see Huprich, 2012); indeed, much of the molecular genetic research on schizotypy views it as an endophenotype for schizophrenia. Others suggest research should focus more strongly on examining endophenotypes for PDs, as the PDs are chronic and enduring difficulties that may be particularly appropriate for this approach (Siever, 2005). One suggested tactic may be to start with the dimensional trait structure underlying PDs as a basis for identifying more low-level physiological, biological, neurological, or anatomical markers. Others, however, are more pessimistic that the highly complex pathways leading to PDs can be reduced to tractable endophenotypes (Paris, 2011).

As reviewed elsewhere, most research to date on possible endophenotypes for PDs has focused on only a few disorders (antisocial, borderline, schizotypal) and a few potential markers (Paris, 2011; Siever, 2005). Whether this work can be successful in finding endophenotypes that have stronger and more consistent associations with gene variants than the PD constructs remains to be seen. In one example, Stefanis et al. (2008) attempted to find associations between SNPs in the G-protein signaling 4 (*RGS4*) gene and endophenotypic markers for schizotypy; although there were associations between the SNPs and self-reported schizotypy, effects for endophenotypes were largely nonsignificant.

SUMMARY

In this chapter, I have provided an overview of current behavior and molecular genetics techniques and findings from the study of pathological personality and PDs. It is known, based on work done to date, that the *DSM*-defined PDs are at least moderately heritable. Comorbidity between the PDs can be explained, at least in part, by overlapping genetic influences; etiological influences on these disorders also appear to overlap with influences on other types of common mental disorders and with normal personality traits. There are many rich avenues for future research on the behavior genetics of pathological personality, particularly as *DSM–5* includes both the categorical PD diagnoses (carried over from *DSM–IV*) and a trait dimensional system as an area for future study (American Psychiatric Association, 2013). There are many proponents for the trait dimensional conceptualization of personality pathology who believe this system would better capture how nature is truly structured (e.g., Widiger, 2011); others would argue that PDs are complex entities that perhaps should not be reduced to a trait system (Wakefield, 2008). Behavior and molecular genetic research will be informative as this debate continues.

REFERENCES

American Psychiatric Association. (2000). *Diagnostic and statistical manual of mental disorders* (4th ed., text rev.). Washington, DC: Author.

American Psychiatric Association. (2013). *Diagnostic and statistical manual of mental disorders* (5th ed.). Arlington, VA: Author.

Amin, N., Schuur, M., Gusareva, E. S., Isaacs, A., Aulchenko, Y. S., Kirichenko, A. V., . . . van Duijn, C. M. (2012). A genome-wide linkage study of individuals with high scores on NEO personality traits. *Molecular Psychiatry, 17,* 1031–1041. doi:10.1038/mp.2011.97

Asarnow, R. F., Nuechterlein, K. H., Fogelson, D., Subotnik, K. L., Payne, D. A., Russell, A. T., . . . Kendler, K. A. (2001). Schizophrenia and schizophrenia-spectrum personality disorders in the first-degree relatives of children with schizophrenia: The UCLA Family Study. *Archives of General Psychiatry, 58,* 581–588. doi:10.1001/archpsyc.58.6.581

Avramopoulos, D., Stefanis, N. C., Hantoumi, I., Smyrnis, N., Evdokimidis, I., & Stefanis, C. N. (2002). Higher scores of self-reported schizotypy in healthy young males carrying the COMT high activity allele. *Molecular Psychiatry, 7,* 706–711. doi:10.1038/sj.mp.4001070

Benjamin, J., Greenberg, B., Murphy, D. L., Lin, L., Patterson, C., & Hamer, D. H. (1996). Population and familial association between the D4 dopamine receptor gene and measures of novelty seeking. *Nature Genetics, 12,* 81–84. doi:10.1038/ng0196-81

Bergeman, C. S., Chlpuer, H. M., Plomin, R., Pedersen, N. L., McClearn, G. E., Nesselroade, J. R., . . . McCrae, R. R. (1993). Genetic and environmental effects on openness to experience, agreeableness, and conscientiousness: An adoption/twin study. *Journal of Personality, 61,* 159–179. doi:10.1111/j.1467-6494.1993.tb01030.x

Bleidorn, W., Kandler, C., Riemann, R., Angleitner, A., & Spinath, F. M. (2009). Patterns and sources of adult personality development: Grown curve analyses of the NEO-PI–R scales in a longitudinal twin study. *Journal of Personality and Social Psychology, 97,* 142–155. doi:10.1037/a0015434

Blom, R. M., Samuels, J. F., Riddle, M. A., Bienvenu, O. J., Grados, M. A., Reti, I. M., . . . Nestadt, G. (2011). Association between a serotonin transporter polymorphism (5-HTTLPR) and personality disorder traits in a community sample. *Journal of Psychiatric Research, 45,* 1153–1159. doi:10.1016/j.jpsychires.2011.03.003

Blonigen, D. M., Carlson, M. D., Hicks, B. M., Krueger, R. F., & Iacono, W. G. (2008). Stability and change in personality traits from late adolescence to early adulthood: A longitudinal twin study. *Journal of Personality, 76,* 229–266. doi:10.1111/j.1467-6494.2007.00485.x

Bouchard, T. J., Jr., & Loehlin, J. C. (2001). Genes, evolution, and personality. *Behavior Genetics, 31,* 243–273. doi:10.1023/A:1012294324713

Cadoret, R. J., Yates, W., Troughton, E., Woodworth, G., & Stewart, M. A. (1995). Genetic–environmental interaction in the genesis of aggressivity and conduct disorders. *Archives of General Psychiatry, 52,* 916–924. doi:10.1001/archpsyc.1995.03950230030006

Caspi, A., McClay, J., Moffitt, T., Mill, J., Martin, J., Craig, I. W., . . . Poulton, R. (2002). Role of genotype in the cycle of violence in maltreated children. *Science, 297,* 851–854. doi:10.1126/science.1072290

Caspi, A., Moffitt, T. E., Cannon, M., McClay, J., Murray, R., Harrington, H., . . . Craig, I. W. (2005). Moderation of the effect of adolescent-onset cannabis use on adult psychosis by a functional polymorphism in the catechol-O-methyltransferase gene: Longitudinal evidence of a gene × environment interaction. *Biological Psychiatry, 57,* 1117–1127. doi:10.1016/j.biopsych.2005.01.026

Caspi, A., Sugden, K., Moffitt, T. E., Taylor, A., Craig, I. W., Harrington, H., . . . Poulton, R. (2003). Influence of life stress on depression: Moderation by a polymorphism in the 5-HTT gene. *Science, 301*, 386–389. doi:10.1126/science.1083968

Clark, L. A. (2005). Stability and change in personality pathology: Revelations of three longitudinal studies. *Journal of Personality Disorders, 19*, 524–532. doi:10.1521/pedi.2005.19.5.524

Cloninger, C. R., Svrakic, D. M., & Przybeck, T. R. (1993). A psychobiological model of temperament and character. *Archives of General Psychiatry, 50*, 975–990. doi:10.1001/archpsyc.1993.01820240059008

Coolidge, F. L., Thede, L. L., & Jang, K. L. (2001). Heritability of personality disorders in childhood: A preliminary investigation. *Journal of Personality Disorders, 15*, 33–40. doi:10.1521/pedi.15.1.33.18645

Costa, P. T., Jr., & McCrae, R. R. (1992). *Revised NEO Personality Inventory (NEO-PI–R) and NEO Five-Factor Inventory (NEO-FFI) professional manual.* Odessa, FL: Psychological Assessment Resources.

Cuartas Arias, J. M., Palacio Acosta, C. A., Valencia, J. G., Montoya, G. J., Arango Viana, J. C., Nieto, O. C., . . . Ruiz-Linares, A. (2011). Exploring epistasis in candidate genes for antisocial personality disorder. *Psychiatric Genetics, 21*, 115–124. doi:10.1097/YPG.0b013e3283437175

de Moor, M. H. M., Costa, P. T., Terracciano, A., Krueger, R. F., de Geus, E. J. C., Toshiko, T., . . . Boomsma, D. I. (2012). Meta-analysis of genome-wide association studies for personality. *Molecular Psychiatry, 17*, 337–349. doi:10.1038/mp.2010.128

Dick, D. M. (2011). Gene–environment interaction in psychological traits and disorders. *Annual Review of Clinical Psychology, 7*, 383–409. doi:10.1146/annurev-clinpsy-032210-104518

Distel, M. A., Willemsen, G., Ligthart, L., Derom, C. A., Martin, N. G., Neale, M. C., . . . Boomsma, D. I. (2010). Genetic covariance structure of the four main features of borderline personality disorder. *Journal of Personality Disorders, 24*, 427–444. doi:10.1521/pedi.2010.24.4.427

Dolan-Sewell, R. T., Krueger, R. F., & Shea, M. T. (2001). Co-occurrence with syndrome disorders. In W. J. Livesley (Ed.), *Handbook of personality disorders: Theory, research, and treatment* (pp. 84–104). New York, NY: Guilford Press.

Douglas, K., Chan, G., Gelernter, J., Arias, A. J., Anton, R. F., Poling, J., . . . Kranzler, H. R. (2011). 5-HTTLPR as a potential moderator of the effects of adverse childhood experiences on risk of antisocial personality disorder. *Psychiatric Genetics, 21*, 240–248. doi:10.1097/YPG.0b013e3283457c15

Eaton, N. R., Krueger, R. F., South, S. C., Simms, L. J., & Clark, L. A. (2011). Contrasting prototypes and dimensions in the classification of personality pathology: Evidence that dimensions, but not prototypes, are robust. *Psychological Medicine, 41*, 1151–1163. doi:10.1017/S0033291710001650

Ebstein, R. P., & Israel, S. (2009). Molecular genetics of personality: How our genes can bring us to a better understanding of why we act the way we do. In Y.-K. Kim (Ed.), *Handbook of behavior genetics* (pp. 239–250). New York, NY: Springer.

Ebstein, R. P., Novick, O., Umansky, R., Priel, B., Osher, Y., Blaine, D., . . . Belmaker, R. H. (1996). Dopamine D4 receptor (D4DR) exon III polymorphism associated with the human personality trait of novelty seeking. *Nature Genetics, 12*, 78–80. doi:10.1038/ng0196-78

Eysenck, H. J. (1991). Dimensions of personality: 16, 5, or 3? Criteria for a taxonomic paradigm. *Personality and Individual Differences, 12*, 773–790. doi:10.1016/0191-8869(91)90144-Z

Eysenck, H. J., & Eysenck, S. B. G. (1975). *Manual of the Eysenck Personality Questionnaire*. San Diego, CA: Educational and Industrial Testing Service.

Falconer, D. S. (1965). The inheritance of liability to certain diseases, estimated from the incidence among relatives. *Annals of Human Genetics, 29*, 51–76. doi:10.1111/j.1469-1809.1965.tb00500.x

Fanous, A. H., Neale, M. C., Gardner, C. O., Webb, B. T., Straub, R. E., O'Neill, F. A., . . . Kendler, K. S. (2007). Significant correlation in linkage signals from genome-wide scans of schizophrenia and schizotypy. *Molecular Psychiatry, 12*, 958–965. doi:10.1038/sj.mp.4001996

Ferguson, C. J. (2010). Genetic contributions to antisocial personality and behavior: A meta-analytic review from an evolutionary perspective. *Journal of Social Psychology, 150*, 160–180. doi:10.1080/00224540903366503

Finkel, D., & McGue, M. (1997). Sex differences and nonadditivity in the heritability of the Multidimensional Personality Questionnaire scales. *Journal of Personality and Social Psychology, 72*, 929–938. doi:10.1037/0022-3514.72.4.929

Garcia, L. F., Aluja, A., Fibla, J., Cuevas, L., & Garcia, O. (2010). Incremental effect for antisocial personality disorder genetic risk combining 5-HTTLPR and 5-HTTVNTR polymorphisms. *Psychiatry Research, 177*, 161–166. doi:10.1016/j.psychres.2008.12.018

Gottesman, I. I., & Gould, T. D. (2003). The endophenotype concept in psychiatry: Etymology and strategic intentions. *The American Journal of Psychiatry, 160*, 636–645. doi:10.1176/appi.ajp.160.4.636

Gottesman, I. I., & Shields, J. (1967). A polygenic theory of schizophrenia. *Proceedings of the National Academy of Sciences, USA, 58*, 199–205. doi:10.1073/pnas.58.1.199

Gunter, T. D., Vaughn, M. G., & Philibert, R. A. (2010). Behavioral genetics in antisocial spectrum disorders and psychopathy: A review of the recent literature. *Behavioral Sciences & the Law, 28*, 148–173. doi:10.1002/bsl.923

Gutknecht, L., Jacob, C., Strobel, A., Kriegebaum, C., Müller, J., Zeng, Y., . . . Lesch, K.-P. (2007). Tryptophan hydroxylase-2 gene variation influences personality traits and disorders related to emotional dysregulation. *International Journal of Neuropsychopharmacology, 10*, 309–320. doi:10.1017/S1461145706007437

Haberstick, B. C., Lessem, J. M., Hewitt, J. K., Smolen, A., Hopfer, C. J., Halpern, C. T., . . . Mullan Harris, K. (2014). MAOA genotype, childhood maltreatment, and their interaction in the etiology of adult antisocial behaviors. *Biological Psychiatry, 75,* 25–30. doi:10.1016/j.biopsych.2013.03.028

Hicks, B. M., Krueger, R. F., Iacono, W. G., McGue, M., & Patrick, C. J. (2004). Family transmission and heritability of externalizing disorders: A twin-family study. *Archives of General Psychiatry, 61,* 922–928. doi:10.1001/archpsyc.61.9.922

Hopwood, C. J., Donnellan, M. B., Blonigen, D. M., Krueger, R. F., McGue, M., Iacono, W. G., . . . Burt, S. A. (2011). Genetic and environmental influences on personality trait stability and growth during the transition to adulthood: A three-wave longitudinal study. *Journal of Personality and Social Psychology, 100,* 545–556. doi:10.1037/a0022409

Huprich, S. K. (2012). Considering the evidence and making the most empirically informed decision about depressive personality disorder in *DSM–5. Personality Disorders: Theory, Research, and Treatment, 3,* 470–482. doi:10.1037/a0027765

Jacob, C. P., Müller, J., Schmidt, M., Hohenberger, K., Gutknecht, L., Reif, A., . . . Lesch, K. P. (2005). Cluster B personality disorders are associated with allelic variation of monoamine oxidase A activity. *Neuropsychopharmacology, 30,* 1711–1718. doi:10.1038/sj.npp.1300737

Jang, K. L., & Livesley, W. J. (1999). Why do measures of normal and disordered personality correlate? A study of genetic comorbidity. *Journal of Personality Disorders, 13,* 10–17. doi:10.1521/pedi.1999.13.1.10

Jang, K. L., Livesley, W. J., Angleitner, A., Riemann, R., & Vernon, P. A. (2002). Genetic and environmental influences on the covariance of facets defining the domains of the five-factor model of personality. *Personality and Individual Differences, 33,* 83–101. doi:10.1016/S0191-8869(01)00137-4

Jang, K. L., Livesley, W. J., & Vernon, P. A. (1996). Heritability of the Big Five personality dimensions and their facets: A twin study. *Journal of Personality, 64,* 577–592. doi:10.1111/j.1467-6494.1996.tb00522.x

Jang, K. L., Livesley, W. J., Vernon, P. A., & Jackson, D. N. (1996). Heritability of personality disorder traits: A twin study. *Acta Psychiatrica Scandinavica, 94,* 438–444. doi:10.1111/j.1600-0447.1996.tb09887.x

Jang, K. L., McCrae, R. R., Angleitner, A., Riemann, R., & Livesley, W. J. (1998). Heritability of facet-level traits in a cross-cultural twin study: Support for a hierarchical model of personality. *Journal of Personality and Social Psychology, 74,* 1556–1565. doi:10.1037/0022-3514.74.6.1556

John, O. P., Naumann, L. P., & Soto, C. J. (2008). Paradigm shift to the integrative Big Five trait taxonomy: History, measurement, and conceptual issues. In O. P. John, R. W. Robins, & L. A. Pervin (Eds.), *Handbook of personality: Theory and research* (pp. 114–158). New York, NY: Guilford Press.

Johnson, W., & Krueger, R. F. (2004). Genetic and environmental structure of adjectives describing the domains of the Big Five model of personality: A nationwide

U.S. twin study. *Journal of Research in Personality, 38*, 448–472. doi:10.1016/j.jrp.2003.11.001

Joyce, P. R., McHugh, P. C., McKenzie, J. M., Sullivan, P. F., Mulder, R. T., Luty, S. E., . . . Kennedy, M. A. (2006). A dopamine transporter polymorphism is a risk factor for borderline personality disorder in depressed patients. *Psychological Medicine, 36*, 807–813. doi:10.1017/S0033291706007288

Joyce, P. R., Rogers, G. R., Miller, A. L., Mulder, R. T., Luty, S. E., & Kennedy, M. A. (2003). Polymorphisms of DRD4 and DRD3 and risk of avoidant and obsessive personality traits and disorders. *Psychiatry Research, 119*, 1–10. doi:10.1016/S0165-1781(03)00124-0

Keller, M. C., Coventry, W. L., Heath, A. C., & Martin, N. G. (2005). Widespread evidence for non-additive genetic variation in Cloninger's and Eysenck's personality dimensions using a twin plus sibling design. *Behavior Genetics, 35*, 707–721. doi:10.1007/s10519-005-6041-7

Kendler, K. S., Aggen, S. H., Czajkowski, N., Røysamb, E., Tambs, K., Torgersen, S., . . . Reichborn-Kjennerud, T. (2008). The structure of genetic and environmental risk factors for *DSM–IV* personality disorders. *Archives of General Psychiatry, 65*, 1438–1446. doi:10.1001/archpsyc.65.12.1438

Kendler, K. S., Aggen, S. H., Knudsen, G. P., Roysamb, E., Neale, M. C., & Reichborn-Kjennerud, T. (2011). The structure of genetic and environmental risk factors for syndromal and subsyndromal common *DSM–IV* Axis I and all Axis II disorders. *The American Journal of Psychiatry, 168*, 29–39. doi:10.1176/appi.ajp.2010.10030340

Kendler, K. S., Czajkowski, N., Tambs, K., Torgersen, S., Aggen, S. H., Neal, M. S., . . . Reichborn-Kjennerud, T. (2006). Dimensional representation of *DSM–IV* Cluster A personality disorders in a population-based sample of Norwegian twins: A multivariate study. *Psychological Medicine, 36*, 1583–1591. doi:10.1017/S0033291706008609

Kendler, K. S., McGuire, M., Gruenberg, A. M., O'Hare, A., Spellman, M., & Walsh, D. (1993). The Roscommon Family Study: III. Schizophrenia-related personality disorders in relatives. *Archives of General Psychiatry, 50*, 781–788. doi:10.1001/archpsyc.1993.01820220033004

Kendler, K. S., Myers, J., Torgersen, S., Neale, M. C., & Reichborn-Kjennerud, T. (2007). The heritability of Cluster A personality disorders assessed by both personal interview and questionnaire. *Psychological Medicine, 37*, 655–665. doi:10.1017/S0033291706009755

Kim-Cohen, J., Caspi, A., Taylor, A., Williams, B., Newcombe, R., Craig, I. W., & Moffitt, T. E. (2006). MAOA, maltreatment, and gene–environment interaction predicting children's mental health: New evidence and a meta-analysis. *Molecular Psychiatry, 11*, 903–913. doi:10.1038/sj.mp.4001851

Kircher, T., Markov, V., Krug, A., Eggermann, T., Zerres, K., Nöthen, M. M., . . . Rietschel, M. (2009). Association of the DTNBP1 genotype with cognition and personality traits in healthy subjects. *Psychological Medicine, 39*, 1657–1665. doi:10.1017/S0033291709005388

Kotov, R., Ruggero, C. J., Krueger, R. F., Watson, D., Yuan, Q., & Zimmerman, M. (2011). New dimensions in the quantitative classification of mental illness. *Archives of General Psychiatry, 68,* 1003–1011. doi:10.1001/archgenpsychiatry.2011.107

Krueger, R. F. (2005). Continuity of Axis I and Axis II: Toward a unified theory of personality, personality disorders, and clinical disorders. *Journal of Personality Disorders, 19,* 233–261. doi:10.1521/pedi.2005.19.3.233

Krueger, R. F., Derringer, J., Markon, K. E., Watson, D., & Skodol, A. E. (2012). Initial construction of a maladaptive personality trait model and inventory for *DSM–5*. *Psychological Medicine, 42,* 1879–1890. doi:10.1017/S0033291711002674

Krueger, R. F., Hicks, B. M., Patrick, C. J., Carlson, S. R., Iacono, W. G., & McGue, M. (2002). Etiologic connections among substance dependence, antisocial behavior, and personality: Modeling the externalizing spectrum. *Journal of Abnormal Psychology, 111,* 411–424. doi:10.1037/0021-843X.111.3.411

Krueger, R. F., & Markon, K. (2006). Reinterpreting comorbidity: A model-based approach to understanding and classifying psychopathology. *Annual Review of Clinical Psychology, 2,* 111–133. doi:10.1146/annurev.clinpsy.2.022305.095213

Krueger, R. F., Skodol, A. E., Livesley, W. J., Shrout, P. E., & Huang, Y. (2007). Synthesizing dimensional and categorical approaches to personality disorders: Refining the research agenda for *DSM–V* Axis II. *International Journal of Methods in Psychiatric Research, 16,* S65–S73. doi:10.1002/mpr.212

Krueger, R. F., South, S. C., Johnson, W., & Iacono, W. (2008). The heritability of personality is not always 50%: Gene–environment interactions and correlations between personality and parenting. *Journal of Personality, 76,* 1485–1522. doi:10.1111/j.1467-6494.2008.00529.x

Lesch, K.-P., Bengel, D., Heils, A., Sabol, S. Z., Greenberg, B. D., Petri, S., . . . Murphy, D. L. (1996). Association of anxiety-related traits with a polymorphism in the serotonin transporter gene regulatory region. *Science, 274,* 1527–1531. doi:10.1126/science.274.5292.1527

Levy, F., Hay, D. A., McStephen, M., Wood, C., & Waldman, I. D. (1997). Attention-deficit hyperactivity disorder: A category or continuum? Genetic analysis of a large-scale twin study. *Journal of the American Academy of Child & Adolescent Psychiatry, 36,* 737–744. doi:10.1097/00004583-199706000-00009

Li, D., Zhao, H., Kranzler, H. R., Oslin, D., Anton, R. F., Farrer, L. A., & Gelernter, J. (2012). Association of *COL25A1* with comorbid antisocial personality disorder and substance dependence. *Biological Psychiatry, 71,* 733–740. doi:10.1016/j.biopsych.2011.12.011

Light, K. J., Joyce, P. R., Luty, S. E., Mulder, R. T., Frampton, C. M. A., Joyce, L. R. M., . . . Kennedy, M. A. (2006). Preliminary evidence for an association between a dopamine D3 receptor gene variant and obsessive-compulsive personality disorder in patients with major depression. *American Journal of Medical Genetics, Part B: Neuropsychiatric Genetics, 141,* 409–413. doi:10.1002/ajmg.b.30308

Lin, H.-F., Liu, Y.-L., Liu, C.-M., Hung, S.-I., Hwu, H.-G., & Chen, W. J. (2005). Neuregulin 1 gene and variations in perceptual aberration of schizotypal personality in adolescents. *Psychological Medicine, 35*, 1589–1598. doi:10.1017/S0033291705005957

Livesley, W. J., & Jackson, D. N. (2001). *Manual for the Dimensional Assessment of Personality Pathology—Basic Questionnaire.* Port Huron, MI: Sigma Press.

Livesley, W. J., & Jang, K. L. (2008). The behavioral genetics of personality disorder. *Annual Review of Clinical Psychology, 4*, 247–274. doi:10.1146/annurev.clinpsy.4.022007.141203

Livesley, W. J., Jang, K. L., Jackson, D. N., & Vernon, P. A. (1993). Genetic and environmental contributions to dimensions of personality disorder. *The American Journal of Psychiatry, 150*, 1826–1831.

Loranger, A. W., Oldham, J. M., & Tulis, E. H. (1982). Familial transmission of *DSM–III* borderline personality disorder. *Archives of General Psychiatry, 39*, 795–799. doi:10.1001/archpsyc.1982.04290070031007

Lyons-Ruth, K., Holmes, B. M., Sasvari-Szekely, M., Ronai, Z., Nemoda, Z., & Pauls, D. (2007). Serotonin transporter polymorphism and borderline or antisocial traits among low-income young adults. *Psychiatric Genetics, 17*, 339–343. doi:10.1097/YPG.0b013e3281ac237e

Manolio, T. A., Collins, F. S., Cox, N. J., Goldstein, B., Hindroff, L. A., Hunter, D. J., . . . Visscher, P. M. (2009, October 8). Finding the missing heritability of complex diseases. *Nature, 461*, 747–753. doi:10.1038/nature08494

Markon, K. E., Krueger, R. F., & Watson, D. (2005). Delineating the structure of normal and abnormal personality: An integrative hierarchical approach. *Journal of Personality and Social Psychology, 88*, 139–157. doi:10.1037/0022-3514.88.1.139

Martin, N. G., Eaves, L. J., Kearsey, M. J., & Davies, P. T. (1978). The power of the classical twin study. *Heredity, 40*, 97–116. doi:10.1038/hdy.1978.10

Maurex, L., Zaboli, G., Ohhman, A., Asberg, M., & Leopardi, R. (2010). The serotonin transporter gene polymorphism (5-HTTLPR) and affective symptoms among women diagnosed with borderline personality disorder. *European Psychiatry, 25*, 19–25. doi:10.1016/j.eurpsy.2009.05.001

McGue, M., Bacon, S., & Lykken, D. T. (1993). Personality stability and change in early adulthood: A behavioral genetic analysis. *Developmental Psychology, 29*, 96–109. doi:10.1037/0012-1649.29.1.96

Miles, D. R., & Carey, G. (1997). Genetic and environmental architecture on human aggression. *Journal of Personality and Social Psychology, 72*, 207–217. doi:10.1037/0022-3514.72.1.207

Morey, L. C. (1991). *The Personality Assessment Inventory: Professional manual.* Odessa, FL: Psychological Assessment Resources.

Neale, M. C., Boker, S. M., Xie, G., & Maes, H. H. (2003). *Mx: Statistical modeling* (6th ed.). Richmond, VA: Department of Psychiatry, Virginia Commonwealth University.

Nemoda, Z., Lyons-Ruth, K., Szekely, A., Bertha, E., Faludi, G., & Sasvari-Szekely, M. (2010). Association between dopaminergic polymorphisms and borderline personality traits among at-risk young adults and psychiatric inpatients. *Behavioral and Brain Functions*, 6, Article 4. doi:10.1186/1744-9081-6-4

Ni, X., Bismil, R., Chan, K., Sicard, T., Bulgin, N., McMain, S., & Kennedy, J. L. (2006). Serotonin 2A receptor gene is associated with personality traits, but not to disorder, in patients with borderline personality disorder. *Neuroscience Letters*, 408, 214–219. doi:10.1016/j.neulet.2006.09.002

Ni, X., Chan, D., Chan, K., McMain, S., & Kennedy, J. L. (2009). Serotonin genes and gene–gene interactions in borderline personality disorder in a matched case-control study. *Progress in Neuro-Psychopharmacology & Biological Psychiatry*, 33, 128–133. doi:10.1016/j.pnpbp.2008.10.022

Ni, X., Chan, K., Bulgin, N., Sicard, T., Bismil, R., McMain, S., & Kennedy, J. L. (2006). Association between serotonin transporter gene and borderline personality disorder. *Journal of Psychiatric Research*, 40, 448–453. doi:10.1016/j.jpsychires.2006.03.010

Ni, X., Sicard, T., Bulgin, N., Bismil, R., Chan, K., McMain, S., & Kennedy, J. L. (2007). Monoamine oxidase A gene is associated with borderline personality disorder. *Psychiatric Genetics*, 17, 153–157. doi:10.1097/YPG.0b013e328016831c

Ohi, K., Hashimoto, R., Nakazawa, T., Okada, T., Yasuda, Y., Yamamori, H., . . . Takeda, M. (2012). The *p250GAP* gene is associated with risk for schizophrenia and schizotypal personality traits. *PLoS ONE*, 7(4), e35696. doi:10.1371/journal.pone.0035696

Paris, J. (2011). Endophenotypes and the diagnosis of personality disorders. *Journal of Personality Disorders*, 25, 260–268. doi:10.1521/pedi.2011.25.2.260

Pascual, J. C., Soler, J., Barrachina, J., Campins, M. J., Alvarez, E., Pérez, V., . . . Baiget, M. (2008). Failure to detect an association between the serotonin transporter gene and borderline personality disorder. *Journal of Psychiatric Research*, 42, 87–88. doi:10.1016/j.jpsychires.2006.10.005

Pfohl, B., Blum, N., & Zimmerman, M. (1997). *Structured Interview for DSM–IV Personality (SIDP-IV)*. Washington, DC: American Psychiatric Press.

Plomin, R., Corley, R., Caspi, A., Fulker, D. W., & DeFries, J. C. (1998). Adoption results for self-reported personality: Evidence for nonadditive genetic effects? *Journal of Personality and Social Psychology*, 75, 211–218. doi:10.1037/0022-3514.75.1.211

Purcell, S. (2002). Variance components models for gene–environment interaction in twin analysis. *Twin Research*, 5, 554–571. doi:10.1375/136905202762342026

Raine, A. (1991). The SPQ: A scale for the assessment of schizotypal personality based on *DSM–III–R* criteria. *Schizophrenia Bulletin*, 17, 555–564. doi:10.1093/schbul/17.4.555

Reichborn-Kjennerud, T., Czajkowski, N., Neale, M. S., Ørstavik, R. E., Torgersen, S., Tambs, K., . . . Kendler, K. S. (2007). Genetic and environmental influences on dimensional representations of *DSM–IV* Cluster C personality disorders: A population-based multivariate twin study. *Psychological Medicine, 37,* 645–653. doi:10.1017/S0033291706009548

Reichborn-Kjennerud, T., Czajkowki, N., Røysamb, E., Ørstavik, R. E., Neale, M. C., Torgersen, S., & Kendler, K. S. (2010). Major depression and dimensional representations of *DSM–IV* personality disorders: A population-based twin study. *Psychological Medicine, 40,* 1475–1484. doi:10.1017/S0033291709991954

Reichborn-Kjennerud, T., Czajkowki, N., Torgersen, S., Neale, M. C., Ørstavik, R. E., Tambs, K., & Kendler, K. S. (2007). The relationship between avoidant personality disorder and social phobia: A population-based twin study. *The American Journal of Psychiatry, 164,* 1722–1728. doi:10.1176/appi.ajp.2007.06101764

Rhee, S. H., & Waldman, I. D. (2002). Genetic and environmental influences on antisocial behavior: A meta-analysis of twin and adoption studies. *Psychological Bulletin, 128,* 490–529. doi:10.1037/0033-2909.128.3.490

Riso, L. P., Klein, D. N., Anderson, R. L., & Ouimette, P. C. (2000). A family study of outpatients with borderline personality disorder and no history of mood disorder. *Journal of Personality Disorders, 14,* 208–217. doi:10.1521/pedi.2000.14.3.208

Roberts, B. W., & DelVecchio, W. F. (2000). The rank-order consistency of personality traits from childhood to old age: A quantitative review of longitudinal studies. *Psychological Bulletin, 126,* 3–25. doi:10.1037/0033-2909.126.1.3

Robins, E., & Guze, S. B. (1970). Establishment of diagnostic validity in psychiatric illness: Its application to schizophrenia. *The American Journal of Psychiatry, 126,* 983–987.

Rosmond, R., Rankinen, T., Chagnon, M., Pérusse, L., Chagnon, Y. C., Bouchard, C., & Björntorp, P. (2001). Polymorphism in exon 6 of the dopamine D(2) receptor gene (DRD2) is associated with elevated blood pressure and personality disorders in men. *Journal of Human Hypertension, 15,* 553–558. doi:10.1038/sj.jhh.1001231

Samuel, D. B., & Widiger, T. A. (2008). A meta-analytic review of the relationships between the five-factor model and *DSM–IV–TR* personality disorders: A facet level analysis. *Clinical Psychology Review, 28,* 1326–1342. doi:10.1016/j.cpr.2008.07.002

Sanislow, C. A., Pine, D. S., Quinn, K. J., Kozak, M. J., Garvey, M. A., Heinssen, R. K., . . . Cuthbert, B. N. (2010). Developing constructs for psychopathology research: Research domain criteria. *Journal of Abnormal Psychology, 119,* 631–639. doi:10.1037/a0020909

Schürhoff, F., Szöke, A., Chevalier, F., Roy, I., Méary, A., Bellivier, F., . . . Leboyer, M. (2007). Schizotypal dimensions: An intermediate phenotype associated with the COMT high activity allele. *American Journal of Medical Genetics, Part B: Neuropsychiatric Genetics, 144B,* 64–68. doi:10.1002/ajmg.b.30395

Sham, P., & McGuffin, P. (2002). Linkage and association. In P. McGuffin, M. J. Owen, & I. I. Gottesman (Eds.), *Psychiatric genetics and genomics* (pp. 55–73). Oxford, England: Oxford University Press.

Siever, L. J. (2005). Endophenotypes in the personality disorders. *Dialogues in Clinical Neuroscience, 7*, 139–151.

Skodol, A. E. (2011). Revision of the personality disorder model for *DSM–5*. *The American Journal of Psychiatry, 168*, 97. doi:10.1176/appi.ajp.2010.10101466

Skodol, A. E., Clark, L. A., Bender, D. S., Krueger, R. F., Morey, L. C., Verheul, R., . . . Oldham, J. M. (2011). Proposed changes in personality and personality disorder assessment and diagnosis for *DSM–5* Part I: Description and rationale. *Personality Disorders: Theory, Research, and Treatment, 2*, 4–22. doi:10.1037/a0021891

South, S. C., & DeYoung, N. (2013). Behavior genetics of personality disorders: Informing classification and conceptualization in *DSM–5*. *Personality Disorders: Theory, Research, and Treatment, 4*, 270–283. doi:10.1037/a0026255

South, S. C., & Krueger, R. F. (2008). Marital quality moderates genetic and environmental influences on the internalizing spectrum. *Journal of Abnormal Psychology, 117*, 826–837. doi:10.1037/a0013499

South, S. C., & Krueger, R. F. (2013). Marital satisfaction and physical health: Evidence for an orchid effect. *Psychological Science, 24*, 373–378. doi:10.1177/0956797612453116

South, S. C., Reichborn-Kjennerud, T., Eaton, N. R., & Krueger, R. F. (2012). Behavior and molecular genetics of personality disorders. In T. A. Widiger (Ed.), *The Oxford handbook of personality disorders* (pp. 143–165). New York, NY: Oxford University Press.

Stefanis, N. C., Os, J. V., Avramopoulos, D., Smyrnis, N., Evdokimidis, I., Hantoumi, I., & Stefanis, C. N. (2004). Variation in catechol-o-methyltransferase val158 met genotype associated with schizotypy but not cognition: A population study in 543 young men. *Biological Psychiatry, 56*, 510–515. doi:10.1016/j.biopsych.2004.06.038

Stefanis, N. C., Trikalinos, T. A., Avramopoulos, D., Smyrnis, N., Evdokimidis, I., Ntzani, E. E., . . . Stefanis, C. N. (2008). Association of *RGS4* variants with schizotypy and cognitive endophenotypes at the population level. *Behavioral and Brain Functions, 4*, Article 46. doi:10.1186/1744-9081-4-46

Tadić, A., Baskaya, O., Victor, A., Lieb, K., Höppner, W., & Dahmen, N. (2008). Association analysis of SCN9A gene variants with borderline personality disorder. *Journal of Psychiatric Research, 43*, 155–163. doi:10.1016/j.jpsychires.2008.03.006

Tadić, A., Elsäber, A., Victor, A., von Cube, R., Baakaya, O., Wagner, S., . . . Dahmen, N. (2009). Association analysis of serotonin receptor 1B (HTR1B) and brain-derived neurotrophic factor gene polymorphisms in borderline personality disorder. *Journal of Neural Transmission, 116*, 1185–1188. doi:10.1007/s00702-009-0264-3

Taylor, A., & Kim-Cohen, J. (2007). Meta-analysis of gene–environment interactions in developmental psychopathology. *Development and Psychopathology, 19*, 1029–1037. doi:10.1017/S095457940700051X

Tellegen, A., Lykken, D. T., Bouchard, T. J., Jr., Wilcox, K. J., Segal, N. L., & Rich, S. (1988). Personality similarity in twins reared apart and together. *Journal of Personality and Social Psychology, 54,* 1031–1039. doi:10.1037/0022-3514.54.6.1031

Tellegen, A., & Waller, N. G. (in press). *Exploring personality through test construction: Development of the Multidimensional Personality Questionnaire (MPQ).* Minneapolis: University of Minnesota Press.

Tielbeek, J. J., Medland, S. E., Benyamin, B., Byrne, E. M., Heath, A. C., Madden, P. A. F., . . . Verweij, K. J. H. (2012). Unraveling the genetic etiology of adult antisocial behavior: A genome-wide association study. *PLoS ONE, 7*(10), e45086. doi:10.1371/journal.pone.0045086

Torgersen, S., Czajkowski, N., Jacobson, K., Reichborn-Kjennerud, T., Røysamb, E., Neale, M. S., & Kendler, K. S. (2008). Dimensional representations of *DSM–IV* Cluster B personality disorders in a population-based sample of Norwegian twins: A multivariate study. *Psychological Medicine, 38,* 1617–1625. doi:10.1017/S0033291708002924

Torgersen, S., Lygren, S., Øien, P. A., Skre, I., Onstad, S., Edvardsen, J., . . . Kringlen, E. (2000). A twin study of personality disorders. *Comprehensive Psychiatry, 41,* 416–425. doi:10.1053/comp.2000.16560

Turkheimer, E. (2000). Three laws of behavior genetics and what they mean. *Current Directions in Psychological Science, 9,* 160–164. doi:10.1111/1467-8721.00084

Tuvblad, C., Grann, M., & Lichtenstein, P. (2006). Heritability for adolescent antisocial behavior differs with socioeconomic status: Gene–environment interaction. *Journal of Child Psychology and Psychiatry, 47,* 734–743. doi:10.1111/j.1469-7610.2005.01552.x

Wakefield, J. C. (2008). The perils of dimensionalization: Challenges in distinguishing negative traits from personality disorders. *Psychiatric Clinics of North America, 31,* 379–393. doi:10.1016/j.psc.2008.03.009

Walters, J. T. R., & Owen, M. J. (2007). Endophenotypes in psychiatric genetics. *Molecular Psychiatry, 12,* 886–890. doi:10.1038/sj.mp.4002068

Warner, M. B., Morey, L. C., Finch, J. F., Gunderson, J. G., Skodol, A. E., Sanislow, C. A., . . . Grilo, C. M. (2004). The longitudinal relationship of personality traits and disorders. *Journal of Abnormal Psychology, 113,* 217–227. doi:10.1037/0021-843X.113.2.217

Widiger, T. A. (2011). A shaky future for personality disorders. *Personality Disorders: Theory, Research, and Treatment, 2,* 54–67. doi:10.1037/a0021855

Widiger, T. A., & Costa, P. T., Jr. (2002). Five-factor model personality disorder research. In P. T. Costa & T. A. Widiger (Eds.), *Personality disorders and the five-factor model of personality* (2nd ed., pp. 59–87). Washington, DC: American Psychological Association.

Widiger, T. A., & Mullins-Sweatt, S. N. (2009). Five-factor model of personality disorder: A proposal for *DSM–V. Annual Review of Clinical Psychology, 5,* 197–220. doi:10.1146/annurev.clinpsy.032408.153542

Widiger, T. A., & Samuel, D. B. (2005). Diagnostic categories or dimensions? A question for the *Diagnostic and Statistical Manual of Mental Disorders— Fifth Edition. Journal of Abnormal Psychology, 114*, 494–504. doi:10.1037/ 0021-843X.114.4.494

Widiger, T. A., & Simonsen, E. (2005). Alternative dimensional models of personality disorder: Finding a common ground. *Journal of Personality Disorders, 19*, 110–130. doi:10.1521/pedi.19.2.110.62628

Widiger, T. A., & Trull, T. J. (2007). Plate tectonics in the classification of personality disorder: Shifting to a dimensional model. *American Psychologist, 62*, 71–83. doi:10.1037/0003-066X.62.2.71

Wilson, S. T., Stanley, B., Brent, D. A., Oquendo, M. A., Huang, Y., & Mann, J. J. (2009). The tryptophan hydroxylase-1 A218C polymorphism is associated with diagnosis, but not suicidal behavior, in borderline personality disorder. *American Journal of Medical Genetics, Part B: Neuropsychiatric Genetics, 150B*, 202–208. doi:10.1002/ajmg.b.30788

Yamagata, S., Suzuki, A., Ando, J., Ono, Y., Kijima, N., Yoshimura, K., . . . Jang, K. L. (2006). Is the genetic structure of human personality universal? A cross-cultural twin study from North America, Europe, and Asia. *Journal of Personality and Social Psychology, 90*, 987–998. doi:10.1037/0022-3514.90.6.987

Yasuda, Y., Hashimoto, R., Ohi, K., Fukumoto, M., Umeda-Yano, S., Yamamori, H., . . . Takeda, M. (2011). Impact on schizotypal personality trait of a genome-wide supported psychosis variant of the ZNF804A gene. *Neuroscience Letters, 495*, 216–220. doi:10.1016/j.neulet.2011.03.069

Zanarini, M. C., Barison, L. K., Frankenburg, F. R., Reich, B., & Hudson, J. I. (2009). Family history study of the familial coaggregation of borderline personality disorder with Axis I and nonborderline dramatic cluster axis II disorders. *Journal of Personality Disorders, 23*, 357–369. doi:10.1521/pedi.2009.23.4.357

8

OBJECT RELATIONS THEORIES AND PERSONALITY DISORDERS: INTERNAL REPRESENTATIONS AND DEFENSE MECHANISMS

CALEB SIEFERT AND JONATHAN H. PORCERELLI

Object relations (OR) theories are often employed to characterize, diagnose, and treat personality disorders (PDs; Blatt, 2008, Kernberg, 1984). OR theories focus on how early experiences influence the formation, organization, and functioning of mental capacities needed to adaptively navigate adult life. They also emphasize the role of defensive processes in adaptive and pathological personalities. The OR literature provides clinicians with a framework for conceptualizing personality development that can be used for characterizing personality pathology. OR research has provided clinicians with tools that can aid in identifying, diagnosing, and conceptualizing patients with PDs.

In this chapter, we focus on how the OR and defense mechanism literatures (a) contribute to how the field defines and conceptualizes PDs and (b) contribute to how clinicians diagnose and characterize individual patients with PDs. We begin with an overview of OR theories as they relate to PDs.

http://dx.doi.org/10.1037/14549-009
Personality Disorders: Toward Theoretical and Empirical Integration in Diagnosis and Assessment,
S. K. Huprich (Editor)

We next discuss contributions from OR in recent field-wide conversations regarding how to best define and classify PDs. We conclude the chapter with a review of measures tapping OR and defensive functioning and note how clinicians can use these measures in clinical assessment and treatment planning.

OBJECT RELATIONS THEORIES, PERSONALITY, AND PERSONALITY DISORDERS

According to OR theories, an individual's personality can be thought of in both structural and functional terms. Understanding an individual's personality requires one to understand how its structure relates to the functioning of various parts. The interrelationship of structures and specific functions can be observed when comparing cars. Although all cars have motors, some differences across cars are due to the motor's structure (e.g., a Lamborghini can accelerate much faster than a Ford Focus) and the specific functioning of various mechanisms (e.g., a Toyota Matrix with an exhaust problem does not function as well as a Toyota Matrix without an exhaust problem). Thus, the individual's personality structure sets limits on the range of his functioning across situations, and the workings of mental capacities within this structure determine functioning within specific situations.

OR theories view personality development as occurring largely during early childhood. Children experiencing a "good enough" early development will leave early childhood with a foundation for developing (a) a coherent sense of self and (b) relationships with others. These achievements coincide with the formation and development of mental capacities necessary for adaptively navigating life. For example, the capacity for empathy, the capacity to desire connection, and the capacity to hold reasonably stable views of others are all necessary for forming close, sustainable relationships (Kernberg, 1984, 2012). Likewise, a balanced view of the self, intact reality testing, and self–other differentiation are mental capacities necessary to begin forming an emerging identity that is adaptive (Blatt, 2008; Westen, 1993). The functioning of mental capacities is ultimately determined by how experiences with others are internalized and organized within the individual. Ultimately, thousands of internalized experiences are grouped together into internal representations (IRs). Once IRs are established, individuals rely on them to organize and respond to the world.

The content, complexity, and integration of experiences within representations shape the functioning of mental capacities and determine the strength of children's foundations for forming an identity and functioning interpersonally. It is both unlikely and unnecessary for development to result in all mental capacities functioning optimally; a "good enough" level of function is all that is required to form an adaptive personality (Winnicott, 1953). However, notable functional deficits in these capacities or heavy reliance on primitive defenses increases risk for identity diffusion and/or interpersonal difficulties. These can make navigating the ups and downs of life challenging and make personality pathology more likely (Kernberg, 2012).

From an OR perspective, PDs emerge when the dual goals of early development are not met or are met to an insufficient degree. A failure to achieve a strong foundation for identity formation and interpersonal functioning is typically due to deficits in mental capacities. Individuals with less mild deficits in a narrow range of capacities are likely to have a reasonably adaptive personality structure (i.e., normal/neurotic). Individuals with PDs, however, may experience a severe deficit in a small range of capacities or moderate to severe deficits across several capacities. The former is associated with pathology that tends to be limited to a more narrow range of life, and the latter involves challenges that are likely to cut across many situations, relationships, and settings. Thus, from a clinical perspective, most OR approaches to PD assessment encourage clinicians to assess patients' (a) personality structure (by assessing basic functions, nature and severity of difficulties, and the quality of IRs); (b) mental capacity functioning (e.g., capacity to invest in relationships; capacity for empathy; capacity for anxiety tolerance); and (c) defensive functioning. To appreciate OR theories' approach to PD diagnosis, one must understand the "expected" developmental trajectory in which internalized experiences become connected and grouped in a manner that ultimately gives rise to IRs that promote adaptive mental capacity functioning.

The Formation of Internal Representations and Personality Functioning

In the early stages of development, infants take in their experiences. These are the basic building blocks of personality and, for most individuals, will ultimately be grouped to form IRs. Two types of experiences are internalized: (a) frequently repeated interactions with others (real or imagined) are taken in (Stern, 1985); (b) traumatic or emotionally powerful experiences are internalized, even if their occurrence is rare (Kernberg, 1984). Internalizations do not perfectly mirror actual events. Instead, the child's subjective experience is internalized. How events are experienced hedges on a number of factors (e.g., developmental stage, temperament, past experience). Thus, from an OR perspective, personality ultimately stems from how biological predispositions interact with the environment to shape one's experience of the world.

During early development, each internalized experience exists independently from others. As the child develops, experiences become more connected. At first, children group experiences involving similar affects together (e.g., negative emotional experiences are grouped) and find it difficult to integrate internalizations containing conflicting emotional tones (Kernberg, 1984). With development, however, grouping becomes increasingly complex as internalized experiences become increasingly connected (e.g., experiences involving an angry parent are linked with experiences involving a happy parent). This is the beginning of the ability to understand others as complex and multifaceted. Increased integration changes how the child experiences others. For example, at this stage, when the child is experiencing a parent (who is typically experienced in a positive manner) as frustrating, she can now access other internalized experiences (e.g., times when the parent was gratifying). This may reduce distress experienced by the child and may alter how she acts on these feelings.

As one becomes better able to integrate internalized experiences of others (e.g., positive and negative), one also becomes increasingly able to conceptualize the self-in-relation-to-others and ultimately the self-as-separate-from-others (i.e., self-differentiation). At this point, internalized experiences can be grouped not only at the emotional valence level (e.g., good/bad) but also at the person level (e.g., self/others, self-with-others, self alone). The child can now tolerate holding opposing views and feelings about the self (e.g., I am mostly good but sometimes bad). This increased integration alters how the child experiences and relates to the self (e.g., when feeling shame, one can remember experiences in which one felt pride).

Throughout early development, internalized experiences are increasingly integrated and grouped into two types of representations: self-representations and other representations. Individuals ultimately rely on representations to rapidly shape their experience and response to a given situation. Thus, representations act as road maps that help us make sense of where we are and what we should do. When representations are complex, multiple pieces of information are organized to shape one's immediate experience of others or the self in a given situation. Further, when the content of representations for the self is reasonably positive, realistic, and stable, there is a greater sense of stability and more acceptance of occasional, situational shifts away from one's desired or "ideal" way of being. Thus, occasional failures to live up to one's standards can occur without one losing one's sense of self. Similarly, when representations for others are stable and contain reasonably positive content, there is greater capacity to accept others' minor shortcomings, tolerate deviations from what we wish others to be, and manage negative or aggressive feelings directed toward them.

Defenses and Personality Development

The formation of complex, coherent, and reasonably positive self- and other representations is needed to create the foundations necessary for establishing identity and functioning interpersonally in early childhood (Blatt, 2008; Kernberg, 1984). However, it is unlikely that one will experience a perfect environment–person match during development. Additionally, throughout the course of development, children experience a number of impulses, feelings, and thoughts that are difficult to integrate (e.g., aggression and love) or that provoke considerable anxiety. Defense mechanisms are used by children to manage anxiety or conflicting impulses. All defenses alter the experience of reality, and this is not in and of itself problematic. In fact, defenses often distort reality in a manner that fosters aspects of development (e.g., maintaining a positive view of others or the self even when feeling negatively) or protects the child from harm (Vaillant, 2000). That said, some defenses are more "primitive" in that they distort reality to a greater degree than others (Perry, 1990; Vaillant, 1994).

It is developmentally normal for young children to rely on primitive defenses that would not be adaptive in adulthood. For example, a child who is very frustrated or angry at a parent (who is typically well loved by the child) may in the heat of anger yell something to the effect of "You're terrible and you're not my Daddy/Mommy!" Such behavior is a developmentally normative form of "splitting" that, as most parents know, tends to be temporary. After strong emotions pass, it is common for children to reexperience desires for connection (which appeared temporarily quashed by feelings of aggression) and to seek rapprochement with the once "terrible" parent. Similarly, it may be hard for young children to tolerate strong negative feelings about themselves or feelings triggered by excessive punitive, aggressive, abandoning, or hostile behaviors of others. Defensive processes (e.g., denial, projection) may distort reality to restrict awareness and reduce consciously experienced anxiety.

As their internalized experiences become increasingly integrated, children are more capable of viewing others and the self in complex ways and better able to make use of coping skills or defenses that distort reality to a lesser degree. Greater organization of internalized experiences and cognitive development also increase anxiety tolerance. Increased anxiety tolerance can reduce the need to significantly distort reality, allowing for the use of more adaptive defenses. Even young children may be capable of using highly adaptive defenses (e.g., humor) to repair relationships or to maintain a sense of coherence (Vaillant, 1994, 2000).

Even with developmental advances, some children rely heavily on primitive defenses. This can be due to biological predispositions that exacerbate anxiety or limit one's ability to tolerate anxiety (Kernberg, 1984, 2012). Alternatively, children lacking predispositions for poor anxiety tolerance may nonetheless find themselves in environments that routinely produce strong anxiety and negative affect (e.g., abuse). Such children may also come to rely more frequently on primitive defenses in an effort to cope with excessive environmental demands. Poor environment–person fits (e.g., anxious child and rejecting parents) can make it difficult for the child to integrate representations or may expose the child to strong affects that are hard to mitigate without primitive defenses. Considerable or repeated trauma produces similar effects. When primitive defenses are adopted as "go to" approaches for managing anxiety or coping with stress, they become increasingly crystalized into stable, trait-like behavioral patterns (as opposed to transient, situation-specific attempts to cope) that shape the way the world is experienced. In addition to being problematic of its own accord, this can harm other developmental processes.

The use of defenses does not occur in a vacuum separate from the formation of IRs. In fact, excessive reliance on primitive defenses in early development is problematic precisely because frequent or significant distortions of reality may result in internalizations that are more malevolent and harder to integrate with other internalizations. This can result in less stable and poorly integrated IRs. In adulthood, individuals possessing IRs that are not sufficiently stable experience rapid shifts in how the self and others are experienced emotionally (Blatt, 2008). Similarly, when representations contain high levels of malevolent content, relationships with the self or others are more simplistic, rigid, and hostile. Further, as noted above, the process through which internalizations are integrated gives rise to mental capabilities necessary for interacting productively with others and forming a coherent identity. Thus, if defensive functioning limits integration within representations, important capacities may not develop or function sufficiently for adaptation.

Translating Theory to Practice: The Contributions of Kernberg and Blatt

Kernberg and Blatt have both developed OR theories applicable for clinical practice (e.g., diagnosis, case conceptualization, psychotherapy). Their roles in developing psychotherapies for PDs are beyond the scope of this chapter; however, their contributions to the diagnosis and characterization of patients with PDs are of central importance.

Kernberg's approach (1984) to PD assessment involves examining patients' personality structure and determining the severity of pathology on the one hand, while trying to understand patients' unique dynamics on the other. This is generally done in two interrelated steps. First, a patient's personality organization (i.e., structure of personality/severity of pathology) is assessed on a three-level continuum: normal/neurotic, borderline, and psychotic. Levels are differentiated on the basis of stability of representations, capacity for reality testing, and the quality of frequently utilized defenses.

Intact reality testing, reasonably stable representations, and more adaptive defenses are suggestive of normal/neurotic organizations. At the opposite end are psychotic organizations, which involve compromised reality testing, overly rigid or highly unstable representations, and frequent use of defensive dysregulation level defenses.

Individuals with borderline organizations are most likely to receive a PD diagnosis, though certain types of PD (e.g., obsessive-compulsive) may occur at neurotic organizations and others (e.g., schizotypal) at psychotic organizations. Borderline organizations involve reasonably intact reality testing (though transient problems may occur when distressed). Though they rarely employ defensive dysregulation level defenses, they rely on more primitive defenses from the action level and major image distorting level (e.g., splitting). Finally, individuals with borderline organizations tend to possess IRs that are unstable and that contain excessive malevolent content. Their experience of the self, others, or both tends to be inconsistent, affectively charged, and problematic.

Assessing personality organization helps clinicians conceptualize the limits of a patient's typical functioning and aids in establishing risk for PD. The second step involves assessing mental capacities (i.e., ego and superego capacities) and basic dispositions (e.g., introversion/internalizing problems vs. extraversion/externalizing problems) to more specifically clarify the nature of any pathology. Because the ego and superego cannot be analyzed directly, Kernberg encourages assessment of their functioning. Clinicians are encouraged to assess aggression management, anxiety tolerance, internalization of moral standards, and capacity for adaptively viewing the self and others. Kernberg also encourages assessment of introversion-extraversion. Some PDs are characterized by higher levels of extroversion and externalizing problems (e.g., antisocial), and others involve more introversion and internalizing problems (e.g., schizoid).

Blatt has also advanced conceptualizations of PDs by clarifying how specific developmental deficits in mental functions contribute to two categories of problems in adulthood (e.g., Blatt, 2008; Blatt & Auerbach, 2003). Blatt argues that in a "good enough" developmental process, individuals become (a) increasingly capable of forming mature and mutually satisfying relationships (i.e., relatedness) and (b) increasingly engaged in the process of self-creation (i.e., self-definition; Blatt & Levy, 1999). Further, they become better able to use coping strategies and defenses that promote (rather than negate) these two aims (Blatt, 2008).

Blatt views children as inherently motivated to seek out experiences that cultivate self-definition and relatedness. Though these lines are conceptually distinct, Blatt views them as complementary (Blatt, 2008; Luyten & Blatt, 2011). Further, self-definition begins as a relational process, as we first define ourselves through relational experiences (Bender, Morey, & Skodol, 2011). Thus, we are first motivated to form attachments with others and actualize relatedness. However, with increasing self–other differentiation we become more motivated to further define ourselves as autonomous individuals. In early development, the child alternates between developing relatedness capacities and self-definition capacities. As the child ages, he or she will begin to be capable of seeking experiences that promote both endeavors.

In Blatt's model, individuals with PDs experience stagnated development with regard to relatedness, self-definition, or both. This may result from biological predispositions, disruptive environments, or poor environment–person fit. The earlier in development that disruptions occur, the more severe personality pathology is likely to be. Blatt and Levy (1999) stated,

> On occasion, severe and repeated untoward events disrupt the complex, normal, dialectic developmental process. Some individuals . . . attempt to compensate for these serious developmental disruptions by exaggerating one developmental line, fixating either on relatedness or on the sense of self. (p. 88)

When "fixation" or preoccupation with one line occurs, the child is more likely to adopt behavior patterns that fail to promote or actively inhibit development in the other line. If no corrective experiences occur, repetition of these behavior patterns consolidates into typical ways of responding to the world. Though problematic, these behaviors may become chronic if, at some level, the individual continues to experience the original motivation leading to the preoccupation (Luyten & Blatt, 2011).

Blatt's approach to PD assessment involves first assessing overall severity of personality pathology by exploring difficulties in both domains. Relatedness is explored by assessing interpersonal skills, the quality of relationships, and the stability and complexity of other representations. Self-definition is assessed by examining the extent to which the individual has developed a coherent sense of identity; engages in purposeful, productive, and argentic activity; and represents the self in stable and complex ways. Functioning deficits or unstable representations are suggestive of personality pathology. Blatt encourages clinicians to assess deficits contributing to problems (Blatt, 2008; Luyten & Blatt, 2011) to clarify the specific nature of the difficulties. Some forms of PD (e.g., paranoid, obsessive-compulsive, narcissistic) involve preoccupation with self-definition (to the detriment of relatedness), and others involve preoccupation with relatedness (e.g., histrionic, dependent, borderline). Research supports Blatt's contention that PDs can be organized as experiencing deficits that involve relatedness and self-definition (Luyten & Blatt, 2011). Blatt encourages clinicians to explore the functioning of mental capacities and defenses after they have considered a client's standing on these two global dimensions. The specific constellation of deficits and defenses is unique to each disorder, though they all share preoccupation with the self-definition domain (Blatt & Levy, 1999).

CONTRIBUTIONS OF OBJECT RELATIONS AND DEFENSES FOR DEFINING PERSONALITY DISORDERS

The theoretical and empirical OR literatures have helped to shape how PDs are defined. How these disorders are defined is a question that has received increased attention in light of the recent development of the *Psychodynamic Diagnostic Manual* (*PDM*; PDM Task Force, 2006) and in anticipation of the fifth edition of the *Diagnostic and Statistical Manual of Mental Disorders* (*DSM–5*; American Psychiatric Association, 2013). In this section, we focus on how the OR literature has influenced those tasked with defining the nature of PDs.

The literature on OR and defense mechanisms had some influence on the fourth edition of the *DSM* (*DSM–IV*; American Psychiatric Association, 1994). Here, PDs were defined in terms of general and specific criteria. Criterion A of the general criteria defined PDs as involving enduring difficulties with cognition, affectivity, interpersonal functioning, and impulse control that negatively impact functioning in a range of situations over time. When patients fulfill the general criteria, clinicians should assess the specific criteria for the 10 PDs. Some specific criteria reflect the influence of OR. For example, the criteria for Borderline PD include "frantic efforts to avoid real or imagined abandonment." Similarly, criteria for Histrionic PD include "shows self-dramatization, theatricality, and exaggerated expression of emotion" and criteria for Borderline PD include "a pattern of unstable and intense interpersonal relationships characterized by alternating between extremes of idealization and devaluation." These criteria are similar to defenses (e.g., splitting). The *DSM–IV* also contains a scale for consideration that specifically quantified defensive functioning.

In the development of *DSM–5* (American Psychiatric Association, 2013), the Personality and Personality Disorders Work Group (PPDWG) was assembled to refine PD diagnosis. In proposing the revised system, the group reviewed research from several theories of personality (e.g., interpersonal theory, attachment theory), including studies dealing with OR and defenses (see Skodol et al., 2011). Though the PD system from *DSM–IV* was ultimately retained in *DSM–5*, the PPDWG recommended many changes. Major changes to the general criteria were suggested (see Section III of *DSM–5*; American Psychiatric Association, 2013, p. 761). Criterion A was rephrased to read "Moderate or greater impairment in personality (self/interpersonal) functioning" (American Psychiatric Association, 2013, p. 761). This phrasing is a notable departure from the current criterion, which conceptualizes PDs as impairment with two of four domains (cognition, affectivity, impulsivity, and interpersonal function). This change is especially consistent with the models of Blatt and Kernberg (Kernberg, 2012; Luyten & Blatt, 2011) in viewing an adaptive personality as one that promotes identity and relatedness. Indeed, in his review and critique of the changes suggested for *DSM–5*, Kernberg (2012) stated,

> The major innovative contribution and strength of the *DSM–V* proposal resides in the belated recognition of the essential nature of experience of the self and of relationships with significant others in the assessment of normality or degree of pathology of personality. (p. 236)

The PPDWG split both domains into elements. Self-functioning is split into *identity* and *self-direction*, and interpersonal functioning is split into *empathy* and *intimacy*. Specific capacities for each element are also provided (American Psychiatric Association, 2013, p. 762). Thus, as in OR, an individual's global functioning is viewed as resulting from more basic mental capacities (e.g., empathy) that foster adaptive functioning in a specific area. The specific functional capacities clinicians are encouraged to assess within each element share many similarities with mental capacities emphasized by OR theories. For example, to characterize a patient's functioning for the identity element, clinicians examine whether the patient (a) possesses a reasonably stable self-view, (b) can experience the self as separate from others, and (c) balances needs to view the self positively with needs to form accurate self-views (for a list of capacities, see American Psychiatric Association, 2013, p. 762). These are highly similar to the OR mental capacities of identity coherence, self–other differentiation, and the quality and complexity of self-representation.

Although it juxtaposes interpersonal functioning with self-functioning, the proposed system clearly places more emphasis on interpersonal experiences regarding the development of PD. Somewhat ironically, this increased emphasis is most pronounced in the self-functioning domain. For example, consider the ability to self-reflect productively (which is listed as a functional capacity under the self-direction element). A number of studies have shown that the ability to engage in productive reflection (i.e., reflective functioning) is related to the quality of one's childhood relationships with caregivers (Fonagy & Luyten, 2009; Mikulincer & Shaver, 2007). The capacity to differentiate self from others and the ability to view the self in a reasonably positive and stable manner are also on the identity element of self-functioning (Blatt, 2008; Kernberg, 1984, 2012). Again, several studies have demonstrated that these capacities develop in large part through relational interactions during development (Blatt, 2008; Kernberg, 2012; Mikulincer & Shaver, 2007). Thus, deficits in these self-functioning areas would be expected to result from relational experiences during development.

The PPDWG's revised model has potential to aid in how clinicians characterize defenses as adaptive or not. Consider a patient with borderline PD who relies heavily on splitting. Within the revised system, this defense is viewed as problematic if it impairs a self-function (e.g., productive self-reflection) and/or when it impairs an interpersonal function (e.g., understanding and appreciating others motives). Even defenses that are typically adaptive (e.g., self-observation, humor) may be characterized in complex ways within this system. For example, a patient who employs self-observation in a manner that fosters productivity (a self-function) or in a manner to better understand the self in relation to others for the purpose of improving relationships (an interpersonal function) would be said to be using the defense adaptively. However, patients with obsessive-compulsive PD or avoidant PD who engage in an excessive self-observation would likely be doing so in a manner that would inhibit self- or interpersonal functioning.

The diagnostic system that overlaps most clearly with OR is the *PDM*. The *PDM* does not have a specific definition for PDs, but it does have a clear approach for assessing them. Using the *PDM* framework for PD assessment, clinicians rate Personality Patterns and Disorders (P Axis) by first assessing level of personality organization (healthy-neurotic-borderline). If a patient exhibits signs of personality pathology or possesses a borderline organization, the clinician then determines fit with a PD type (PDM Task Force, 2006, p. 32). If a patient's maturational problems, central tensions/preoccupations, central affects, pathogenic self–other beliefs, and primary defenses match those of a known type, a PD type diagnosis is given. Thus, one patient may possess a borderline organization and fit the Paranoid PD type, and another patient may possess a borderline organization and fit the Masochistic PD type.

Although it is obviously impossible to separate the assessment of mental capacities from the assessment of personality organization and PD type fit, the second axis of the *PDM*, the Profile of Mental Functioning Axis (M Axis), is used to characterize the functioning of mental capacities. Full discussion of the nature of these capacities is beyond the scope of this chapter; however, we do wish to note that many of the capacities listed involve assessment of constructs considered important by OR theories. For example, the M Axis includes capacity for relationships and intimacy; capacity to construct or use internal standards and ideals; development of self-observing capacities; and capacity for affective experience, expression, and communication. The *PDM* also encourages assessment of "defensive patterns and capacities" on this axis. The *PDM* actively encourages the use of quantifiable assessment tools, such as the Object Relations Inventory (Blatt & Auerbach, 2001), for characterizing capacities.

The OR literature has been a part of field-wide discussions regarding the nature of PDs. Inclusion of these literatures in such discussions is due in large part to the pioneering efforts of several scholar–practitioners who developed psychometrically sound, clinically sophisticated measures of OR and defenses (Azim, Piper, Segal, Nixon, & Duncan, 1991; Bell, Billington, & Becker, 1986; Bers, Blatt, Sayward, & Johnston, 1993; Hilsenroth, Stein, & Pinsker, 2004; Perry, 1990). Although many therapists are familiar with this research, they may not realize that these tools can also be used clinically in PD assessment and case conceptualization (Bender et al., 2011; Huprich & Greenberg, 2003).

OBJECT RELATIONS AND DEFENSE MECHANISM MEASURES FOR PERSONALITY DISORDERS

The *DSM–5* suggests a two-step approach to identifying PDs. Both the *PDM* and the recent model proposed by the PPDWG encourage clinicians to determine PD status by assessing global functioning, fit with a PD type, and specific mental capacities. Many OR theorists encourage assessment of personality at the level of organization/severity/structure, followed by assessing capacities and functioning. Here we focus on clinically rated tools clinicians can leverage toward these aims. We limit our review to measures that have been specifically explored or utilized with samples containing at least some patients with PD and to instruments that are clinician rated (as excellent reviews including self-report measures of OR and defenses already exist; see Bender et al., 2011; Davidson & MacGregor, 1998; Huprich & Greenberg, 2003). For clarity, we refer to efforts to assess personality organization and severity as Step 1 and efforts to assess fit with a PD type and patient-specific characteristics (e.g., mental capacities) as Step 2. At Step 1, clinicians seek to determine risk for PD and severity of dysfunction. Step 2 assessment involves clarifying the unique dynamics involved. As noted below, assessing defenses is useful for both aims.

The Personality Organization Diagnostic Form—II (PODF–II; Gamache et al., 2009) is an OR measure that can be used for Step 1. It can be used to reliably rate clinical encounters (e.g., intake evaluations) and/or narratives provided patients (Gamache et al., 2009). Five dimensions are rated on the PODF–II: identity coherence, use of primitive defenses, use of mature defenses, reality testing, and quality of OR. Combining dimension scores produces two factor scores (a neurotic-to-borderline dimension and a psychotic dimension [not present–more present]). Lower PODF–II ratings and organizations (e.g., borderline) are associated with greater symptom severity and life problems (Gamache et al., 2009). Studies with an earlier version of the PODF also suggested that patients with lower personality organizations on the PODF-II experience more severe dysfunction (Diguer et al., 2004). Thus, this measure may be useful in determining a patient's personality structure and identifying risk for PD.

Another interview-based measure is the Quality of Object Relations Scale (QORS; Piper, McCallum, & Joyce, 1993). To rate the QORS, an interviewer must conduct a semistructured interview with the patient over the course of two sessions (1 hour each). Thus, some training and familiarity with the QORS is necessary. In the interview, information regarding patients' relational history, such as the quality of adult sexual relationships, the quality of nonsexual adult relationships, and the presence of a stable relationship, is gathered (Høglend, Dahl, Hersoug, Lorentzen, & Perry, 2011). Ratings are made for four dimensions: affect regulation, self-image, the quality of relational patterns, and antecedent events (e.g., past experiences or relationships that influence current functioning). Dimension ratings are aggregated to provide an index of personality pathology. The psychometric properties of the QORS ratings and overall index scores have been found to range from adequate to excellent (Piper & Duncan, 1999). A handful of studies support the utility of the QORS for assessing personality pathology. For example, in a sample of patients with and without PD, Piper and Duncan (1999) found that patients with PDs had lower QORS scores. Further, lower QORS scores were related to greater dysfunction (i.e., severity).

The Social Cognitions and Object Relations Scale (SCORS; Westen, 1993) can aid in both Step 1 and Step 2 assessment. The most recent version of the SCORS, the SCORS-Global (Hilsenroth et al., 2004), has a publicly available manual that clinicians can use to achieve reliability. The SCORS-G can be used to code narrative data (e.g., stories told to Thematic Apperception Task cards [TAT; Murray, 1943], therapy transcripts, early memories). Eight mental capacities are assessed: complexity of representations, affective tone of relationships, emotional investment in relationships, emotional investment in moral standards, social causality, self-esteem, management of aggressive impulses, and identity cohesion. A global score can be calculated by aggregating ratings across dimensions. The validity of the global score for Step 1 assessments has recently been demonstrated. Using a clinical sample (containing patients with and without PD), Peters, Hilsenroth, Eudell-Simmons, Blagys, and Handler (2006) found that patients with PDs had lower global scores than did patients without PD. Global scores were also associated with clinician-rated indicators of severity, such as symptom severity, occupational dysfunction, and intensity of interpersonal problems. Specific SCORS-G scales can also be used in Step 1 assessments. For example, the identity coherence dimension alone was predictive of PD severity in the study by Peters et al. (2006). Similarly, using the original SCORS to assess a sample of patients with PD, Hibbard, Hilsenroth, Hibbard, and Nash (1995) found that lower affective tone scores were linked to greater personality pathology (i.e., severity).

At times, as part of Step 1 assessment, clinicians may be attempting to determine the extent to which a patient's distress is more or less personality driven. For some forms of PD, the SCORS can be particularly useful for this purpose. For example, Huprich, Porcerelli, Binienda, Karana, and Kamoo (2007) found SCORS ratings of TAT stories differentiated patients with dysthymia from those with depressive PD. Across studies, the most common dimensions differentiating patients with borderline PD from others are low scores on investment in relationships, affective tone, and complexity of representations for self and others (Nigg, Lohr, Westen, Gold, & Silk, 1992; Westen, Lohr, Silk, Gold, & Kerber, 1990; Westen, Ludolph, et al., 1990).

Because SCORS-G ratings are made at the level of specific mental capacities, they can also be employed to clarify the specific nature of a patient's pathology at Step 2. Ackerman, Clemence, Weatherill, and Hilsenroth (1999) demonstrated that each Cluster B PD could be differentiated on the basis of its SCORS-G profiles. Further, profiles also differentiated Cluster B PDs from Cluster C PDs in this study. Such findings suggest that the SCORS can aid clinicians in clarifying fit with specific PD types. Even within diagnostic categories, SCORS profiles can help discriminate among different subgroups. For example, Tramantano, Javier, and Colon (2003) used the SCORS to differentiate subgroups of patients with borderline PD. Such findings suggest that SCORS dimensions provide fine-grained analyses of a patient's mental capacities that permit clinicians to conceptualize cases in a manner that is more specific than diagnosis alone.

The Mutuality of Autonomy Scale (MOA; Urist, 1977) is a system for coding early memory protocols, TAT stories, or Rorschach responses involving interactions in a reliable manner (Fowler, Hilsenroth, & Handler, 1996). This tool can be useful for clinicians who utilize the Rorschach or early memory protocols. Thus far, studies with the MOA have primarily focused on identifying specific forms of PD. For example, MOA ratings of Rorschach responses differentiate patients with borderline PD from normal controls and patients with depression but without PD (Stuart et al., 1990). In this study, high levels of malevolent content and hostile interactions were suggestive of borderline PD. Rosenberg, Blatt, Oxman, McHugo, and Ford (1994) replicated these findings, again finding MOA ratings to differentiate patients with Borderline PD from patients without PD.

Assessment of defensive functioning is also central to personality assessments. The Defensive Functioning Scale (DFS) of *DSM–IV* (American

Psychiatric Association, 1994) provides a means for reliably assessing defensive functioning in a manner that is easily integrated into clinical practice (see Perry et al., 1998). The DFS contains seven levels (each with three to five defenses) ordered in a hierarchical fashion from most adaptive to least adaptive (High Adaptive Level, Mental Inhibition Level, Minor Image Distorting Level, Disavowal Level, Major Image Distorting Level, Action Level, and Level of Defensive Dysregulation). To score the DFS, clinicians rank order the frequency of defenses used by a patient during an evaluation. Thus, the scale is easily integrated into intake procedures. Based on these rankings, a patient's overall defensive functioning score (ODF) is calculated. This score can range from 1 (*severely maladaptive*) to 7 (*very adaptive*; Hilsenroth, Callahan, & Eudell, 2003). Scores can also be calculated for each defense level. The reliability of the DFS, at the ODF level and level-specific scores, is well established (Blais, Conboy, Wilcox, & Norman, 1996; DeFife & Hilsenroth, 2005; Perry et al., 1998; Porcerelli, Cogan, Kamoo, & Miller, 2010; Porcerelli, Cogan, Markova, Miller, & Mickens, 2011).

ODF scores are particularly useful in Step 1 assessment. ODF scores from the DFS have been shown to differentiate patients with PDs from patients without PDs, and they appear to do so better than self-report approaches (Perry & Høglend, 1998). More recently, Perry, Presniak, and Olson (2013) examined defensive functioning in a large sample ($n = 107$) of patients with schizotypal, borderline, antisocial, and narcissistic PDs. All four PDs had higher rates of immature defenses (as compared with mature defenses), including heavier reliance on defenses from the minor image distorting level, disavowal level, major image distorting level, action level defenses, and level of defensive dysregulation. Vaillant (1994) reported similar findings, concluding that patients with PDs rely heavily on immature defenses and that patients functioning within the healthy or neurotic levels do so less. The pattern of findings in these studies seems to indicate that frequent use of immature defenses (e.g., major image distorting defense, action-level defenses) is associated with risk for PD. This is consistent with OR theories' emphasis on assessing defenses as part of determining a patient's personality organization.

DFS specific-level scores can also help clinicians determine the severity of personality pathology. Using a sample of 110 women seeking primary care at a university-based clinic, Porcerelli et al. (2006) found that higher Adaptive Level scores were linked with more positive OR; higher scores for the Major Image Distortion Level and Action Level were associated with greater symptomatic distress, history of abuse, and negative ORs. This study provides some support that specific level scores may also aid in determining severity of personality pathology at Step 1.

The DFS also provides information that can help clarify the specific nature of patients' personality pathology during Step 2. There is some empirical support suggesting that specific forms of PD are linked to certain DFS defense levels in theoretically predicted manners. For example, in the study by Perry et al. (2013) described above, findings supported hypothesized disorder-defense constellations for the four types of PDs included. For example, image distorting defenses, such as splitting, were strongly associated with borderline PD, and disavowal defenses (e.g., denial) were associated with antisocial PD. Using a different approach, Blais et al. (1996) reported similar findings. In this study, 100 clinicians (psychiatrists, psychologists, and social workers) used the DFS to rate a patient with PD. Higher Adaptive Level defenses predicted less severe forms of PD (e.g., obsessive–compulsive PD), and Major Image Distorting level scores predicted more severe forms of PD (e.g., borderline; schizoid PDs). Some forms of PD were notable for elevations at multiple levels. For example, higher Major Image Distorting Level and Disavowal Level scores predicted histrionic PD, but higher Mental Inhibition Level and Major Image Distorting scores predicted dependent PD. These studies provide some support for the notion that assessment of specific defensive levels can aid clinicians in clarifying the precise nature of a given patient's PD.

The DFS can also assist in another aspect of Step 2 assessments: the detection of strengths. When a patient with PD is evaluated, it is important to assess the entire range of defenses utilized. Even if the relative use of immature defenses in comparison with less pathological defenses (i.e., mental inhibition level and high adaptive level) is high, noting what adaptive defenses the patient uses can be important because it can point to unique strengths. Mental health training often gives less weight to the assessment of patient strengths, emphasizing instead a focus on symptoms and difficulties (Vaillant, 2000). However, assessing strengths in those with PDs, such as the adaptive use of defenses, can aid the clinician in identifying personality characteristics that can be leveraged in and outside of the treatment. For example, helping the patient recognize and more frequently use healthy defenses he or she already employs can be a way for the clinician to include a focus on the patient's more positive aspects. Discussing the patient's use of healthy defenses, such as affiliation (the ability to share problems with others without burdening them), altruism (gains pleasure from giving to others what they would like to receive), and humor, can be a way for patient and therapist to explore situations and relationships in which the patient has been effective or felt satisfied. Further, clinicians may be able to leverage this information to help the patient identify adaptive strategies for coping with distress or problems in life.

INTERNAL REPRESENTATIONS, DEFENSE MECHANISMS, AND TREATMENT OUTCOME FOR PERSONALITY DISORDERS

Many measures of OR and defenses can also be used to monitor treatment gains with individuals with PD. The Object Relations Inventory (ORI; Bers et al., 1993) can be used to rate narrative descriptions of self and others. Using the ORI in a single-case design, Gruen and Blatt (1990) examined changes in the internal representations of an adolescent inpatient with borderline features. This patient was asked to write descriptions of her parents and self at the beginning of treatment and at 6-month intervals. Narratives were scored with the ORI. Changes in the patient's Global Assessment of Functioning scores over the course of treatment were significantly related to changes in the conceptual level of representations (i.e., descriptions of self and parents become more differentiated and complex). In other words, global functioning improved as the adolescent developed more positive and complex representations for the self and other and demonstrated a greater self–other differentiation.

Diamond, Blatt, Stayner, and Kaslow (1991) developed the Self–Other Differentiation Scale for the ORI. Diamond, Kaslow, Coonerty, and Blatt (1990) used this scale to study four adolescent girls with borderline PD. Patients wrote self-descriptions and descriptions of their mother, father, and therapist at the beginning of treatment and at 6-month intervals; these were scored with the Self–Other Differentiation Scale. Increased self–other differentiation and greater positivity for self-representations occurred from admission to the conclusion of the first year of treatment for all four patients. These changes were associated with functional improvements, suggesting that changes in internal representations occurred in parallel with other improvements in functioning.

Like the ORI, the SCORS can be used to assess changes in internal representations and identity coherence as a function of treatment. Porcerelli et al. (2006) used the SCORS to compare young adult inpatients at the beginning and end of intensive (15 months on average) inpatient treatment for severe personality pathology. Changes were observed across multiple SCORS dimensions: complexity of representations, affective tone of relationships, capacity for emotional investment in relationships, and understanding social causality. The results of these studies suggest that the ORI and the SCORS are sensitive to the complex changes that occur as a result of treatment. Both are likely to have utility for assessing treatment outcome in patients with PDs.

Because defense mechanisms are held to partially mediate the relationship between stress and symptom development, one would expect changes in defenses (i.e., a lessening of the use of immature defenses and an increase

in the use of mature defenses) to precede or accompany symptom improvement. Some empirical evidence suggests that this is the case (Perry & Bond,
2012). Two methodologically rigorous case studies of long-term psychoanalytic therapy of patients with PDs reported that treatment resulted in changes
in the use of defense mechanisms. Lingiardi, Gazzillo, and Waldron (2010)
reported changes in defense mechanisms over the course of a 2-year treatment in a female patient with histrionic PD. Presniak, Olson, Porcerelli,
and Dauphin (2010) reported such changes at a 1-year follow up of a 5-year
treatment of a male with avoidant PD. In both cases, treatment increased
the use of adaptive defenses, and this increase was associated with significant
decreases in personality pathology and symptoms, as well as improvements
in functioning.

CONCLUSION

OR theories have made many contributions to the field's understanding and approach for working with individuals with PD. Clinical, theoretical, and empirical advances have broadened the number of individuals
integrating OR theories into their practices. Although the use of measures
tapping OR and defenses is increasing among researchers (Bender et al.,
2011; Huprich & Greenberg, 2003), in our experience these measures tend
to be used sparingly by clinicians. This is unfortunate, as a broadening
literature suggests that such measures may be particularly helpful to clinicians working with PDs. These measures are also capable of quantifying
fine-grained, patient-specific information in a manner that goes beyond
diagnoses. Like the *PDM*, which complements other diagnostic systems,
these tools provide clinicians with the means to assess OR from multiple
vantage points.

REFERENCES

Ackerman, S. J., Clemence, A. J., Weatherill, R., & Hilsenroth, M. J. (1999). Use
of TAT in the assessment of *DSM–IV* Cluster B personality disorders. *Journal of
Personality Assessment, 73*, 422–448. doi:10.1207/S15327752JPA7303_9

American Psychiatric Association. (1994). *Diagnostic and statistical manual of mental
disorders* (4th ed.). Washington, DC: Author.

American Psychiatric Association. (2013). *Diagnostic and statistical manual of mental
disorders* (5th ed.). Washington, DC: Author.

Azim, H. F., Piper, W. E., Segal, P. M., Nixon, G. W. H., & Duncan, S. (1991). The
Quality of Object Relations Scale. *Bulletin of the Menninger Clinic, 55*, 323–343.

Bell, M., Billington, R., & Becker, B. (1986). A scale for the assessment of object relations: Reliability, validity, and factorial invariance. *Journal of Clinical Psychology, 42,* 733–741. doi:10.1002/1097-4679(198609)42:5<733::AID-JCLP2270420509>3.0.CO;2-C

Bender, D. S., Morey, L. C., & Skodol, A. E. (2011). Toward a model for assessing level of personality functioning in *DSM–5,* Part I: A review of theory and methods. *Journal of Personality Assessment, 93,* 332–346. doi:10.1080/00223891.2011.583808

Bers, S. A., Blatt, S. J., Sayward, H. K., & Johnston, R. S. (1993). Normal and pathological aspects of self-descriptions and their change over long-term treatment. *Psychoanalytic Psychology, 10,* 17–37. doi:10.1037/h0079432

Blais, M. A., Conboy, C. A., Wilcox, N., & Norman, D. K. (1996). An empirical study of the *DSM–IV* Defensive Functioning Scale in personality disordered patients. *Comprehensive Psychiatry, 37,* 435–440. doi:10.1016/S0010-440X(96)90027-9

Blatt, S. J. (2008). *Polarities of experience: Relatedness and self-definition in personality development, psychopathology, and the therapeutic process.* Washington, DC: American Psychological Association.

Blatt, S. J., & Auerbach, J. S. (2001). Mental representation, severe psychopathology, and the therapeutic process. *Journal of the American Psychoanalytic Association, 49,* 113–159.

Blatt, S. J., & Auerbach, J. S. (2003). Psychodynamic measures of therapeutic change. *Psychoanalytic Inquiry, 23,* 268–307. doi:10.1080/07351692309349034

Blatt, S. J., & Levy, K. N. (1999). A psychodynamic approach to the diagnosis of psychopathology. In J. W. Barron (Ed.), *Making diagnosis meaningful: Enhancing evaluation and treatment of psychological disorders* (pp. 73–109). Washington, DC: American Psychological Association.

Davidson, K., & MacGregor, M. W. (1998). A critical appraisal of self-report defense mechanism measures. *Journal of Personality, 66,* 965–992. doi:10.1111/1467-6494.00039

DeFife, J. A., & Hilsenroth, M. J. (2005). Clinical utility of the Defensive Functioning Scale in the assessment of depression. *Journal of Nervous and Mental Disease, 193,* 176–182. doi:10.1097/01.nmd.0000154839.43440.35

Diamond, D., Blatt, S., Stayner, D., & Kaslow, N. (1991). *The Differentiation-Relatedness Scale of Self and Object Representations.* Unpublished research manual, Yale University.

Diamond, D., Kaslow, N., Coonerty, S., & Blatt, S. J. (1990). Changes in separation–individuation and intersubjectivity in long-term treatment. *Psychoanalytic Psychology, 7,* 363–397. doi:10.1037/h0079215

Diguer, L., Pelletier, S., Hébert, E., Descôteaux, J.-P., Rousseau, P., & Daoust, J.-P. (2004). Personality organizations, psychiatric severity, and self and object representations. *Psychoanalytic Psychology, 21,* 259–275. doi:10.1037/0736-9735.21.2.259

Fonagy, P., & Luyten, P. (2009). A developmental, mentalization-based approach to the understanding and treatment of borderline personality disorder. *Development and Psychopathology, 21*, 1355–1381. doi:10.1017/S0954579409990198

Fowler, C., Hilsenroth, M. J., & Handler, L. (1996). A multimethod approach to assessing dependency: The Early Memory Dependency Probe. *Journal of Personality Assessment, 67*, 399–413. doi:10.1207/s15327752jpa6702_13

Gamache, D., Laverdière, O., Diguer, L., Hébert, E., Larochelle, S., & Descôteaux, J. (2009). Personality Organization Diagnostic Form (PODF): Psychometric properties of a revised version. *Journal of Nervous and Mental Disease, 197*, 368–377. doi:10.1097/NMD.0b013e3181a2097

Gruen, R. J., & Blatt, S. J. (1990). Change in self and object representation during long-term dynamically oriented treatment. *Psychoanalytic Psychology, 7*, 399–422. doi:10.1037/h0079216

Hibbard, S., Hilsenroth, M. J., Hibbard, J. K., & Nash, M. R. (1995). A validity study of two projective object representations measures. *Psychological Assessment, 7*, 432–439. doi:10.1037/1040-3590.7.4.432

Hilsenroth, M. J., Callahan, K. L., & Eudell, E. M. (2003). Further reliability, convergent and discriminant validity of overall defensive functioning. *Journal of Nervous and Mental Disease, 191*, 730–737.

Hilsenroth, M., Stein, M., & Pinsker, J. (2004). *Social Cognition and Object Relations Scale: Global Rating Method (SCORS–G)*. Unpublished manuscript, Derner Institute of Advanced Psychological Studies, Adelphi University.

Høglend, P., Dahl, H. S., Hersoug, A. G., Lorentzen, S., & Perry, J. C. (2011). Long-term effects of transference interpretation in dynamic psychotherapy of personality disorders. *European Psychiatry, 26*, 2418–2424. doi:10.1016/j.eurpsy.2010.05.006

Huprich, S. K., & Greenberg, R. P. (2003). Advances in the assessment of object relations in the 1990s. *Clinical Psychology Review, 23*, 665–698. doi:10.1016/S0272-7358(03)00072-2

Huprich, S. K., Porcerelli, J. H., Binienda, J., Karana, D., & Kamoo, R. (2007). Parental representations, object relations, and their relationship to depressive personality disorder and dysthymia. *Personality and Individual Differences, 43*, 2171–2181. doi:10.1016/j.paid.2007.06.030

Kernberg, O. (1984). *Severe personality disorders: Psychotherapeutic strategies.* New Haven, CT: Yale University Press.

Kernberg, O. F. (2012). Overview and critique of the classification of personality disorders proposed for *DSM–V. Swiss Archives of Neurology and Psychiatry, 163*, 234–238.

Lingiardi, V., Gazzillo, F., & Waldron, S. (2010). An empirically supported psychoanalysis: The case of Giovanna. *Psychoanalytic Psychology, 27*, 190–218. doi:10.1037/a0019418

Luyten, P., & Blatt, S. J. (2011). Integrating theory-driven and empirically-derived models of personality development and psychopathology: A proposal for *DSM V*. *Clinical Psychology Review, 31*, 52–68. doi:10.1016/j.cpr.2010.09.003

Mikulincer, M., & Shaver, P. R. (2007). *Attachment in adulthood: Structure, dynamics and change.* New York, NY: Guilford Press.

Murray, H. A. (1943). *Thematic Apperception Test manual.* Cambridge, MA: Harvard University Press.

Nigg, J., Lohr, N. E., Westen, D., Gold, L., & Silk, K. R. (1992). Malevolent object representations in borderline personality disorder and major depression. *Journal of Abnormal Psychology, 101*, 61–67. doi:10:1037/0021-843X.101.1.61

PDM Task Force. (2006). *Psychodynamic diagnostic manual.* Silver Spring, MD: Alliance of Psychoanalytic Organizations.

Perry, J. C. (1990). *The Defense Mechanism Rating Scales* (5th ed.). Cambridge, MA: Cambridge Hospital.

Perry, J. C., & Bond, M. (2012). Change in defense mechanisms during long-term dynamic psychotherapy and five-year outcome. *The American Journal of Psychiatry, 169*, 916–925.

Perry, J. C., & Høglend, P. (1998). Convergent and discriminant validity of overall defensive functioning. *Journal of Nervous and Mental Disorders, 186*, 529–535.

Perry, J. C., Høglend, P., Shear, K., Vaillant, G. E., Horowitz, M., Kardos, M. E., . . . Kagen, D. (1998). Field trial of a diagnostic axis for defense mechanisms for *DSM–IV*. *Journal of Personality Disorders, 12*, 56–68. doi:10.1521/pedi.1998.12.1.56

Perry, J. C., Presniak, M. D., & Olson, T. R. (2013). Defense mechanisms in schizotypal, borderline, antisocial, and narcissistic personality disorders. *Psychiatry: Interpersonal and Biological Processes, 76*, 32–52. doi:10.1521/psyc.2013.76.1.32

Peters, E. J., Hilsenroth, M. J., Eudell-Simmons, E. M., Blagys, M. D., & Handler, L. (2006). Reliability and validity of the Social Cognition and Object Relations Scale in clinical use. *Psychotherapy Research, 16*, 617–626. doi:10.1080/10503300600591288

Piper, W. E., & Duncan, S. C. (1999). Object relations theory and short-term dynamic psychotherapy: Findings from the Quality of Object Relations Scale. *Clinical Psychology Review, 19*, 669–685. doi:10.1016/S0272-7358(98)00080-4

Piper, W. E., McCallum, M., & Joyce, A. S. (1993). *Manual for assessment of quality of object relations.* Unpublished manuscript, University of British Columbia, Vancouver, Canada.

Porcerelli, J. H., Cogan, R., Kamoo, R., & Miller, K. (2010). Convergent validity of the Defense Mechanisms Manual and the Defensive Functioning Scale. *Journal of Personality Assessment, 92*, 432–438. doi:10.1080/00223891.2010.497421

Porcerelli, J. H., Cogan, R., Markova, T., Miller, K., & Mickens, L. (2011). The *Diagnostic and Statistical Manual of Mental Disorders, Fourth Edition* Defensive

Functioning Scale: A validity study. *Comprehensive Psychiatry, 52*, 225–230. doi:10.1016/j.comppsych.2010.06.003

Porcerelli, J. H., Shahar, G., Blatt, S. J., Ford, R. Q., Mezza, J. A., & Greenlee, L. M. (2006). Social Cognition and Object Relations Scale: Covergent validity and changes following intensive inpatient treatment. *Personality and Individual Differences, 41*, 407–417. doi:10.1016/j.paid.2005.10.027

Presniak, M. D., Olson, T. R., Porcerelli, J. H., & Dauphin, V. B. (2010). Changes in defensive functioning in a case of avoidant personality disorder. *Psychotherapy: Theory, Research, Practice, Training, 47*, 134–139. doi:10.1037/a0018838

Rosenberg, S. D., Blatt, S. J., Oxman, T. E., McHugo, G. J., & Ford, R. Q. (1994). Assessment of object relations through lexical content analysis of the TAT. *Journal of Personality Assessment, 63*, 345–362. doi:10.1207/s15327752jpa6302_13

Skodol, A. E., Clark, L. A., Bender, D. S., Krueger, R. F., Morey, L. C., Verheul, R., . . . Oldham, J. M. (2011). Proposed changes in personality and personality disorder assessment and diagnosis for *DSM–5* Part I: Description and rationale. *Personality Disorders: Theory, Research, and Treatment, 2*, 4–22. doi:10.1037/a0021891

Stern, D. N. (1985). *The psychological world of the infant*. New York, NY: Basic Books.

Stuart, J., Westen, D., Lohr, N., Benjamin, J., Becker, S., Vorus, N., & Silk, K. (1990). Object relations in borderlines, depressives, and normals: An examination of human responses on the Rorschach. *Journal of Personality Assessment, 55*, 296–318. doi:10.1207/s15327752jpa5501&2_28

Tramantano, G., Javier, R. A., & Colon, M. (2003). Discriminating among subgroups of borderline personality disorder: An assessment of object representations. *American Journal of Psychoanalysis, 63*, 149–175. doi:10.1023/A:1024079115405

Urist, J. (1977). The Rorschach test and the assessment of object relations. *Journal of Personality Assessment, 41*, 3–9. doi:10.1207/s15327752jpa4101_1

Vaillant, G. E. (1994). Ego mechanisms of defense and personality psychopathology. *Journal of Abnormal Psychology, 103*, 44–50. doi:10.1037/0021-843X.103.1.44

Vaillant, G. E. (2000). Adaptive mental mechanisms: Their role in a positive psychology. *American Psychologist, 55*, 89–98. doi:10.1037/0003-066X.55.1.89

Westen, D. (1993). *The Social Cognition and Object Relations Scale: Q-sort for projective stories*. Unpublished manuscript, Harvard Medical School.

Westen, D., Lohr, N., Silk, K. R., Gold, L., & Kerber, K. (1990). Object relations and social cognition in borderlines, major depressives, and normals: A Thematic Apperception Test analysis. *Psychological Assessment, 2*, 355–364. doi:10.1037/1040-3590.2.4.355

Westen, D., Ludolph, P., Silk, K., Kellam, A., Gold, L., & Lohr, N. (1990). Object relations in borderline adolescents and adults: Developmental differences. *Adolescent Psychiatry, 17*, 360–384.

Winnicott, D. W. (1953). Transitional objects and transitional phenomena. *International Journal of Psycho-Analysis, 34*, 89–97.

9

INTEGRATING CLINICAL AND EMPIRICAL PERSPECTIVES ON PERSONALITY: THE SHEDLER–WESTEN ASSESSMENT PROCEDURE (SWAP)

JONATHAN SHEDLER

> It is well known that [Paul Meehl] not only thinks it important for a psychologist to work as a responsible professional with real-life clinical problems but, further, considers the purely "theoretical" personality research of academic psychologists to be unusually naïve and unrealistic when the researcher is not a seasoned, practicing clinician. (Meehl, 1973)

One of the greatest challenges facing psychology and psychiatry is the schism between science and practice. The schism is especially pronounced when it comes to understanding personality. For skilled clinical practitioners, personality assessment generally means *clinical case formulation*: understanding the patterns of thinking, feeling, fantasizing, desiring, fearing, coping, defending, attaching, relating, experiencing self and others, and so on, that make a person unique and (if he is in treatment) underlie his suffering. Understanding personality in this way requires skill. Sophisticated clinicians consider a range of information, attending not only to what patients say but also to how they say it, drawing inferences from patients' accounts of their lives and relationships, from their manner of interacting with the clinician, and from their own emotional reactions

This chapter contains ideas first published in Shedler & Westen, 2006. Address e-mail correspondence to jonathan@shedler.com.

http://dx.doi.org/10.1037/14549-010
Personality Disorders: Toward Theoretical and Empirical Integration in Diagnosis and Assessment,
S. K. Huprich (Editor)
Copyright © 2015 by Jonathan Shedler.

to the patient (Betan, Heim, Conklin, & Westen, 2005; McWilliams, 2011; Peebles, 2012).

For example, clinicians generally do not assess lack of empathy, a central feature of narcissistic personality, by administering self-report questionnaires or asking direct questions. A moment's reflection reveals the futility of doing so: It would be a rare narcissistic patient who could report his own lack of empathy. More likely, the patient would describe himself as a caring person and a wonderful friend. An initial sign of lack of empathy on the part of the patient may be a subtle sense on the part of the clinician of being interchangeable or replaceable, or of being treated as a sounding board rather than as a person, or of feeling put down (Betan et al., 2005; Kernberg, 1975, 1984; McWilliams, 2011). Lack of empathy is something clinicians *infer*.

In other words, the clinician's subjective experience of the patient is a source of data and a vehicle for hypothesis generation. The clinician might go on to consider whether she often feels this way with this patient and whether such feelings are characteristic for her in her role as therapist. She might then become aware that the patient tends to describe other people more in terms of the functions they serve or needs they fulfill than in terms of who they are as people. She might further consider how these observations dovetail with the facts the patient has provided about his life and the problems that brought him to treatment. This kind of thinking lies at the heart of clinically sophisticated approaches to personality.

It is just such clinical judgment and inference that research approaches have eschewed. With respect to descriptive psychiatry, successive editions of the *Diagnostic and Statistical Manual of Mental Disorders* (*DSM*) have minimized the role of clinical inference and treated personality diagnosis as a largely technical task of tabulating signs and symptoms (for a discussion of the limitation of *DSM* personality disorder diagnosis, see Shedler & Westen, 2007).

With respect to academic psychology, personality research has focused on dimensional trait models derived from factor analysis of questionnaire data, notably the five-factor model (FFM) and its variants (e.g., Widiger & Simonsen, 2005). Although they derive from different traditions, academic psychology and descriptive psychiatry have both sought to minimize if not eliminate clinical inference and deduction. Indeed, the FFM was developed without input from clinical practitioners or theorists. It derives instead from questionnaire responses of laypersons describing themselves and their social acquaintances. Although the model is valuable for certain purposes, many experienced clinicians see it as quite removed from their clinical needs (Kernberg, 1996; Rottman, Ahn, Sanislow, & Kim, 2009; Shedler et al., 2010; Spitzer,

First, Shedler, Westen, & Skodal, 2008). Proposals by academic psychologists to replace clinical personality concepts with the FFM betray a devaluing attitude toward clinical knowledge and exemplify the science–practice schism. This is what Paul Meehl decried in the epigraph that begins this chapter.

ON THE SCIENCE–PRACTICE SCHISM

There is no inherent reason why the mental health professions must choose between clinical depth and scientific rigor. Good clinical work depends on scientific thinking and reasoning; it is characterized by an ongoing, cyclical process of data collection, hypothesis generation, hypothesis testing, and hypothesis revision. Empirical research rests (one hopes) on psychologically sophisticated human judgment from beginning to end, starting with judgments about what psychological phenomena are important to study, through judgments about how to conceptualize and operationalize them, to judgments about how to revise hypotheses as new information emerges.

Thus, good science and good clinical work involve a reciprocal interplay between the observations and judgments that lead to sound hypotheses and the investigation necessary to test them (in the language of philosopher of science Hans Reichenbach, 1938, a *context of discovery* and a *context of justification*). At its worst, clinical personality theory can seem a context of discovery without a credible context of justification—in other words, psychologically rich inference and conjecture without a credible basis for sifting sound from unsound ideas. At its worst, academic personality research can seem a context of justification without a credible context of discovery—in other words, sophisticated methodological tools applied to psychologically vacuous ideas.

Diagnosis and Case Formulation, Clinical and Statistical

The solution to the science–practice schism cannot be to turn back the clock and abandon scientific advances of the past decades, nor can it be to ignore more than a century of cumulative clinical observation and knowledge. Efforts to eliminate clinical observation and inference from empirical personality research may, inadvertently, exclude psychological phenomena of paramount importance (Cousineau & Shedler, 2006; Shedler, Mayman, & Manis, 1993).

The approach to personality described in this chapter, based on the Shedler–Westen Assessment Procedure (SWAP), bridges clinical and empirical approaches to personality and seeks to integrate the strengths of each. The approach relies on clinicians to do what clinicians do well: observe and describe individual patients or clients they know. It relies on statistical methods to do what they do well: combine information in optimal ways to derive maximally valid information (Meehl, 1954; Sawyer, 1966; Westen & Weinberger, 2004). The goal is to provide a means of conceptualizing and assessing personality that is both clinically relevant and scientifically sound.

The remainder of this chapter (a) discusses the challenges of using clinical observation and inference in research, (b) describes the development of the SWAP as a method for systematizing clinical observation and understanding, (c) illustrates its use for diagnosis and clinical case formulation, and (d) describes a new taxonomy for personality diagnosis that is both empirically based and clinically relevant.

The Challenge of Clinical Data

It has become a truism that "clinical judgment is unreliable," but truisms are not truths. In fact, the problem with clinical observation and inference is not that they are unreliable, as many investigators are happy to repeat (for a review, see Westen & Weinberger, 2004). The problem, rather, is that they come in a form that is difficult to work with. Rulers measure in inches and scales measure in pounds, but what metric do clinicians share? Consider three clinicians describing the same case. One might speak of schemas and beliefs, another of learning and conditioning, and the third, perhaps, of conflict and defense. It is not readily apparent whether the clinicians can or cannot make the same observations and inferences. There are three possibilities: (a) They may be observing the same thing but using different language and metaphor systems to describe it; (b) they may be attending to different aspects of the clinical material, as in the parable of the elephant and the blind men; or (c) they may not be able to make the same observations at all. To find out whether the clinicians can make the same observations and inferences, investigators must first ensure that they are speaking the same language and attending to the same spectrum of clinical phenomena.

DEVELOPING A STANDARD VOCABULARY FOR CASE DESCRIPTION

The SWAP is a tool for personality diagnosis and clinical case formulation that provides clinicians of all theoretical orientations with a standard vocabulary for clinical case description (Shedler & Westen, 2004a, 2004b, 2007; Westen & Shedler, 1999a, 1999b; Westen, Shedler, Bradley, & DeFife,

2012). The vocabulary consists of 200 personality-descriptive statements, each of which may describe a given patient very well, somewhat, or not at all. The clinician describes a patient by ranking the statements into eight categories, from most descriptive of the patient (scored 7) to not descriptive or irrelevant (scored 0). Thus, the SWAP yields a score from 0 to 7 for 200 personality-descriptive variables.

The major editions of the SWAP instrument are the SWAP-200 and the newer, revised SWAP-II (their precursor was the SWAP-167; Shedler & Westen, 1998). In this chapter, I use the acronym SWAP to refer to concepts and findings that apply to both major editions; I specify SWAP-200 or SWAP-II when a finding applies to a specific edition. The instrument can be obtained from http://www.SWAPassessment.org.[1]

The "standard vocabulary" of the SWAP allows clinicians to provide comprehensive, in-depth psychological descriptions of patients in a form that is systematic and quantifiable, and it ensures that all clinicians attend to the same spectrum of clinical phenomena. SWAP statements stay close to the clinical data (e.g., "Tends to get into power struggles" or "Is capable of sustaining meaningful relationships characterized by genuine intimacy and caring"), and statements that require inference or deduction are written in clear, jargon-free language (e.g., "Tends to express anger in passive and indirect ways [e.g., may make mistakes, procrastinate, forget, become sulky, etc.]" or "Tends to see own unacceptable feelings or impulses in other people instead of in him/herself").

SWAP Item Set

The initial SWAP item pool was drawn from a wide range of sources, including the clinical literature on personality pathology written over the past 50 years (e.g., Kernberg, 1975, 1984; Kohut, 1971; Linehan, 1993; Shapiro, 1965); DSM Axis II diagnostic criteria included in of the third through fourth editions of the DSM (American Psychiatric Association, 1980, 1994); selected DSM Axis I criteria that could reflect enduring dispositions (e.g., depression and anxiety); research on coping, defense, and affect regulation (e.g., Perry & Cooper, 1987; Shedler et al., 1993; Vaillant, 1992; Westen, Muderrisoglu, Fowler, Shedler, & Koren, 1997); research on interpersonal functioning in patients with PDs (e.g., Westen, 1991; Westen, Lohr, Silk, Gold, & Kerber, 1990); research on personality traits in nonclinical populations (e.g., Block,

---

[1]Versions of the SWAP have been developed for adolescent personality assessment as well (e.g., Westen, Dutra, & Shedler, 2005; Westen, Shedler, Durrett, Glass, & Martens, 2003), but discussion of adolescent personality and its assessment is beyond the scope of this chapter.

1971; John, 1990; McCrae & Costa, 1990); research on personality pathology conducted since the development of *DSM* Axis II (see, e.g., Livesley, 1995); pilot studies in which observers watched videotaped interviews of patients with personality pathology and described them using draft versions of the SWAP item set; and the clinical experience of the SWAP authors.

Perhaps most important, the current SWAP item set is the product of a 12-year iterative item revision process that incorporated the feedback of more than 2,000 clinician-consultants of all theoretical orientations who used earlier versions of the instrument to describe their patients. We asked each clinician-consultant one crucial question: "Were you able to describe the things you consider psychologically important about your patient?" We added, rewrote, and revised items based on this feedback, then asked new clinician-consultants to describe new patients. We repeated this process over many iterations, until most clinicians could answer "yes" most of the time (Westen et al., 2012).

The methods used to develop and refine the SWAP item set ensured the inclusion of clinically crucial concepts that are absent from other personality item sets. For example, clinical theorists have identified the phenomena of *splitting* and *projective identification* as central, defining features of borderline personality (Clarkin, Yeomans, & Kernberg, 2006; Gabbard, 2005; Kernberg, 1975, 1984; McWilliams, 2011). These concepts are notably absent both from the *DSM* and from dimensional trait models of personality. The SWAP–II addresses splitting with items like "When upset, has trouble perceiving both positive and negative qualities in the same person at the same time (e.g., may see others in black or white terms, shift suddenly from seeing someone as caring to seeing him/her as malevolent and intentionally hurtful, etc.)" and "Expresses contradictory feelings or beliefs without being disturbed by the inconsistency; has little need to reconcile or resolve contradictory ideas." It addresses projective identification with items like "Manages to elicit in others feelings similar to those s/he is experiencing (e.g., when angry, acts in such a way as to provoke anger in others; when anxious, acts in such a way as to induce anxiety in others)" and "Tends to draw others into scenarios, or 'pull' them into roles, that feel alien or unfamiliar (e.g., being uncharacteristically insensitive or cruel, feeling like the only person in the world who can help, etc.)."

I provide these examples of SWAP items only to illustrate that it is possible to conduct empirical research without sacrificing clinical richness and complexity and to operationalize clinical (in this instance, psychodynamic) concepts and theories that many investigators dismiss as not lending themselves to empirical investigation. I am not (yet) addressing the question of whether the theories are correct. Rather, I am making the point that such concepts, which reflect the accrued experience of generations of skilled clinical observers, deserve to be taken seriously, as hypotheses to test. Neither

DSM-based structured interviews nor FFM instruments could ever confirm or disconfirm these hypotheses *because they make no attempt to address them*.

The methods used to develop and refine the SWAP item set were successful in creating a relatively comprehensive vocabulary for clinical case description. In a sample of 1,201 psychologists and psychiatrists who used the SWAP–II to describe a current patient, 84% "agreed" or "strongly agreed" that "the SWAP–II allowed me to express the things I consider important about my patient's personality" (fewer than 5% disagreed).

Scoring the SWAP

The SWAP is based on the Q-sort method, which requires assessors to assign each score (0–7) a specified number of times (i.e., there is a "fixed" score distribution). The fixed score distribution is asymmetric, with many items receiving low scores and progressively fewer items receiving higher scores (the shape of the fixed distribution mirrors the naturally occurring distribution in the population; for a discussion of this and other psychometric issues, see Westen & Shedler, 2007). Use of a fixed distribution has psychometric advantages and reduces measurement error or "noise" inherent in standard rating scales.[2] The method maximizes the opportunity to observe statistical relations where they exist but does not, as some have mistakenly speculated, inflate or otherwise impact reliability or validity coefficients. Both Monte Carlo simulations and empirical data demonstrate that the shape of the SWAP fixed score distribution has no effect on the magnitude of correlation coefficients (Blagov, Bi, Shedler, & Westen, 2012). The psychometric rationale for the Q-sort method has been described in detail by Block (1961/1978).

When the SWAP is used in the context of psychotherapy, an experienced clinician can score the instrument after a minimum of 6 clinical contact hours with a patient. If a patient or subject is seen for assessment only—for example, in research, forensic, or personnel assessment contexts—the SWAP can be scored on the basis of the Clinical Diagnostic Interview (CDI), which systematizes and compresses into an approximately 2.5-hour time frame the kind of interviewing most skilled clinicians engage in during the initial hours of patient contact to assess personality (Westen, 2004; Westen & Muderrisoglu, 2003; Westen & Weinberger, 2004). The SWAP

---

[2]One way it does so is by ensuring that raters are calibrated with one another. Consider the situation with rating scales, where raters can use any value as often as they wish. Inevitably, certain raters gravitate toward extreme values (e.g., values of 0 and 7 on a 0–7 scale) and others toward middle values (e.g., values of 4 and 5). Thus, scores reflect not only the characteristics of the patients but also the calibration of the raters. The Q-sort method, with its fixed distribution, eliminates this source of measurement error, because all clinicians must assign each score the same number of times. If use of a standard item set gives clinicians a common vocabulary, use of a fixed score distribution can be said to give them a "common grammar" (Block, 1961/1978).

can also be scored reliably from other, comparably psychologically rich interview sources (e.g., Marin-Avellan, McGauley, Campbell, & Fonagy, 2005).

Capturing Clinical Nuance

Just as academic researchers tend to be skeptical regarding clinical observation and inference, clinicians sometimes express skepticism that any structured assessment instrument could do justice to the richness, complexity, and uniqueness of human psychological functioning. However, SWAP statements can be combined in virtually infinite patterns to capture complex, nuanced psychological phenomena and convey meanings that transcend the content of the individual items. The whole is greater than the sum of its parts. (The mathematically inclined reader might consider that the number of possible orderings of SWAP statements vastly exceeds the earth's population.)

By way of illustration, consider the meaning of the SWAP item "Tends to be sexually seductive or provocative." If a patient receives a high score on this item along with high scores on the items "Has an exaggerated sense of self-importance (e.g., feels special, superior, grand, or envied)" and "Seems to treat others primarily as an audience to witness own importance, brilliance, beauty, etc.," a portrait begins to emerge of a narcissistically organized person who may seek sexual attention to bolster a sense of being special and uniquely desirable. If this same patient also receives high scores on the items "Tends to feel s/he is not his/her true self with others; may feel false or fraudulent" and "Tends to feel s/he is inadequate, inferior, or a failure," a more complex portrait begins to emerge. The items, in combination, indicate that grandiosity coexists with painful feelings of inadequacy and serves to mask or compensate for them. This duality lies at the heart of narcissistic personality pathology (Russ, Bradley, Shedler, & Westen, 2008).

Alternatively, if the SWAP item describing sexual seductiveness is combined with the items "Tends to fear s/he will be rejected or abandoned," "Appears to fear being alone; may go to great lengths to avoid being alone," and "Tends to be ingratiating or submissive (e.g., consents to things s/he does not want to do, in the hope of getting support or approval)," a portrait begins to emerge of a person with a dependent personality style, who may rely on sexuality as a desperate means of maintaining attachments in the face of feared abandonment.

If the sexual seductiveness item is instead combined with the items "Tends to act impulsively (e.g., acts without forethought or concern for consequences)," "Takes advantage of others; has little investment in moral values (e.g., puts own needs first, uses or exploits people with little regard for their feelings or welfare, etc.)," and "Experiences little or no remorse for harm or injury caused to others," a portrait begins to emerge of a person with a psychopathic personality style who seeks immediate need gratification and has no qualms about exploiting others sexually.

These examples illustrate how SWAP items can be combined to communicate complex clinical concepts and how a single SWAP item can convey a range of meanings depending on the items that surround and contextualize it. I will further illustrate this with a case example (see Bridging Diagnosis and Clinical Case Formulation, below).

Diagnosis, Syndromal and Dimensional

The SWAP-200 generates 37 diagnostic scale scores organized into three score profiles.[3] The score profiles provide (a) dimensional scores for *DSM–IV* and *DSM–5* (American Psychiatric Association, 2013) personality disorder diagnoses, (b) dimensional scores for an alternative set of personality syndromes identified empirically through SWAP research (see An Improved Taxonomy for Personality Diagnosis, below), and (c) dimensional trait scores derived via factor analysis of the SWAP item set (Shedler & Westen, 2004a). The SWAP also generates a Psychological Health Index, which measures adaptive psychological resources and capacities, or ego strengths. The SWAP National Security Edition includes the Dispositional Indicators of Risk Exposure (DIRE) scale, which was developed in collaboration with agencies of the United States federal government to assess the potential for destructive or high-risk behavior in personnel employed in, or being evaluated for, sensitive positions such as those requiring access to classified information (Shechter & Lang, 2011).

SWAP diagnostic scores are expressed as T-scores ($M = 50$, $SD = 10$) and graphed to create score profiles, as shown in Figure 9.1.[4] SWAP-200 personality disorder scales measure the similarity or "match" between a patient and diagnostic prototypes representing each *DSM* personality disorder in its pure or "ideal" form (e.g., a prototypical patient with paranoid personality disorder). Thus, personality disorders are assessed on a continuum: Low scores indicate that the patient does not resemble or match the diagnostic prototype, and high scores indicate a strong match.

Where categorical diagnosis is desired (e.g., to facilitate clinical communication or for "backward compatibility" with the categorical approach

---

[3]SWAP-200 is available for clinical use at the time of this writing (see Shedler, 2009). SWAP-II will be available in the future and will similarly provide score profiles for *DSM* diagnoses, empirically identified personality syndromes, and factor-analytically derived trait dimensions. Computational algorithms for SWAP-II differ from those of SWAP-200 (see Westen et al., 2012, 2014).

[4]For descriptions of scale construction methods for SWAP-200, see Shedler and Westen (2004b) and Westen and Shedler (1999a, 1999b). For descriptions of scale construction methods for SWAP-II, see Westen et al. (2012, 2014).

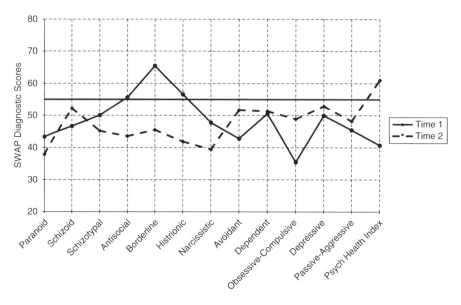

Figure 9.1. SWAP-200 Personality Disorder Score Profile (*DSM–5* diagnoses).

of *DSM*), a cut-score of T ≥ 60 provides a threshold for assigning a categorical diagnosis and a score of T ≥ 55 warrants a diagnosis of traits or features of a PD. Thus, the patient represented by the solid line in Figure 9.1 would receive a *DSM* diagnosis of "borderline personality disorder with antisocial and histrionic traits."

This approach to dimensional diagnosis preserves a *syndromal* understanding of personality. That is, it views personality as a configuration of functionally interrelated psychological processes (encompassing, for example, patterns of thinking, feeling, motivation, interpersonal functioning, coping, and defending). *Functionally related* means that the personality processes are interdependent, are causally linked, and form a coherent, recognizable configuration or whole (cf. Ahn, 1999; Cantor & Genero, 1986; Kim & Ahn, 2002).

Dimensional diagnosis follows from the recognition that all personality syndromes fall on a continuum from relatively healthy through severely disturbed. For example, a relatively healthy person with an obsessional personality style might be precise, orderly, logical, more comfortable with ideas than feelings, a bit more concerned than most with authority and control, and somewhat rigid in certain areas of thought and behavior. Toward the more disturbed end of the obsessional spectrum are individuals who are rigidly dogmatic. They have little conscious access to affect, are preoccupied with control, and misapply logic in ways that lead them to "miss the forest for the trees." Such individuals might properly be described as having a "disorder," but the threshold for diagnosing a disorder is a cut-point on a continuum (similar to many diagnoses in medicine, where variables such as blood pressure are measured on a continuum but physicians refer to certain ranges as "borderline" or "high").

Although I am emphasizing here the utility of a syndromal approach to personality, SWAP also provides dimensional trait scores, derived via factor analysis of the SWAP item set. Factor analysis of the SWAP item sets yields clinically and empirically coherent personality factors, 12 in the case of SWAP-200 (Shedler & Westen, 2004a) and 14 in the case of SWAP-II (Westen, Waller, Shedler, & Blagov, 2014). These dimensional trait or factor scores provide an additional source of information to supplement syndromal diagnosis.

Syndromal and trait models of personality serve different purposes. Among other things, the former is *person-centered* (focusing on kinds of people) and the latter is *variable-centered* (focusing on kinds of variables). Elsewhere, I have suggested that a diagnostic system is like a good map in that it must accurately depict the territory (Shedler et al., 2010). However, sometimes one requires a road map, sometimes a topographical map depicting elevations, and sometimes a political map. A road map, regardless of its validity, is of little use to a mountaineer, and a topographical map will be of little use to a motorist. One consequence of the science–practice schism is that there has been virtually no constructive discussion in the field about what kind of map is useful when. Instead, different constituencies have simply lobbied for maps that serve their own purposes, citing reliability and validity but failing to recognize that the wrong reliable and valid map can leave a different kind of traveler stranded on a cliff.

BRIDGING DIAGNOSIS AND CLINICAL CASE FORMULATION

Diagnosis and clinical case formulation are often viewed as separate activities. SWAP bridges these activities, allowing clinicians and investigators to both make psychiatric diagnoses and derive detailed clinical case formulations from the same item set.[5] I will illustrate with a clinical case example.

---

[5]This section contains ideas first published in Lingiardi, Shedler, and Gazzillo (2006). See the original publication for a more complete description of the case, treatment methods, and findings. The narrative description presented here incorporates some items from the revised SWAP-II and therefore differs slightly from the description in the original publication.

Background

"Melanie" is a 30-year-old woman with chief complaints of substance abuse and an inability to extricate herself from an abusive relationship. She was diagnosed with substance abuse, based on the Structured Clinical Interview for *DSM–IV* Axis I Disorders (SCID), and with Borderline Personality Disorder with histrionic traits, based on the SCID-II. She received a Global Assessment of Functioning (GAF) score of 45 at intake, indicating significant impairment in functioning.

Melanie's early family environment was one of neglect and family strife. A recurring scenario is illustrative: Melanie's mother would scream at her husband and say she was leaving him, then lock herself in her room, leaving Melanie frightened and in tears. Both parents would then ignore Melanie and often forget to feed her. By adolescence, Melanie was skipping school and spending her days sleeping or wandering the streets. At age 18 she left home and began "life on the streets," entering a series of chaotic sexual relationships, abusing street drugs, and engaging in petty theft. In her mid-20s, she moved in with her boyfriend, a small-time drug dealer. She periodically prostituted herself to obtain money or drugs for him.

Melanie began psychodynamic therapy at a frequency of three sessions per week. The first 10 sessions were recorded and transcribed. Two clinicians, blind to other data, reviewed the transcripts and scored the SWAP-200 based on the session transcripts. The SWAP-200 scores were averaged across the two clinical judges to enhance reliability and obtain a single SWAP description. After 2 years of psychotherapy, 10 consecutive psychotherapy sessions were again recorded and transcribed and the SWAP evaluation was repeated.

Descriptive Diagnosis

The solid line in Figure 9.1 (Time 1) shows Melanie's SWAP-200 scores profile for *DSM–IV/DSM–5* personality disorder diagnoses. Higher scale scores indicate more severe disturbance. The Psychological Health Index, which reflects clinicians' consensual understanding of healthy personality functioning (Westen & Shedler, 1999a), is graphed as well. Higher scores on the Psychological Health Index indicate greater psychological strengths and resources.

Melanie's score profile shows a marked elevation for borderline personality (T = 65, or one and a half standard deviations above the reference sample mean), with secondary elevations for histrionic personality disorder (T = 57) and antisocial personality disorder (T = 56). After application of the recommended cut-scores of T ≥ 60 for making a categorical personality disorder diagnosis and T ≥ 55 for diagnosing traits or features, Melanie's *DSM* diagnosis at the start of treatment (Time 1) is "borderline personality disorder with histrionic and antisocial traits." Also noteworthy is the low T-score of 41 on the Psychological Health Index, nearly a standard deviation below the mean in a reference sample of patients with personality disorder diagnoses. The low score indicates significant psychological deficit and impairment.

Narrative Case Description

Clinicians can move from diagnosis to individualized case description by shifting focus from diagnostic scale scores to individual SWAP items. A narrative description can be created simply by selecting and listing the 30 SWAP items with the highest scores (i.e., those scored 5, 6, or 7) or (preferably) arranging them in paragraph form to create a narrative description.

The narrative description for Melanie, below, illustrates this approach. The description is constructed exclusively from the 30 SWAP items with scores of 5 or above. To aid the flow of the text, I have grouped conceptually related items, made minor grammatical edits, and added some topic sentences and connecting text (italicized).

Melanie experiences severe depression and dysphoria. She tends to feel unhappy, depressed, or despondent, appears to find little or no pleasure or satisfaction in life's activities, feels life is without meaning, and tends to feel like an outcast or outsider. She tends to feel guilty, and to feel inadequate, inferior, or a failure. Her behavior is often self-defeating and self-destructive. She appears inhibited about pursuing goals or successes, is insufficiently concerned with meeting her own needs, and seems not to feel entitled to get or ask for things she deserves. She appears to want to "punish" herself by creating situations that lead to unhappiness or actively avoiding opportunities for pleasure and gratification. *Specific self-destructive tendencies include* getting drawn into and remaining in relationships in which she is emotionally or physically abused, abusing illicit drugs, and acting impulsively and without regard for consequences. She shows little concern for consequences generally.

Melanie has personality features associated specifically with borderline personality. Her relationships are unstable, chaotic, and rapidly changing. She has little empathy and seems unable to understand or respond to others' needs and feelings unless they coincide with her own. Moreover, she tends to confuse her own thoughts, feelings, and personality traits with those of others. She often acts in such a way as to elicit her own feelings in other people (e.g., provoking anger when she herself is angry, inducing anxiety in others when she herself is anxious), and she tends to draw people into scenarios or pull them into roles that they experience as alien and unfamiliar (e.g., being uncharacteristically cruel, feeling like the only person in the world who can help).

When upset, Melanie has difficulty perceiving positive and negative qualities in the same person at the same time (e.g., she sees others in black or white terms and may shift suddenly from seeing someone as caring to seeing them as malevolent). She expresses contradictory feelings without being disturbed by the inconsistency and seems to have little need to reconcile or resolve contradictory ideas. She lacks a stable image of who she is or would like to become (e.g., her attitudes, values, goals, and feelings about self are unstable and changing), and she tends to feel empty inside. *Her affect regulation is poor:* She tends to become irrational when strong emotions are stirred up and shows a noticeable decline from her customary level of functioning. She seems unable to soothe or comfort herself when distressed and requires the involvement of another person to help her regulate affect. Both her living arrangements and her work life tend to be chaotic and unstable.

Finally, Melanie's attitudes toward men and sexuality are problematic and conflictual. She tends to be hostile toward members of the opposite sex (whether consciously or unconsciously), and she associates sexual activity with danger (e.g., injury or punishment). She appears afraid of commitment to a long-term love relationship, instead choosing partners who seem inappropriate in terms of age, status (e.g., social, economic, intellectual), or other factors.

This narrative case description provides an in-depth portrait of a troubled patient with borderline personality pathology, highlighting personality features such as splitting, projective identification, identity diffusion, and affect dysregulation. The description illustrates the difference between descriptive psychiatry (aimed at establishing a diagnosis) and clinical case formulation (aimed at understanding the psychological makeup of an individual person). However, all the findings presented here are derived from the same quantitative SWAP data.

Melanie's case has a happy ending. The dashed line in Figure 9.1 shows Melanie's PD scores after 2 years of psychotherapy (Time 2). Her scores on the Borderline, Histrionic, and Antisocial dimensions have dropped below T = 50, and she no longer warrants any *DSM* PD diagnosis. Her score on the Psychological Health Index has increased by two standard deviations, from 41 to 61, indicating the development of substantial psychological resources and capacities (for a more complete discussion of this case, see Lingiardi, Shedler, & Gazzillo, 2006).

Reliability and Validity

Interrater reliability of SWAP diagnostic scale scores is above .80 in all studies to date and is often above .90 (Marin-Avellan et al., 2005; Westen & Muderrisoglu, 2003; Westen & Shedler, 2007). Median test–retest reliability of SWAP-II personality disorder scales, over a 4- to 6-month time interval, is .90, with a range of .86 to .96 for individual scales. Median test–retest reliability for SWAP-II factor (dimensional trait) scales is .85, with a range of .77 to .96 (Blagov et al., 2012). Median alpha reliability (Cronbach's alpha) for diagnostic scales for SWAP-II empirically derived personality syndromes (see An Improved Taxonomy for Personality Diagnosis, below) is .79, with a range from .72 to .94. These are strong reliability findings that compare favorably with reliabilities for structured interviews and questionnaires that minimize or eliminate clinical inference.

With respect to validity, SWAP diagnostic scales show predicted relations with an extensive range of external criterion variables in both adult and adolescent samples. These include genetic history variables such as psychosis and substance abuse in first- and second-degree biological relatives; developmental history variables such as childhood physical abuse, sexual abuse, animal torture, fire setting, truancy, and other school-related problems; life events such as psychiatric hospitalizations, suicide attempts, arrests, violent criminal behavior, and perpetrating domestic abuse; ratings of occupational functioning, social functioning, and global adaptive functioning; response to mental health treatment, and numerous other measures (see, e.g., Marin-Avellan et al., 2005; Shedler & Westen, 2004a; Westen & Muderrisoglu, 2003, 2006; Westen & Shedler, 1999a, 1999b, 2007; Westen, Shedler, Durrett, Glass, & Martens, 2003; Westen & Weinberger, 2004). For reviews, see Westen and Shedler (2007) and Blagov et al. (2012).

There is a well-established literature on the limitations of clinical judgment, and it is fair to ask why the SWAP yields strong reliability and validity findings that seem incongruous with this literature. The answers are straightforward. First, studies of clinical judgment have too often asked clinicians to make predictions about things that fall well outside their legitimate expertise (Westen & Weinberger, 2004).[6] In contrast, the SWAP does not ask clinicians to *predict* anything, only to describe patients they know, based on psychological information that is readily available to them. Second, studies of clinical judgment often do not use appropriate psychometric methods to quantify clinical judgment in a reliable way, as the SWAP is designed to do. Third, studies of clinical judgment typically conflate clinicians' ability to provide accurate information about their patients (which they do well) with their ability to combine and weight variables to make predictions (a task necessarily performed better by statistical methods). In fact, a substantial literature documents the reliability and validity of clinical observation and inference when it is quantified and utilized appropriately (see Westen

---

[6]Unfortunately, some clinicians have been all too willing to offer such prognostications.

& Weinberger, 2004). It is unfortunate (and telling) that research on the limitations of clinical judgment is widely cited in academic psychology while compelling research on its strengths is often overlooked.

The SWAP differs from other assessment approaches in that it harnesses clinical judgment with psychometric methods designed for this purpose, then applies statistical and actuarial methods to the resulting quantitative data. In short, it relies on clinicians to do what they do best: describe individual patients they know well. It relies on statistical algorithms to do what they do best: combine data optimally to derive reliable and valid scales and maximize prediction. In the framework of Paul Meehl's (1954) classic text *Clinical Versus Statistical Prediction*, the SWAP would be considered an example of *statistical* prediction.

AN IMPROVED TAXONOMY FOR PERSONALITY DIAGNOSIS

The system for personality diagnosis provided by the *DSM* finds little favor with clinicians or researchers (Shedler & Westen, 2004b, 2007; Westen & Shedler, 1999a). The *DSM–5* Personality and Personality Disorders Work Group attempted to replace it entirely, but ideological disputes prevented the work group from producing a viable alternative. As a result, *DSM–5* defaulted to *DSM–IV* diagnostic categories and criteria, and the opportunity for an improved, officially sanctioned system for personality diagnosis was lost.

An optimal diagnostic system should (a) "carve nature at the joints" as closely as nature reveals them and available research methods permit; (b) provide descriptions of personality syndromes that are clinically useful and relevant—ideally, they should facilitate a level of understanding that can guide treatment decisions; and (c) provide a sound, workable method for making diagnoses in day-to-day clinical practice.

An alternative to developing a diagnostic system by committee (with the unavoidable influences of group dynamics, politics, ideology, and other biases) is to derive a diagnostic taxonomy empirically. Doing so entails conducting comprehensive assessments of personality in large, clinically representative patient samples, then employing statistical methods to identify and describe naturally occurring diagnostic groupings, assuming such groupings exist.

My coinvestigators and I first described a diagnostic system based on such an approach in 1999, identifying naturally occurring diagnostic groupings in a national sample of personality disordered patients assessed with the SWAP-200 (Westen & Shedler, 1999b). In this section, I summarize the findings of newer research using the SWAP-II in a larger, more representative sample ($N = 1,201$) of adult patients (Westen et al., 2012). We used the method of Q-factor analysis to identify naturally occurring diagnostic groupings. Q-factor analysis is computationally identical to factor analysis, with the difference that factor analysis identifies groupings of similar *variables*, whereas Q-factor analysis identifies groupings of similar *cases* or *people*. The resulting diagnostic groupings are data-driven and are not the product of a committee decision process.

Data were provided by 1,201 licensed psychologists or psychiatrists, each of whom used the SWAP-II to describe a single, randomly selected current patient. The clinicians were instructed to describe "an adult patient you are currently treating or evaluating who has enduring patterns of thoughts, feelings, motivation, or behavior—that is, personality patterns—that cause distress or dysfunction." To ensure a clinically representative sample, the instructions emphasized that patients need not have a *DSM* PD diagnosis. The methods are described in our original research report (Westen et al., 2012).

An Empirically Derived Personality Taxonomy

The research identified 10 distinct, empirically and clinically coherent personality syndromes (Q-factors) organized hierarchically under superordinate groupings or broad personality spectra. Figure 9.2 illustrates the hierarchical structure of the empirically derived diagnostic system. At the level of broad superordinate groupings, the analysis identified an internalizing spectrum of personality syndromes, an externalizing spectrum, a borderline-dysregulated spectrum, and a spectrum labeled neurotic styles.

Individuals with syndromes in the *internalizing* spectrum experience chronic painful emotions, especially depression and anxiety. They tend to be emotionally constricted and socially avoidant and tend to blame themselves for their difficulties. The spectrum subsumes the diagnoses of Depressive Personality, Anxious-Avoidant Personality, Dependent-Victimized Personality, and Schizoid-Schizotypal Personality.

Individuals with syndromes in the *externalizing* spectrum are angry or hostile, self-centered, and lacking in empathy. They blame others for their difficulties. The spectrum subsumes the diagnoses of Antisocial-Psychopathic Personality, Narcissistic Personality, and Paranoid Personality.

Individuals in the *borderline-dysregulated* spectrum are qualitatively distinct from stable internalizers or stable externalizers. Their perceptions of self and others are unstable and changeable, and they show impaired ability to regulate emotion. As a result, they tend to oscillate between emotions characteristic of both internalizing and externalizing spectrum pathology (e.g., depression, anxiety, rage). They may best be described as "stably unstable" (Schmideberg, 1959). The salience of affect dysregulation in the clinical

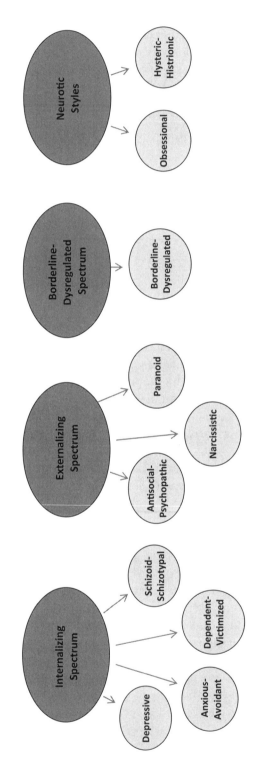

Figure 9.2. Hierarchical structure of personality diagnoses.

picture led my coinvestigators and I to hyphenate the name of the syndrome and add *dysregulated* to the more familiar term *borderline*.

The *neurotic styles* spectrum subsumes the diagnoses of Obsessional Personality and Hysteric-Histrionic Personality. The name of the spectrum reflects the recognition that individuals with these personality syndromes are, on average, higher functioning than those in the other diagnostic groupings and may or may not show a level of impairment that warrants the term *disorder*. The two personality syndromes resemble the character styles or "neurotic styles" described in the clinical literature (e.g., MacKinnon, Michels, & Buckley, 2009; McWilliams, 2011; Shapiro, 1965) more than they resemble *DSM* descriptions of obsessive–compulsive and histrionic personality disorders. The framers of *DSM–III* amplified the level of pathology of these personality syndromes to fit them into a medical-model taxonomy of disorders. Unfortunately, the resulting *DSM* diagnostic criteria described caricatures, not the patients generally seen in real-world practice.

Empirically Derived Descriptions of Personality Syndromes

In addition to identifying naturally occurring personality syndromes, our research method allowed us to generate an empirically-derived description of each personality syndrome. A description of the core, defining features of each diagnostic grouping or syndrome was obtained simply by listing the SWAP items with the highest factor scores for the syndrome. I will use borderline-dysregulated personality for illustration.

Exhibit 9.1 lists the 24 SWAP items with the highest factor scores for borderline-dysregulated personality (the items most central to the syndrome).[7] A number of findings are noteworthy. First, the emergence of this diagnostic grouping in the Q-factor analysis validates the concept of borderline personality as a diagnostic entity. Second, the items describe a psychologically richer and more complex syndrome than described by the *DSM*. Third, the description addresses internal psychological processes and aspects of inner experience that are crucial to understanding and treating this personality syndrome.

The findings also indicate that clinical theories that view splitting, projective identification, and related psychological processes as central to borderline personality are, in fact, accurate. Overall, the empirically-derived personality syndrome more closely resembles the concept of borderline

---

[7]To facilitate understanding of this complex syndrome, I have grouped the items under several broad themes. Another investigator might quibble with my method of organization, but the headings and item groupings serve only to facilitate presentation; they have no bearing on the definition or assessment of the personality syndrome.

EXHIBIT 9.1
Empirically-Derived Description of Borderline-Dysregulated Personality

Affect dysregulation

Emotions tend to change rapidly and unpredictably.

Emotions tend to spiral out of control, leading to extremes of anxiety, sadness, rage, etc.

Tends to become irrational when strong emotions are stirred up; may show a significant decline from customary level of functioning.

Is prone to intense anger, out of proportion to the situation at hand (e.g., has episodes of rage).

Is unable to soothe or comfort him/herself without the help of another person (i.e., has difficulty regulating own emotions).

Tends to "catastrophize"; is prone to see problems as disastrous, unsolvable, etc.

Tends to feel unhappy, depressed, or despondent.

Splitting

When upset, has trouble perceiving both positive and negative qualities in the same person at the same time; sees others in black or white terms (e.g., may swing from seeing someone as caring to seeing him/her as malevolent and intentionally hurtful).

Tends to stir up conflict or animosity between other people (e.g., may portray a situation differently to different people, leading them to form contradictory views or work at cross purposes).

Projective identification

Manages to elicit in others feelings similar to those she/he is experiencing (e.g., when angry, acts in such a way as to provoke anger in others; when anxious, acts in such a way as to induce anxiety in others).

Tends to draw others into scenarios, or pull them into roles, that feel alien or unfamiliar (e.g., being uncharacteristically insensitive or cruel, feeling like the only person in the world who can help).

Identity diffusion

Lacks a stable sense of who she/he is (e.g., attitudes, values, goals, and feelings about self seem unstable or ever-changing).

Is prone to painful feelings of emptiness (e.g., may feel lost, bereft, abjectly alone even in the presence of others).

Insecure attachment

Tends to be needy or dependent.

Appears to fear being alone; may go to great lengths to avoid being alone.

Tends to fear she/he will be rejected or abandoned.

Tends to become attached quickly or intensely; develops feelings, expectations, etc. that are not warranted by the history or context of the relationship.

Tends to feel misunderstood, mistreated, or victimized.

Self-harm (desperate efforts to self-regulate)

Tends to engage in self-mutilating behavior (e.g., self-cutting, self-burning).

Tends to make repeated suicidal threats or gestures, either as a "cry for help" or as an effort to manipulate others.

Struggles with genuine wishes to kill him/herself.

Chaotic lifestyle

Relationships tend to be unstable, chaotic, and rapidly changing.

Work life and/or living arrangements tend to be chaotic or unstable (e.g., job or housing situation seems always temporary, transitional, or ill-defined).

Tends to be impulsive.

personality *organization* described in the clinical literature (e.g., Clarkin et al., 2006; Kernberg, 1975, 1984; McWilliams, 2011) than it does the *DSM* description of borderline personality disorder.

The items or personality features constituting the description of borderline-dysregulated personality (and all of the other empirically-identified syndromes) cannot be explained away as artifacts of clinicians' theoretical preconceptions. They emerged repeatedly when we stratified the sample by the theoretical orientation of the reporting clinicians, with the same items ranked highly by psychodynamic clinicians, cognitive-behavioral clinicians, humanistic clinicians, biologically-oriented clinicians, and so on.

Psychometric Assessment With the SWAP

We developed the SWAP-II diagnostic scales to assess the empirically derived diagnostic syndromes by summing the most descriptive SWAP-II items for each syndrome (thus, the diagnostic scale for borderline-dysregulated personality comprises the 24 items listed in Exhibit 9.1). The number of scale items ranges from a low of 14 (for paranoid personality) to a high of 24 (for borderline-dysregulated personality), with the number of items reflecting the psychological complexity of the syndrome. Alpha reliabilities for the diagnostic scales range from .72 to .94, with a median reliability of .79. All diagnostic scores are scaled as normalized T-scores (M = 50, SD = 10) to facilitate test interpretation.

An empirically derived Psychological Health Index was created by the same method and yielded an additional scale assessing global personality health/dysfunction. All personality syndromes fall on a continuum of functioning, and the score on the Psychological Health Index provides a context for interpreting other SWAP scale scores. An elevated score for a personality syndrome, coupled with a high Psychological Health Index score, indicates that the person is functioning at the healthier end of the health-pathology continuum for that syndrome, and a low score on the Psychological Health Index indicates the opposite. For example, a patient with an elevated score for paranoid personality and a high Psychological Health Index score has meaningful psychological resources (ego strengths) to draw upon and may be able to make constructive use of psychotherapy. A patient with the same paranoid personality score and a low Psychological Health Index score may prove untreatable. Both patients are likely to incorporate the therapist into a paranoid worldview, suspecting the therapist of nefarious motives and intentions. However, the first patient will likely retain a capacity to reflect on his experience of the therapist and call his perceptions into question, whereas the second patient may not.

Diagnosis in Day-to-Day Practice

When maximum psychometric precision is required or where there are challenging diagnostic dilemmas, assessors can describe patients with the SWAP and obtain diagnostic scale scores for all the empirically-derived personality syndromes (as well as for *DSM* personality disorder diagnoses and for SWAP factors or trait dimensions). For day-to-day diagnosis, my coinvestigators and I have proposed a diagnostic system based on *prototype matching*.

In prototype matching diagnosis, the descriptions of the empirically-derived personality syndromes are presented in paragraph rather than list form, to create a narrative description of each personality syndrome. The narrative descriptions constitute *diagnostic prototypes* that describe each syndrome in its "ideal" or "pure" form. The diagnostic prototypes comprise the SWAP-II items that are most defining of each syndrome (the same items used to construct the psychometric scales), organized and edited to create narratively coherent paragraphs. Each prototype description is preceded by a single-sentence summary intended to orient the diagnostician and convey telegraphically the core features of the syndrome.

The diagnostician's task is to consider the prototype description as a whole—that is, as a configuration or gestalt—and rate the overall similarity or match between a patient and the diagnostic prototype. The resulting diagnosis is dimensional (a 1–5 rating), but the scale can be dichotomized when a categorical (present/absent) diagnosis is desired (with ratings ≥ 4 indicating "caseness").

Figure 9.3 illustrates the prototype matching approach to personality diagnosis, with depressive personality used as an example. Despite its omission from the *DSM*, depressive personality appears to be the most prevalent personality syndrome seen in the community (Westen & Shedler, 1999b). Diagnostic prototypes for all of the empirically derived personality syndromes are reproduced in our original research report (Westen et al., 2012) and are available for download from http://www.SWAPassessment.org.

Prototype matching works *with*, rather than against, the naturally occurring cognitive decision processes of diagnosticians. It has considerable advantages over the criterion-counting approach of the *DSM*, leading to improved diagnostic reliability and validity as well as reduced diagnostic comorbidity. In head-to-head comparisons clinicians rated the SWAP prototype matching approach as more clinically useful and relevant than both the *DSM* diagnostic system and dimensional trait models of personality (e.g., Rottman et al., 2009; Spitzer et al., 2008). The conceptual rationale for the prototype matching method and the research evidence supporting it are described in detail elsewhere (see Westen, DeFife, Bradley, & Hilsenroth, 2010; see also Ortigo,

Summary statement: Individuals With Depressive Personality are prone to feelings of depression and inadequacy, tend to be self-critical or self-punitive, and may be preoccupied with concerns about abandonment or loss.

Individuals who match this prototype tend to feel depressed or despondent and to feel inadequate, inferior, or a failure. They tend to find little pleasure or satisfaction in life's activities and to feel life has no meaning. They are insufficiently concerned with meeting their own needs, disavowing or squelching their hopes and desires to protect against disappointment. They appear conflicted about experiencing pleasure, inhibiting feelings of excitement, joy, or pride. They may likewise be conflicted or inhibited about achievement or success (e.g., failing to reach their potential or sabotaging themselves when success is at hand). Individuals who match this prototype are generally self-critical, holding themselves to unrealistic standards and feeling guilty and blaming themselves for bad things that happen. They appear to want to "punish" themselves by creating situations that lead to unhappiness or avoiding opportunities for pleasure and gratification. They have trouble acknowledging or expressing anger and instead become depressed, self-critical, or self-punitive. Individuals who match this prototype often fear that they will be rejected or abandoned, are prone to painful feeling of emptiness, and may feel bereft or abjectly alone even in the presence of others. They may have a pervasive sense that someone or something necessary for happiness has been lost forever (e.g., a relationship, youth, beauty, success).

Please form an overall impression of the type of person described, then rate the extent to which your patient matches or resembles this prototype.

5	very good match (patient ***exemplifies*** this disorder; prototypical case)	**Diagnosis**
4	good match (patient ***has*** this disorder; diagnosis applies)	
3	moderate match (patient has ***significant features*** of this disorder)	**Features**
2	slight match (patient has minor features of this disorder)	
1	no match (description does not apply)	

Figure 9.3. Depressive Personality Prototype.

Bradley, & Westen, 2010; Shedler & Westen, 2004b; Westen, Shedler, & Bradley, 2006).

CONCLUSION: INTEGRATING CLINICAL AND EMPIRICAL PERSPECTIVES

A clinically useful diagnostic system should encompass the spectrum of personality syndromes seen in clinical practice and have meaningful treatment implications. An empirically sound diagnostic system should facilitate reliable and valid diagnoses: Independent clinicians should be able to arrive at the same diagnosis, diagnoses should be distinct, and each diagnosis should be associated with conceptually meaningful correlates, antecedents, and sequelae.

An obstacle to achieving this ideal has been the persistent schism between science and practice in the mental health professions. Too often, empirical research has been conducted in isolation from the crucial data of clinical observation, and clinical theory has developed without regard for empirical credibility. Professional researchers and professional clinicians tend to talk past rather than with one another.

SWAP research represents an effort to bridge the science–practice schism by quantifying clinical observation and expertise, thus making clinical constructs accessible to empirical study. It relies on clinicians to make observations and inferences about individual patients they know and relies on quantitative methods to reveal relationships and combine data in optimal ways.

The SWAP provides a "language" for clinical case description that is both psychometrically sound and clinically rich enough to describe the complexities of real patients. A sizable schism remains between science and practice. Perhaps the SWAP will provide a language all parties can speak.

REFERENCES

Ahn, W.-K. (1999). Effect of causal structure on category construction. *Memory & Cognition, 27,* 1008–1023. doi:10.3758/BF03201231

American Psychiatric Association. (1980). *Diagnostic and statistical manual of mental disorders* (3rd ed.). Washington, DC: Author.

American Psychiatric Association. (1994). *Diagnostic and statistical manual of mental disorders* (4th ed.). Washington, DC: Author.

American Psychiatric Association. (2013). *Diagnostic and statistical manual of mental disorders* (5th ed.). Arlington, VA: Author.

Betan, E., Heim, A. K., Conklin, C. Z., & Westen, D. (2005). Countertransference phenomena and personality pathology in clinical practice: An empirical investigation. *The American Journal of Psychiatry, 162,* 890–898. doi:10.1176/appi.ajp.162.5.890

Blagov, P. S., Bi, W., Shedler, J., & Westen, D. (2012). The Shedler–Westen Assessment Procedure (SWAP): Evaluating psychometric questions about its reliability, validity, and impact of its fixed score distribution. *Assessment, 19,* 370–382. doi:10.1177/1073191112436667

Block, J. (1971). *Lives through time.* Berkeley, CA: Bancroft.

Block, J. (1978). *The Q-sort method in personality assessment and psychiatric research.* Palo Alto, CA: Consulting Psychologists Press. (Original work published 1961)

Cantor, N., & Genero, N. (1986). Psychiatric diagnosis and natural categorization: A close analogy. In T. Millon & G. L. Klerman (Eds.), *Contemporary directions in psychopathology: Toward the DSM–IV* (pp. 233–256). New York, NY: Guilford Press.

Clarkin, J. F., Yeomans, F. E., & Kernberg, O. F. (2006). *Psychotherapy for borderline personality: Focusing on object relations*. Washington, DC: American Psychiatric Publishing.

Cousineau, T. M., & Shedler, J. (2006). Predicting physical health: Implicit mental health measures versus self-report scales. *Journal of Nervous and Mental Disease, 194*, 427–432. doi:10.1097/01.nmd.0000221373.74045.51

Gabbard, G. O. (2005). *Psychodynamic psychiatry in clinical practice* (4th ed.). Washington, DC: American Psychiatric Publishing.

John, O. (1990). The "Big Five" factor taxonomy: Dimensions of personality in the natural language and in questionnaires. In L. Pervin (Ed.), *Handbook of personality: Theory and research* (pp. 66–100). New York, NY: Guilford Press.

Kernberg, O. (1975). *Borderline conditions and pathological narcissism*. New York, NY: Aronson.

Kernberg, O. (1984). *Severe personality disorders*. New Haven, CT: Yale University Press.

Kernberg, O. (1996). A psychoanalytic theory of personality disorders. In J. F. Clarkin & M. F. Lenzenweger (Eds.), *Major theories of personality disorder* (pp. 106–137). New York, NY: Guilford Press.

Kim, N. S., & Ahn, W. (2002). Clinical psychologists' theory-based representations of mental disorders predict their diagnostic reasoning and memory. *Journal of Experimental Psychology: General, 131*, 451–476. doi:10.1037/0096-3445.131.4.451

Kohut, H. (1971). *The analysis of the self*. New York, NY: International Universities Press.

Linehan, M. M. (1993). *Cognitive-behavioral treatment of borderline personality disorder*. New York, NY: Guilford Press.

Lingiardi, V., Shedler, J., & Gazzillo, F. (2006). Assessing personality change in psychotherapy with the SWAP-200: A case study. *Journal of Personality Assessment, 86*, 23–32. doi:10.1207/s15327752jpa8601_04

Livesley, W. J. (Ed.). (1995). *The DSM–IV personality disorders*. New York, NY: Guilford Press.

MacKinnon, R., Michels, R., & Buckley, P. (2009). *The psychiatric interview in clinical practice* (2nd ed.). Washington, DC: American Psychiatric Publishing.

Marin-Avellan, L. E., McGauley, G., Campbell, C., & Fonagy, P. (2005). Using the SWAP-200 in a personality-disordered forensic population: Is it valid, reliable and useful? *Journal of Criminal Behaviour and Mental Health, 15*, 28–45. doi:10.1002/cbm.35

McCrae, R., & Costa, P., Jr. (1990). *Personality in adulthood*. New York, NY: Guilford Press.

McWilliams, N. (2011). *Psychoanalytic diagnosis: Understanding personality structure in the clinical process* (2nd ed.). New York, NY: Guilford Press.

Meehl, P. E. (1954). *Clinical versus statistical prediction: A theoretical analysis and a review of the evidence.* doi:10.1037/11281-000

Meehl, P. E. (1973). Why I do not attend case conferences. In *Psychodiagnosis: Selected papers* (pp. 225–302). Minneapolis: University of Minnesota Press.

Ortigo, K. M., Bradley, B., & Westen, D. (2010). An empirically based prototype diagnostic system for *DSM–V* and *ICD–11*. In T. Millon, R. Krueger, & E. Simonsen (Eds.), *Contemporary directions in psychopathology: Scientific foundations of the* DSM–V *and* ICD–11 (pp. 374–390). New York, NY: Guilford Press.

Peebles, M. J. (2012). *Beginnings: The art and science of planning psychotherapy* (2nd ed.). New York, NY: Routledge.

Perry, J. C., & Cooper, S. H. (1987). Empirical studies of psychological defense mechanisms. In R. Michels & J. O. Cavenar (Eds.), *Psychiatry* (Vol. 1, pp. 1–19). Philadelphia, PA: Lippincott.

Reichenbach, H. (1938). *Experience and prediction.* Chicago, IL: University of Chicago Press.

Rottman, B. M., Ahn, W. K., Sanislow, C. A., & Kim, N. S. (2009). Can clinicians recognize *DSM–IV* personality disorders from five-factor model descriptions of patient cases? *The American Journal of Psychiatry, 166,* 427–433. doi:10.1176/appi.ajp.2008.08070972

Russ, E., Shedler, J., Bradley, R., & Westen, D. (2008). Refining the construct of narcissistic personality disorder: Diagnostic criteria and subtypes. *The American Journal of Psychiatry, 165,* 1473–1481. doi:10.1176/appi.ajp.2008.07030376

Sawyer, J. (1966). Measurement and prediction, clinical and statistical. *Psychological Bulletin, 66,* 178–200. doi:10.1037/h0023624

Schmideberg, M. (1959). The borderline patient. In S. Arieti (Ed.), *American handbook of psychiatry* (Vol. 1, pp. 398–416). New York, NY: Basic Books.

Shapiro, D. (1965). *Neurotic styles.* New York, NY: Basic Books.

Shechter, O. G., & Lang, E. L. (2011). *Identifying personality disorders that are security risks: Field test results* (Tech. Rep. No. 11-05). Retrieved from http://www.dhra.mil/perserec/reports/tr11-05.pdf

Shedler, J. (2009). *Guide to SWAP-200 interpretation.* Retrieved from http://www.SWAPassessment.org

Shedler, J., Beck, A. T., Fonagy, P., Gabbard, G. O., Gunderson, J., Kernberg, O., . . . Westen, D. (2010). Commentary: Personality disorders in *DSM–5. The American Journal of Psychiatry, 167,* 1026–1028. doi:10.1176/appi.ajp.2010.10050746

Shedler, J., Mayman, M., & Manis, M. (1993). The illusion of mental health. *American Psychologist, 48,* 1117–1131. doi:10.1037/0003-066X.48.11.1117

Shedler, J., & Westen, D. (1998). Refining the measurement of Axis II: A Q-sort procedure for assessing personality pathology. *Assessment, 5,* 333–353.

Shedler, J., & Westen, D. (2004a). Dimensions of personality pathology: An alternative to the five-factor model. *The American Journal of Psychiatry, 161,* 1743–1754.

Shedler, J., & Westen, D. (2004b). Refining *DSM–IV* personality disorder diagnosis: Integrating science and practice. *The American Journal of Psychiatry, 161,* 1350–1365.

Shedler, J., & Westen, D. (2006). Personality diagnosis with the Shedler–Westen Assessment Procedure (SWAP): Bridging the gulf between science and practice. In Alliance Task Force (Ed.), *Psychodynamic diagnostic manual* (pp. 573–613). Silver Spring, MD: Alliance of Psychoanalytic Organizations.

Shedler, J., & Westen, D. (2007). The Shedler–Westen Assessment Procedure (SWAP): Making personality diagnosis clinically meaningful. *Journal of Personality Assessment, 89,* 41–55.

Spitzer, R. L., First, M. B., Shedler, J., Westen, D., & Skodal, A. E. (2008). Clinical utility of five dimensional systems for personality diagnosis: A "consumer preference" study. *Journal of Nervous and Mental Disease, 196,* 3567–374. doi:10.1097/NMD.0b013e3181710950

Vaillant, G. (Ed.). (1992). *Ego mechanisms of defense: A guide for clinicians and researchers.* Washington, DC: American Psychiatric Press.

Westen, D. (1991). Social cognition and object relations. *Psychological Bulletin, 109,* 429–455. doi:10.1037/0033-2909.109.3.429

Westen, D. (2004). *Clinical Diagnostic Interview.* Atlanta, GA: Emory University, Departments of Psychology and Psychiatry and Behavioral Sciences.

Westen, D., DeFife, J. A., Bradley, B., & Hilsenroth, M. J. (2010). Prototype personality diagnosis in clinical practice: A viable alternative for *DSM–5* and *ICD-11. Professional Psychology: Research and Practice, 41,* 6, 482–487. doi:10.1037/a0021555

Westen, D., Dutra, L., & Shedler, J. (2005). Assessing adolescent personality pathology: Quantifying clinical judgment. *British Journal of Psychiatry, 186,* 227–238. doi:10.1192/bjp.186.3.227

Westen, D., Lohr, N., Silk, K., Gold, L., & Kerber, K. (1990). Object relations and social cognition in borderlines, major depressives, and normals: A TAT analysis. *Psychological Assessment, 2,* 355–364. doi:10.1037/1040-3590.2.4.355

Westen, D., & Muderrisoglu, S. (2003). Reliability and validity of personality disorder assessment using a systematic clinical interview: Evaluating an alternative to structured interviews. *Journal of Personality Disorders, 17,* 350–368.

Westen, D., & Muderrisoglu, S. (2006). Clinical assessment of pathological personality traits. *The American Journal of Psychiatry, 163,* 1285–1297. doi:10.1076/appi.ajp.163.7.1285

Westen, D., Muderrisoglu, S., Fowler, C., Shedler, J., & Koren, D. (1997). Affect regulation and affective experience: Individual differences, group differences, and measurement using a Q-sort procedure. *Journal of Consulting and Clinical Psychology, 65,* 429–439. doi:10.1037/0022-006X.65.3.429

Westen, D., & Shedler, J. (1999a). Revising and assessing Axis II: I. Developing a clinically and empirically valid assessment method. *The American Journal of Psychiatry, 156*, 258–272.

Westen, D., & Shedler, J. (1999b). Revising and assessing Axis II: II. Toward an empirically based and clinically useful classification of personality disorders. *The American Journal of Psychiatry, 156*, 258–272.

Westen, D., & Shedler, J. (2007). Personality diagnosis with the Shedler–Westen Assessment Procedure (SWAP): Integrating clinical and statistical measurement and prediction. *Journal of Abnormal Psychology, 116*, 810–822. doi:10.1037/0021-843X.116.4.810

Westen, D., Shedler, J., Bradley, B., & DeFife, J. (2012). An empirically derived taxonomy for personality diagnosis: Bridging science and practice in conceptualizing personality. *The American Journal of Psychiatry, 169*, 273–284. doi:10.1176/appi.ajp.2011.11020274

Westen, D., Shedler, J., & Bradley, R. (2006). A prototype approach to personality diagnosis. *The American Journal of Psychiatry, 163*, 846–856. doi:10.1176/appi.ajp.163.5.846

Westen, D., Shedler, J., Durrett, C., Glass, S., & Martens, A. (2003). Personality diagnosis in adolescence: *DSM–IV* Axis II diagnoses and an empirically derived alternative. *The American Journal of Psychiatry, 160*, 952–966. doi:10.1176/appi.ajp.160.5.952

Westen, D., Waller, N. G., Shedler, J., & Blagov, P. S. (2014). Dimensions of personality and personality pathology: Factor structure of the Shedler–Westen Assessment Procedure–II (SWAP-II). *Journal of Personality Disorders, 28*, 281–318. doi:10.1521/pedi_2012_26_059

Westen, D., & Weinberger, J. (2004). When clinical description becomes statistical prediction. *American Psychologist, 59*, 595–613. doi:10.1037/0003-066X-59.7.595

Widiger, T. A., & Simonsen, E. S. (2005). Alternative dimensional models of personality disorders: Finding common ground. *Journal of Personality Disorders, 19*, 110–130. doi:10.1521/pedi.19.2.110.62628

10

ASSESSING EXPLICIT AND IMPLICIT PROCESSES IN PERSONALITY PATHOLOGY

IRVING B. WEINER

This chapter on explicit and implicit approaches to the assessment of personality pathology begins with definitions of personality style, personality pathology, and personality assessment. The text then addresses advantages and limitations of explicit and implicit methods of personality assessment and identifies standardized measures that exemplify these two assessment approaches. The discussion emphasizes the benefits of integrating these explicit and implicit measures in clinical assessment practice.

PERSONALITY STYLE, PERSONALITY PATHOLOGY, AND PERSONALITY ASSESSMENT

Personality style consists of an individual's customary ways of thinking, feeling, and acting. These customary ways of behaving are commonly referred to as *traits*, which can also be defined as abiding dispositions to behave in

http://dx.doi.org/10.1037/14549-011
Personality Disorders: Toward Theoretical and Empirical Integration in Diagnosis and Assessment,
S. K. Huprich (Editor)

certain ways in certain kinds of situations. As further elaborated by Roberts, Donnellan, and Hill (2013), traits are what people automatically think, feel, and do, and they constitute habituated and automatic rather than planned and deliberate patterns of behavior. Although they are habituated and automatic, these behavior patterns do not cause people to respond in the same way at all times, however. Personality styles are individualistic blends of various traits. Depending on the particular mix of their dispositions, people may conduct themselves in one way in some situations and in a different way in other situations, as in being assertive and demanding at home but passive and deferential when at work. By generating similar types of responses in similar situations, personality styles lead people to behave in a distinctive but fairly consistent and predictable manner.

Personality pathology consists of a maladaptive exaggeration of one or more features of an individual's personality style. Personality styles that become pathological or disordered evolve into rigidly entrenched and inflexible patterns of behavior that interfere with an individual's capacities to work productively and relate comfortably to others. Whatever interpersonal problems or behavioral dysfunctions they may have, however, individuals with personality disorders (PDs) seldom attribute them to unwelcome aspects of themselves that should be changed. To the contrary, individuals with PD are usually content with themselves and feel justified in being the way they are. Instead of seeing any need to change, they blame their adjustment difficulties on circumstances outside their control or the actions of others, and they consider these circumstances or other people as what needs to change.

Because people vary in the extent to which they are well or poorly adjusted, flexible or single-minded, and constructively self-critical or unreflectively self-content, the maladaptive behavior, rigidity, and self-satisfaction that characterize PDs are dimensional characteristics. On this basis, numerous authors have presented a compelling rationale for describing and assessing PDs as dimensional rather than categorical phenomena (e.g., Clark, 2007; Huprich & Bornstein, 2007; Trull, Carpenter, & Widiger, 2013; Widiger & Mullins-Sweatt, 2010). Although conceptually sound, this dimensional perspective unavoidably blurs the distinction between personality styles and personality pathology and makes it difficult to draw lines between them. There are no fixed rules for deciding whether a person is showing enough maladjustment, rigidity, and self-satisfaction to warrant diagnosing a PD. In illustrative diagnostic terms, there is no absolute criterion for determining whether features of dependency, narcissism, or compulsivity have become sufficiently exaggerated or pervasive to constitute a dependent, narcissistic, or obsessive–compulsive PD.

Without fixed rules and absolute criteria, deciding whether an individual's personality style has crystallized into a PD usually requires examiners to exercise some judgment. To be sure, available assessment scales and conceptual formulations provide cutoff scores and qualitative criteria that can be helpful in diagnosing PD. However, quantitative scales for identifying PDs and other dimensional phenomena typically offer a range of choices rather than a single cutoff score to be used in every case. Guided by the reference data for a particular scale, examiners must select a cutoff score likely to produce both a high percentage of correct classifications and a desired balance between sensitivity and specificity. Lowering the cutoff score increases the sensitivity of a scale at the expense of its specificity (by producing more false positive classifications), whereas raising the cutoff score makes a scale more specific but less sensitive (by increasing the frequency of false negatives classifications; see Trull, 2005).

Hence, the selection of scale cutoff scores often depends on examiner judgments concerning whether the purposes of an evaluation are better served by maximizing true positive (highly sensitive) or true negative (highly specific) results. Despite any uncertainty in choosing precise scale scores for inferring the presence of a PD, it remains the case that the higher a person's score on these scales or the more clearly the person manifests relevant qualitative criteria, the more likely he or she is to have a PD. To recap the qualitative guideline umbrella for identifying personality pathology, the more an individual's personality style has become maladaptive, the more rigidly it governs the person's life, and the more accepting the individual is of it, the more likely it is that this style has evolved into a PD.

Personality assessment consists of integrating information from diverse sources to identify an individual's personality characteristics. These information sources include interviews with the person who is being assessed and with other people who know the individual well; reviews of health, school, military, and other relevant records concerning the person; observations of the person in certain kinds of natural or contrived situations; and administration to the person of a battery of standardized personality tests (see Butcher, 2009; Harwood, Beutler, & Groth-Marnat, 2011; Weiner & Greene, 2008).

Personality assessment provides descriptions of an individual's personality traits and states. As previously noted, personality traits are abiding dispositions to act in certain ways in certain situations. Personality traits define what people are generally like and how people are likely to behave, and they comprise a broad range of fairly stable characteristics and orientations, such as being generally reserved or demonstrative, altruistic or self-centered, outgoing or reclusive, careful or careless, or caring or callous. *Personality states*, on the other hand, are the current content of a person's thoughts and feelings. They consist of relatively transitory affects and attitudes that arise in response to situational circumstances, such as being happy, angry, anxious, wary, or deeply in thought at the moment.

Personality states are independent of personality traits and are unrelated to personality pathology or disorder. Individuals with a borderline PD can be happy or sad at particular moments in time, for example, but they continue to have a borderline PD during each of these moments. An individual with a narcissistic PD can be anxious or relaxed at various times, but he or she remains a narcissistic person on each of these occasions. As elaborated by Morey and Hopwood (2013), neither personality traits nor PDs are immutable during a person's lifetime, and they may become modified in the course of events. Nevertheless, personality pathology is not a transitory state of the individual, and its assessment must accordingly emphasize the nature and implications of personality traits. Because personality traits and any personality pathology attributable to them are largely stable phenomena, furthermore, psychological test variables or scales intended to assess PD should show good retest reliability.

EXPLICIT AND IMPLICIT APPROACHES IN PERSONALITY ASSESSMENT

The assessment of personality pathology is a two-step process that involves (a) identifying an individual's personality style and (b) deciding whether this style is sufficiently maladaptive, rigidly entrenched, and self-accepted to be considered pathological. Explicit approaches to this assessment process consist of direct inquiries into a person's attitudes, affects, self-perceptions, and life experiences. Among the previously mentioned sources of information in personality assessments, these direct inquiries include behavioral observations, record reviews, interviews, and personality testing with self-report inventories. The following discussion of explicit measures focuses mainly on self-report inventories, in particular the Minnesota Multiphasic Personality Inventory—2 (MMPI–2; Butcher, 2011; Graham, 2006).

Self-report inventories consist of statements on which respondents describe themselves by endorsing a Yes or No answer or by selecting a point on a Likert scale (e.g., alternatives ranging from "Very Much Like Me" to "Not at All Like Me"). Should a person report Yes to MMPI–2 statements assessing the respondent's willingness to let others take charge or to be swayed even after having made a decision, there would be fairly definite basis for inferring the presence of passive-dependent personality characteristics.

In contrast with the directness of an explicit approach to personality assessment, implicit approaches are indirect methods of assessment that infer characteristics of people not from what they say about themselves or what others say about them but from how they perform on various tasks. Implicit assessment is exemplified by the Rorschach Inkblot Method (RIM), in which respondents are asked what a series of inkblots might be (Exner, 2003; Weiner, 2003). In common with most other indirect personality measures, the RIM provides both structural and thematic data. As an illustration of structural data and their implications, Rorschach respondents who report what numerous details of the blots look like but seldom attend to any of the blots in their entirety are likely to be people who generally become preoccupied with the details of situations and fail to grasp their overall significance, as in not seeing the forest for the trees. As an illustration of thematic Rorschach data and their implications, a person who frequently sees the blots as figures with blood on them and as objects that have been damaged or destroyed may be revealing fears of being harmed or feelings of vulnerability to becoming injured or unable to function effectively.

These Rorschach inferences are less definite and more open to alternative implications than would be direct statements by people that they often become preoccupied with details or worry about coming to harm. On the other hand, these illustrative responses may indirectly identify styles and concerns that would not come to light in direct assessments of what people are able and willing to say about themselves. In these respects, both explicit and implicit approaches bring advantages and limitations to the assessment process, as elaborated next.

Advantages and Limitations of Explicit Approaches

Because of their directness, explicit assessments usually provide more definite information than do implicit measures. As noted in the MMPI example just given, a stated preference for having other people make decisions for them warrants fairly definite conclusions about passivity and dependence. In most respects, respondents who describe themselves accurately on direct personality assessment measures are providing reasonably certain and dependable indications of their personality characteristics. By contrast, inferring in the previous Rorschach example that giving responses only to details of the blots indicates a characteristic preoccupation with details poses a reasonable possibility but not a definite certainty. Direct assessments of the person's behavioral style would be necessary to confirm preoccupation with details as a general characteristic of the individual.

In further contrast to explicit assessments, implicit measures often leave examiners with alternative possibilities rather than any single conclusion. In the Rorschach example of bleeding figures and damaged objects suggesting concerns about being harmed or vulnerable to injury, the possibility would have to be considered that the respondent is identifying with the victimizer and not the victim. Were that the case, the blood and damage in the Rorschach responses would be suggesting not a fearful person but an angry or sadistic person who enjoys giving harm to others or observing their harm.

As another Rorschach example, suppose a man describes a human figure in one of the blots as "A woman with her arms up, like she is waving at someone." Does this figure represent the man's mother, or wife, or employer, or teacher, or women in general? Is the woman waving hello or waving goodbye, which would have different implications for what this man expects from this woman, whomever she represents? Some speculative hypotheses could be framed in response to these questions, but direct inquiry would be necessary to provide reasonably definite answers to them. As these examples show, implicit assessment in general and thematic imagery in particular seldom provide adequate basis for statements of certainty but instead generate alternative possibilities and speculative hypotheses. Explicit assessment approaches accordingly have the advantage of going beyond alternative possibilities and speculative hypotheses to arrive at relatively certain statements about personality characteristics.

As a second advantage of self-report inventories, they are easier to administer than performance-based measures. Respondents can work on their own to complete these measures, whether with paper and pencil or on a computer. Examiners need to give instructions, provide some supervision, and be available to answer questions, but they do not otherwise have to be engaged in the administration process. Computerized administration can also record responses, calculate scores and scales, and print out results, thereby sparing examiners from having to devote time to these tasks. Software programs are available for some performance-based measures as well (e.g., Exner & Weiner, 2003), but these programs produce printouts only after an examiner has administered the measure, coded the responses in some fashion, and entered the response codes into a computer template.

This ease of administration gives self-report inventories a related third advantage over performance-based measures, which is the relative simplicity of conducting research with them. A pencil-and-paper administration allows groups of virtually any size to take a self-report inventory simultaneously, and dozens or even hundreds of test protocols can be collected in a single session, depending on the size of the room. Researchers find it much more demanding to include some personality characteristics among their variables if they use performance-based rather than self-report measures. Validating research on personality assessment methods is consequently more extensive for self-report than for performance-based measures. This does not mean that performance-based measures are necessarily less valid than self-report measures, but only that having to administer them to one research participant at a time has restricted the collection of validating data concerning them. Nonetheless, recent reviews of performance-based measures, such as the Rorschach, have documented their validity and clinical utility (Mihura, Meyer, Dumitrascu, & Bombel, 2013).

The main limitation of explicit approaches to personality assessment is their dependence on what people are able and willing to say when asked to describe themselves. With respect to what they are able to self-report, people vary in how correctly they perceive themselves and in the extent of their self-awareness. For example, respondents who endorse Yes on MMPI–2 items indicating that they are well liked and emotionally calm may not in fact be as well liked or as emotionally resilient as they perceive themselves to be, and research studies have documented conspicuous inaccuracy in self-assessments of one's characteristics and competencies (Dunning, Heath, & Suls, 2004). As for their self-awareness, respondents may not be fully mindful of interpersonal problems or behavioral difficulties they have had. Most people have feelings and attitudes that are outside their conscious awareness, and most people have had life experiences that they recall vaguely or not at all.

With respect to their willingness to describe themselves, most people are aware of personal characteristics and past actions that they would rather not disclose, whether because of embarrassment or possible unwelcome consequences of the disclosure. Unwilling respondents try to limit their revelations and restrict what examiners can learn about them. Even when such respondents cooperate with explicit assessment procedures by answering all of the questions they are asked and responding to every test item, their guardedness can compromise the accuracy and dependability of the information they provide.

In addition to having limitations resulting from the inability or unwillingness of people to describe themselves fully and accurately, explicit assessments are vulnerable to uncertainty caused by disagreement among sources of information. Research findings have confirmed common clinical experience that people may describe themselves on self-report inventories or during an interview differently from how they are observed to behave, how others describe them, and what historical documents say about them. As noted by Ganellen (2007) and Trull et al. (2013), examiners faced with these disagreements often find it difficult to determine which of these information sources is most dependable. Disagreements have been found to arise not only among but within these direct information sources. Research reviewed by Widiger and Boyd (2009) showed generally good agreement among several self-report measures of PDs but also some instances of minimal convergent validity. As for collateral reports, informants frequently differ in how well they know the person they are describing, how accurately they perceive this person, and personal reasons they may have for describing the person in glowing or uncomplimentary terms.

A further limitation of self-report inventories is the lack of opportunity their administration provides for behavioral observation. Whereas interviews and performance-based assessments involve examiners in ongoing face-to-face interaction with people they are evaluating, self-report administration is largely an impersonal procedure in which, as already noted, examinees work by themselves. Self-report administrations consequently provide less information than interviews and performance-based assessments about a respondent's interpersonal style, general demeanor, energy level, and expectations of doing well or poorly. Item endorsements on self-administered questionnaires can contribute to identifying these personality characteristics, but they do not carry the weight of observing manifestations of these characteristics firsthand.

Advantages and Limitations of Implicit Approaches

As indirect measures in which people are asked not to describe themselves but to perform various tasks, implicit approaches to personality assessment are more likely than interviews or self-report inventories to elicit clues to personal characteristics and behavioral tendencies of which individuals are not fully aware or that they are reluctant to divulge. The indirect nature and lack of obvious item content in performance-based measures can be particularly helpful in evaluating respondents who are reluctant to admit their shortcomings or hesitant to report difficulties they are having when asked about these directly. Faced with the relatively ambiguous test stimuli (e.g., inkblots) and minimal instructions (e.g., "What might this be?") of performance-based measures, guarded respondents typically find it difficult to decide how to respond, and they may consequently provide more information about their personal problems and characteristics than was their intent.

Similarly, with regard to the extent of a person's self-awareness, indirect measures can often provide glimpses of an inner life of attitudes and concerns of which an individual being examined is not fully conscious and is therefore unable to report directly. Because performance-based assessments generate alternative possibilities and speculative hypotheses, as previously noted, they often raise as many questions as they answer. However, this disadvantage relative to direct assessments can also prove advantageous in the assessment process, because alternatives and speculations may reveal what is beneath the surface and lead examiners to consider and explore attitudes and concerns that might otherwise go unrecognized.

As a related advantage of implicit approaches in personality assessment, the minimal face validity of performance-based measures makes them relatively resistant to impression management. On the MMPI–2, respondents can easily recognize that Yes answers on items having to do with "feeling blue" or a lack of self-confidence are indications of depressed affect and low self-esteem, respectively. By contrast, examinees asked what inkblots look like have little way of knowing what their responses signify. Those who want to appear more psychologically troubled or disturbed than is actually the case, or who want to present a deceptively positive picture of their psychological soundness and well-being, will have considerably more difficulty tailoring their responses to create their desired impression on performance-based measures than when they are answering direct questions about their mental state and behavior patterns. Likely in this regard is a direct relationship between the face validity of a measure and its fakability (Bornstein, Rossner, Hill, & Stepanian, 1994; McDaniel, Beier, Perkins, Goggin, & Frankel, 2009).

This difference between explicit and implicit approaches does not mean that self-report inventories are commonly compromised by impression management and performance-based measures are immune to them. To the contrary, most self-report inventories provide validity scales that help to identify overreporting or underreporting of psychological difficulties and personal attributes (see Ben-Porath, 2013). As for performance-based measures, misleading results are difficult but not impossible for respondents to achieve. Although this possibility cannot be ruled out, contemporary concerns that online information about presumably "good" and "bad" responses to give on the Rorschach has undercut its resistance to impression management appear overblown. The effects of this information exposure have been found to be minimal, and there are available guidelines by which Rorschach examiners can usually detect examinee efforts to appear psychologically better or worse off than they are (Schultz & Brabender, 2013; Weiner, 2013).

The main limitation of implicit approaches in personality assessment is that, unlike interviews, records, and self-report inventories, they provide little information about an individual's life history, current behavior patterns, and psychological symptom formation. Lack of this information makes it particularly difficult to decide solely on the basis of performance-based assessments whether a respondent's personality style has become a diagnosable PD. Other limitations of implicit assessment are counterpoint to the previously identified advantages of explicit approaches. Whereas the direct nature of self-report inquiries can generate definite conclusions, the indirect nature of performance-based measures results in alternative possibilities and sometimes even strong likelihoods but rarely any certainties. Performance-based measures require more training and time to administer and score than do self-report inventories, which makes them less efficient in clinical practice and more difficult to include in research studies.

STANDARDIZED PERSONALITY ASSESSMENT MEASURES

Psychology in the United States has had a long tradition of behaviorism, largely as the legacy of John Watson and B. F. Skinner. From the perspective of behaviorism, all that matters in psychology is what can be observed. Skinner was adamant that understanding and predicting behavior consisted of identifying connections between stimuli and responses, and he had no interest in unseen "black-box" processes that might mediate these connections. As a reflection of this behaviorist perspective, assessment in mainstream psychology emphasized explicit methods, and those who endorsed or practiced implicit assessments were pejoratively labeled "soft-headed" to contrast them with presumably more respectable "hard-headed" psychologists.

Interestingly, however, Skinner (1953) also made the uncharacteristic observation that behavior related to ambiguous stimuli can "reveal variables which the individual himself cannot identify" (p. 289). This observation anticipated an influential article in which McClelland, Koestner, and Weinberger (1989) conceptualized differences between self-attributed and implicit motives. The McClelland et al. conceptualization expanded awareness of the advantages of implicit assessment in clinical practice, enhanced the respectability of indirect measurement, and extended the application of implicit approaches from clinical practice to many fields of psychological research (see Fazio & Olson, 2003; Gawronski & Payne, 2010; Rudman, 2011).

Both explicit and implicit approaches have generated standardized personality assessment measures that facilitate clinical practice and enrich research studies. Many of these measures have proved helpful in recognizing personality pathology as well as personality style. The discussion that follows identifies some widely used measures of these kinds and their implications for assessing personality pathology.

Explicit Measures of Personality Pathology

Explicit assessments of personality pathology include interview schedules, omnibus self-report inventories, and focused questionnaires for measuring one or more specific PD. Among available diagnostic interview schedules, the one most suitable for assessing personality pathology is the Structured Clinical Interview for *DSM–IV* Axis II Personality Disorders (SCID–II;

First & Gibbon, 2004). The SCID–II is semistructured, in that interviewers can ask respondents to clarify their answers, but the items themselves are based directly on *Diagnostic and Statistical Manual of Mental Disorders* (DSM; American Psychiatric Association, 2013) criteria for PDs. The SCID–II is commonly used as the criterion against which the validity of other measures of PD is judged.

Among the four most widely used omnibus self-report inventories, the previously referenced MMPI–2 can be scored for some PD scales, but these scales have received scant attention in the literature. On the other hand, textbook discussions of the most commonly occurring MMPI–2 code types list PDs that should be considered or ruled out for each of them (Weiner & Greene, 2008, pp. 150–186). As for the other three widely studied and applied personality self-report inventories, the Millon Clinical Multiaxial Inventory–III (Craig, 2008) includes 14 scales for specific PDs, whereas the Personality Assessment Inventory (Morey & Hopwood, 2006), despite its breadth in other respects, includes only two such scales, one for borderline features and one for antisocial features. The NEO Personality Inventory— Revised (NEO-PI–R; Costa & McCrae, 2008) was designed to measure dimensions of personality and was not intended to identify psychopathology. Nevertheless, a procedure developed by Widiger and Lowe (2007) for diagnosing PD from the perspective of the five-factor model on which the NEO-PI–R is based is showing considerable utility in this regard (Widiger & Costa, 2013). An extensive body of research has validated these four self-report inventories as measures of personality and has found sufficient retest reliability to qualify them as useful measures of personality pathology as well.

Frequently used questionnaires specifically designed to identify a range of personality disorders include the Personality Disorder Questionnaire–4 (Bagby & Farvolden, 2004), the Coolidge Axis II Inventory (Coolidge & Merwin, 1992), the Dimensional Assessment of Personality Pathology (Livesley, 2006), and the Schedule for Nonadaptive and Adaptive Personality (Simms & Clark, 2006). The items in these questionnaires are based either on *DSM* criteria for the various PDs or on descriptions in the literature of traits characteristic of these disorders. These questionnaires correlate reasonably well with SCID–II classification and have demonstrated good retest reliability.

A more recently developed personality pathology questionnaire, the General Assessment of Personality Disorder (GAPD), is intended to transcend variability across specific PDs and assess instead PD as a general type of psychopathology (Hentschel & Livesley, 2013). The GAPD comprises scales for self-pathology and interpersonal pathology, both of which correlate significantly with most of the SCID–II PD scores. Also frequently mentioned in the literature are four scales designed to identify specific disorders: the Borderline Personality Inventory (Leichsenring, 1999), the Depressive Personality Inventory (DPI; Huprich & Roberts, 2012), the Pathological Narcissism Inventory (Pincus, 2013), and the Psychopathic Personality Inventory–Revised (Edens & McDermott, 2010). Each of these scales has been validated against appropriate criteria, but the DPI is the only one for which retest correlations have so far been reported.

Two other personality measures bridge explicit and implicit assessment by consisting of descriptive statements that are rated by clinicians on the basis of their knowledge of the person being evaluated. The Shedler–Westen Assessment Procedure (SWAP) asks clinicians to describe the person by sorting 200 statements considered characteristic of various PDs into eight piles ranging from those that most accurately to those that least accurately describe the individual (Blagov, Bi, Shedler, & Westen, 2012; see also Chapter 9, this volume). The Psychopathy Checklist—Revised (PCL–R) is focused more narrowly than the SWAP on a single PD, psychopathy, but it similarly calls on clinicians to use information they have gained from various sources to rate the extent of 20 characteristics of the individual that are likely to occur in a psychopathic PD (Hare & Neuman, 2006). The SWAP and the PCL–R have been extensively validated, and both measures have demonstrated good to excellent retest reliability. Additional information concerning these and other standardized measures of personality pathology is provided in a review by Widiger and Boyd (2009).

Implicit Measures of Personality Pathology

The best known implicit personality assessment measures are the previously referenced RIM and a variety of storytelling, figure-drawing, and sentence completion tests, commonly used examples of which are the Thematic Apperception Test, the Draw-a-Person, and the Rotter Incomplete Sentences Blank (Hogan, 2005; Weiner & Greene, 2008). Except for the RIM, these indirect measures are used mainly to measure personality dynamics rather than personality pathology. As such, they identify underlying attitudes and concerns but provide only incidental information about PD. As for the RIM, it shares with explicit assessment methods the difficulty of drawing clear lines between personality style and PD, and the extensive quantification of Rorschach data in Exner's (2003) Comprehensive System (CS) does not include any PD scales.

However, the Rorschach CS does provide some well-validated indices of personality characteristics that correspond to *DSM* criteria for particular PDs. The RIM additionally contains some indices of personality stability, rigidity, and self-satisfaction that can help to identify the exaggeration of a personality style into a diagnosable PD. Some advantages of assessing PD with the

RIM are elaborated by Huprich and Ganellen (2006), and Rorschach clinicians have formulated guidelines for utilizing this measure in the evaluation of a broad range of specific PDs (see Huprich, 2006).

In addition to clinical instruments, other kinds of implicit assessment procedures have been developed for research purposes. Notable among these are association tasks that monitor reaction time to, memory for, or evaluation of (e.g., good–bad, pleasant–unpleasant) certain words, statements, or pictures. The most widely researched of these instruments is the Implicit Association Test (Olson & Fazio, 2004; Yovel & Friedman, 2013), and performance on conditional reasoning problems is also proving useful as an implicit measure of personality characteristics (James & LeBreton, 2012). Similarly, there have been recent advances in developing reliable and valid Thematic Apperception Test scales (Jenkins, 2008).Whether these measures can contribute to the assessment of personality pathology is a question for future research.

INTEGRATING EXPLICIT AND IMPLICIT APPROACHES

Whether undertaken to identify PD or for any other diagnostic or treatment planning purpose, personality assessment is most effective when the obtained data provide thorough and dependable information about the person being evaluated. The dependability of assessment information is greatest when the information comprises what people are able and willing to say about themselves, clues to dispositions and inner thoughts and feelings that are outside of conscious awareness, and indications of efforts at impression management. This statement recaps the discussion in this chapter of the advantages and limitations of explicit and implicit approaches to assessing PD. Explicit approaches provide definite information and are relatively easy to administer, but they are relatively insensitive to underlying personality characteristics and relatively susceptible to underreporting and underreporting. Implicit approaches are relatively attuned to a person's inner life and resistant to impression management, but they provide little information about a respondent's personal history and actual life behavior and often warrant only speculative inferences. However, combining these approaches, particularly in the form of an integrated test battery, compensates for their limitations and maximizes the dependability and consequent utility of a PD assessment.

This value of multimethod assessment has been recognized since the publication of Campbell and Fiske's (1959) seminal article about it, and assessment psychologists generally concur that integrating data from different types of tests will paint a fuller and more accurate picture of an individual's personality functioning than will testing only with self-report inventories or performance-based measures. The Psychological Assessment Work Group, a task force appointed by the American Psychological Association Board of Professional Affairs to examine the utility of psychological assessment methods, similarly concluded that conjoint testing with self-report and performance-based instruments is how "practitioners have historically used the most efficient means at their disposal to maximize the validity of their judgments about individual clients" (Meyer et al., 2001, p. 150). With specific respect to the two most widely used personality assessment measures, the self-report MMPI–2 and the performance-based RIM, there have been abundant conceptualizations and empirical confirmation going back many years of the incremental validity provided by their joint use (Ganellen, 1996; Weiner, 1993). This incremental validity of combining direct indirect measures has been demonstrated in experimental personality research as well as clinical practice (Back, Schmulke, & Egloff, 2009). In light of the requisites for effective assessment and the comparisons presented here between explicit and implicit approaches, clinicians are well advised to include both self-report and performance-based measures in their personality test batteries.

REFERENCES

American Psychiatric Association. (2013). *Diagnostic and statistical manual of mental disorders* (5th ed.). Arlington, VA: Author.

Back, M. D., Schmulke, S. C., & Egloff, B. (2009). Predicting actual behavior from the explicit and implicit self-concept of personality. *Journal of Personality and Social Psychology, 97*, 533–548. doi:10.1037/a0016229

Bagby, R. M., & Farvolden, P. (2004). The Personality Diagnostic Questionnaire–4 (PDQ-4). In M. J. Hilsenroth & D. L. Segal (Eds), *Comprehensive handbook of psychological assessment* (Vol. 2, pp. 122–133). Hoboken, NJ: Wiley.

Ben-Porath, Y. S. (2013). Self-report inventories: Assessing personality and psychopathology. In I. B. Weiner (Series Ed.), J. R. Graham (Vol. Ed.), & J. A. Naglieri (Vol. Ed.), *Handbook of psychology: Vol. 10. Assessment psychology* (2nd ed., pp. 622–644). Hoboken, NJ: Wiley.

Blagov, P. S., Bi, W., Shedler, J., & Westen, D. (2012). The Shedler–Westen Assessment Procedure (SWAP): Evaluating psychometric questions about its reliability, validity, and impact of its fixed score distribution. *Assessment, 19*, 370–382. doi:10.1177/1073191112436667

Bornstein, R. F., Rossner, S. C., Hill, E. L., & Stepanian, M. L. (1994). Face validity and fakability of objective and projective measures of dependency. *Journal of Personality Assessment, 63*, 363–386. doi:10.1207/s15327752jpa6302_14

Butcher, J. N. (Ed.). (2009). *Oxford handbook of personality assessment*. New York, NY: Oxford University Press.

Butcher, J. N. (2011). *A beginner's guide to the MMPI–2* (3rd ed.). Washington, DC: American Psychological Association.

Campbell, D. T., & Fiske, D. W. (1959). Convergent and discriminant validation by the multitrait-multimethod matrix. *Psychological Bulletin, 56*, 81–105. doi:10.1037/h0046016

Clark, L. A. (2007). Assessment and diagnosis of personality disorder: Perennial issues and an emerging reconceptualization. *Annual Review of Psychology, 58*, 227–257. doi:10.1146/annurev.psych.57.102904.190200

Costa, P. T., Jr., & McCrae, R. R. (2008). The revised NEO Personality Inventory (NEO-PI–R). In G. J. Boyle, G. Matthews, & D. H. Saklofske (Eds.), *The SAGE handbook of personality theory and assessment: Vol. 2. Personality measurement and testing* (pp. 179–198). Thousand Oaks, CA: Sage.

Coolidge, F. L., & Merwin, M. M. (1992). Reliability and validity of the Coolidge Axis II Inventory. *Journal of Personality Assessment, 59*, 223–238.

Craig, R. J. (2008). Essentials of MCMI-III assessment. In R. P. Archer & J. R. Smith (Eds.), *Personality assessment* (pp. 135–165). New York, NY: Routledge.

Dunning, D., Heath, C., & Suls, J. M. (2004). Flawed self-assessment: Implications for health, education, and the workplace. *Psychological Science in the Public Interest, 5*, 69–106. doi:10.1111/j.1529-1006.2004.00018.x

Edens, J. F., & McDermott, B. E. (2010). Examining the construct validity of the Psychopathic Personality Inventory—Revised: Preferential correlates of fearless dominance and self-centered impulsivity. *Psychological Assessment, 22*, 32–42. doi:10.1037/a0018220

Exner, J. E., Jr. (2003). *The Rorschach: A comprehensive system* (4th ed.). Hoboken, NJ: Wiley.

Exner, J. E., Jr., & Weiner, I. B. (2003). *Rorschach Interpretation Assistance Program (RIAP 5)*. Odessa, FL: Psychological Assessment Resources.

Fazio, R. H., & Olson, M. A. (2003). Implicit measures in social cognition research: Their meaning and use. *Annual Review of Psychology, 54*, 297–327. doi:10.1146/annurev.psych.54.101601.145225

First, M. B., & Gibbon, M. (2004). The Structured Clinical Interview for *DSM–IV* Axis I Disorders (SCID–I) and the Structured Clinical Interview for *DSM–IV* Axis II Disorders (SCID–II). In M. J. Hilsenroth, D. L. Segal, & M. Hersen (Eds), *Comprehensive handbook of psychological assessment: Vol. 2. Personality assessment* (pp. 134–143). New York, NY: Wiley.

Ganellen, R. J. (1996). *Integrating the Rorschach and the MMPI–2 in personality assessment*. Hillsdale, NJ: Erlbaum.

Ganellen, R. J. (2007). Assessing normal and abnormal personality functioning: Strengths and weaknesses of self-report, observer, and performance-based methods. *Journal of Personality Assessment, 89*, 30–40. doi:10.1080/00223890701356987

Gawronski, B., & Payne, B. K. (Eds.). (2010). *Handbook of implicit social cognition: Measurement, theory, and applications*. New York, NY: Guilford Press.

Graham, J. R. (2006). *MMPI–2: Assessing personality and psychopathology*. New York, NY: Oxford University Press.

Hare, R. D., & Neuman, C. S. (2006). The PCL–R assessment of psychopathy: Development, structural properties, and new directions. In C. J. Patrick (Ed.), *Handbook of psychopathy* (pp. 58–88). New York, NY: Guilford Press.

Harwood, T. M., Beutler, L. E., & Groth-Marnat, G. (2011). *Integrative assessment of adult personality* (3rd ed.). New York, NY: Guilford Press.

Hentschel, A. G., & Livesley, W. J. (2013). The General Assessment of Personality Disorder (GAPD): Factor structure, incremental validity of self-pathology, and relations to *DSM–IV* personality disorders. *Journal of Personality Assessment, 95,* 479–485. doi:10.1080/00223891.2013.778273

Hogan, T. P. (2005). Fifty widely used psychological tests. In G. P. Koocher, J. C. Norcross, & S. S. Hill III (Eds.), *Psychologists' desk reference* (2nd ed., pp. 101–104). New York, NY: Oxford University Press.

Huprich, S. K. (Ed.). (2006). *Rorschach assessment of the personality disorders*. Mahwah, NJ: Erlbaum.

Huprich, S. K., & Bornstein, R. F. (2007). An overview of issues related to categorical and dimensional models of personality disorder assessment. *Journal of Personality Assessment, 89,* 3–15. doi:10.1080/00223890701356904

Huprich, S. K., & Ganellen, R. J. (2006). The advantages of assessing personality disorders with the Rorschach. In S. K. Huprich (Ed.), *Rorschach assessment of the personality disorders* (pp. 27–56). Mahwah, NJ: Erlbaum.

Huprich, S. K., & Roberts, C. R. D. (2012). The two-week and five-week dependability and stability of the Depressive Personality Inventory and its association with current depressive symptoms. *Journal of Personality Assessment, 94,* 205–209. doi:10.1080/00223891.2011.645930

James, L. R., & LeBreton, J. M. (2012). *Assessing the implicit personality through conditional reasoning*. Washington, DC: American Psychological Association.

Jenkins, S. R. (2008). *A handbook of clinical scoring systems for thematic apperceptive techniques*. Mahwah, NJ: Erlbaum.

Leichsenring, F. (1999). Development and first results of the Borderline Personality Inventory: A self-report instrument for assessing borderline personality organization. *Journal of Personality Assessment, 73,* 45–63. doi:10.1207/S15327752JPA730104

Livesley, W. J. (2006). The Dimensional Assessment of Personality Pathology (DAPP). In S. Strack (Ed.), *Differentiating normal and abnormal personality* (2nd ed., pp. 401–429). New York, NY: Springer.

McClelland, D. C., Koestner, R., & Weinberger, J. (1989). How do self-attributed and implicit motives differ? *Psychological Review, 96,* 690–702. doi:10.1037/0033-295X.96.4.690

McDaniel, M. J., Beier, M. E., Perkins, A. W., Goggin, S., & Frankel, B. (2009). An assessment of the fakability of self-report and implicit personality measures. *Journal of Research in Personality, 43*, 682–685.

Meyer, G. J., Finn, S. E., Eyde, L. D., Kay, G. G., Moreland, K. L., Dies, R. R., . . . Reed, G. M. (2001). Psychological testing and psychological assessment: A review of evidence and issues. *American Psychologist, 56*, 128–165. doi:10.1037/0003-066X.56.2.128

Mihura, J. L., Meyer, G. J., Dumitrascu, N., & Bombel, G. (2013). The validity of individual Rorschach variables: Systematic reviews and meta-analyses of the Comprehensive System. *Psychological Bulletin, 139*, 548–605. doi:10.1037/a0029406

Morey, L. C., & Hopwood, C. J. (2006). The Personality Assessment Inventory. In R. P. Archer (Ed.), *Forensic uses of clinical assessment instruments* (pp. 89–120). Mahwah, NJ: Erlbaum.

Morey, L. C., & Hopwood, C. J. (2013). Stability and change in personality disorders. *Annual Review of Clinical Psychology, 9*, 499–528.

Olson, M. A., & Fazio, R. H. (2004). Reducing the influence of extrapersonal associations on the Implicit Association Test: Personalizing the IAT. *Journal of Personality and Social Psychology, 86*, 653–667. doi:10.1037/0022-3514.86.5.653

Pincus, A. L. (2013). The Pathological Narcissism Inventory. In J. S. Ogrodniczuk (Ed.), *Understanding and treating pathological narcissism* (pp. 93–110). Washington, DC: American Psychological Association.

Roberts, B. W., Donnellan, M. B., & Hill, P. L. (2013). Personality trait development in adulthood. In I. B. Weiner (Series Ed.), H. Tennen (Vol. Ed.), & J. Suls (Vol. Ed.), *Handbook of psychology: Vol. 5. Personality and social psychology* (2nd ed., pp. 183–196). Hoboken, NJ: Wiley.

Rudman, L. A. (2011). *Implicit measures for social and personality psychology.* Thousand Oaks, CA: Sage.

Schultz, D. S., & Brabender, V. M. (2013). More challenges since Wikipedia: The effect of exposure to Internet information about the Rorschach on selected Comprehensive System variables. *Journal of Personality Assessment, 95*, 149–158. doi:10.1080/00223891.2012.725438

Simms, L. J., & Clark, L. A. (2006). The Schedule for Nonadaptive and Adaptive Personality (SNAP): A dimensional measure of traits relevant to personality and personality pathology. In S. Strack (Ed.), *Differentiating normal and abnormal personality* (2nd ed., pp. 431–450). New York, NY: Springer.

Skinner, B. F. (1953). *Science and human behavior.* New York, NY: Macmillan.

Trull, T. J. (2005). Dimensional models of personality disorder: Coverage and cut-offs. *Journal of Personality Disorders, 19*, 262–282. doi:10.1521/pedi.2005.19.3.262

Trull, T. J., Carpenter, R. W., & Widiger, T. A. (2013). Personality disorders. In I. B. Weiner (Series Ed.), G. Stricker (Vol. Ed.), & T. A. Widiger (Vol. Ed.), *Handbook of psychology: Vol. 8: Clinical psychology* (2nd ed., pp. 94–120). Hoboken, NJ: Wiley.

Weiner, I. B. (1993). Clinical considerations in the conjoint use of the Rorschach and MMPI. *Journal of Personality Assessment, 60,* 148–152. doi:10.1207/s15327752jpa6001_12

Weiner, I. B. (2003). *Principles of Rorschach interpretation* (2nd ed.). Mahwah, NJ: Erlbaum.

Weiner, I. B. (2013). The Rorschach inkblot method. In R. P. Archer & E. M. A. Wheeler (Eds.), *Forensic uses of clinical assessment instruments* (2nd ed., pp. 202–229). New York, NY: Routledge.

Weiner, I. B., & Greene, R. L. (2008). *Handbook of personality assessment.* Hoboken, NJ: Wiley.

Widiger, T. A., & Boyd, S. E. (2009). Personality disorder assessment instruments. In J. N. Butcher (Ed.), *Oxford handbook of personality assessment* (pp. 336–363). New York, NY: Oxford University Press.

Widiger, T. A., & Costa, P. T., Jr. (Eds.). (2013). *Personality disorders and the five-factor model of personality* (3rd ed.). Washington, DC: American Psychological Association.

Widiger, T. A., & Lowe, J. (2007). Five-factor model assessment of personality disorder. *Journal of Personality Assessment, 89,* 16–29. doi:10.1080/00223890701356953

Widiger, T. A., & Mullins-Sweatt, S. N. (2010). Clinical utility of a dimensional model of personality disorder. *Professional Psychology: Research and Practice, 41,* 488–494. doi:10.1037/a0021694

Yovel, I., & Friedman, A. (2013). Bridging the gap between explicit and implicit measurement of personality: The questionnaire-based implicit association test. *Personality and Individual Differences, 54,* 76–80. doi:10.1016/j.paid.2012.08.015

11

PROCESS-FOCUSED ASSESSMENT OF PERSONALITY PATHOLOGY

ROBERT F. BORNSTEIN

Across the decades, a curious circularity has characterized the conceptualization and assessment of personality pathology. Early models of personality dysfunction (e.g., those of Kraepelin, Schneider, and others) tended to be rooted in biology, emphasizing the physiological substrates of disordered behavior (see Millon, 2011). Although there were no formal, psychometrically sound instruments for the assessment of personality disorders (PDs) when these early models were in ascendance, one might imagine that—had such instruments existed—they would have focused on linking the neurological underpinnings of personality pathology with the trait patterns and surface behaviors characteristic of different PDs. With the National Institute of Mental Health (NIMH) now emphasizing the role of endophenotypes and aberrant neural processes in the etiology and dynamics of mental disorders (including PDs), the stage is set for a return to a more biological conceptualization of personality

http://dx.doi.org/10.1037/14549-012
Personality Disorders: Toward Theoretical and Empirical Integration in Diagnosis and Assessment,
S. K. Huprich (Editor)

dysfunction, albeit one that draws upon contemporary neuroimaging methods (e.g., fMRI) and more precise genetic markers (see Insel & Wang, 2010; NIMH, 2008).

In the interim, PD research has taken quite a detour: When Bornstein (2003) examined PD screening measures and outcome variables in published studies of personality pathology between 1991 and 2000 he found that 81% of these investigations relied exclusively on self-report data, both to assess PDs and to quantify their correlates. This situation has not changed (for updated findings, see Bornstein, 2011; Cizek, Rosenberg, & Koons, 2008; Hogan & Agnello, 2004). Moreover, regardless of their preferred methodology and theoretical allegiance, clinical investigators generally agree that for the past several decades PD research has been dominated by interviews and self-report scales (see Rogers, 2003; Widiger & Samuel, 2005).

Structured interviews and questionnaires have several advantages in assessing personality pathology. Questionnaires are efficient and cost-effective, allowing for rapid assessment in clinical settings and large-scale data collection in laboratory and community studies. Structured clinical interviews—though less efficient than questionnaires with respect to time and cost—allow the interviewer's clinical skill and experience to enter into the assessment process and enable the assessor to revise and adjust the flow of questions as information accumulates. Life history information and behavioral observations obtained during the interview can be incorporated into the assessment and help guide the interviewer's conclusions as well.

As clinical researchers have noted (e.g., Huprich, Bornstein, & Schmitt, 2011), questionnaires and interviews also have some significant limitations in the assessment of personality pathology. By design, most PD questionnaires yield substantial numbers of false positives (Rogers, 2003). Interviews can be comparatively costly and time consuming, and myriad studies have shown that, no matter how well-trained or well-intentioned interviewers are, their conclusions are invariably tainted by information-processing heuristics that allow extraneous information (e.g., gender, age, ethnicity) to influence their inferences and conclusions (Garb, 1998). Perhaps most important, interviews and self-report tests rely primarily (sometimes exclusively) on patients' self-reports. A plethora of studies in cognitive and social psychology have shown that self-attributions are unreliable sources of information regarding past and present behavior even under the best of circumstances (Fernández, 2013; von Hippel & Trivers, 2011). When patients with PD—people who are known a priori to have limited insight—are assessed, these problems are compounded exponentially.

SOME UNINTENDED CONSEQUENCES
OF RELIANCE ON SELF-REPORTS

Clearly, assessing personality pathology by asking individuals with limited insight to describe their intra- and interpersonal dynamics and then taking these reports at face value is unwarranted. In addition, overreliance on interview and questionnaire methods has had several unintended negative effects. These are discussed in the following sections.

Excessive PD Comorbidity

People who perceive themselves as having personality problems typically describe these problems as emerging in multiple domains and affecting multiple areas of life (e.g., friendships, romantic relationships, work relationships; see Crawford, Koldobsky, Mulder, & Tyrer, 2011). As a result, when PDs are assessed via traditional self-report measures, most patients acknowledge symptoms from multiple PD categories. The number of differential diagnoses per PD in the *Diagnostic and Statistical Manual of Mental Disorders* (4th ed., text rev. [*DSM–IV–TR*]; American Psychiatric Association, 2000) ranges from 3 (Dependent, Obsessive-Compulsive) to 7 (Paranoid), with the mean number of differential diagnoses per category being 4.5. When Ekselius, Lindstrom, Knorring, Bodlund, and Kullgren (1994) calculated correlations among Structured Clinical Interview for *DSM–IV* Axis II Disorders (SCID-II) scores for *DSM* (4th ed.) PDs in a heterogeneous sample of psychiatric inpatients and nonclinical participants, they obtained a mean interscale correlation (*r*) of .41 and statistically significant interscale correlations in 41 of 45 comparisons (see also Wise, 1996, for parallel findings). Similar results were obtained by Cox, Clara, Worobec, and Grant (2012).

Failure to Capture Underlying PD Dynamics

Because measures that rely primarily on self-reports reflect how people perceive and present themselves, they do not allow clinicians and researchers to assess aspects of PDs that are not easily verbalized (e.g., underlying conflicts, implicit motives, defenses; see Huprich, 2011). Few patients with Narcissistic PD describe themselves as grandiose, and few psychopaths describe themselves as callous and cruel. Evidence confirms that in the absence of other types of data, self-reports provide limited information regarding whether a withdrawn, detached patient is schizoid or avoidant (McWilliams, 2006), or whether high levels of interpersonal dependency reflect underlying dependent or histrionic pathology (Blais & Baity, 2006). These dynamics must be documented with measures that go beyond self-description.

Inattention to Situational Variability in PD-Related Responding

Although clinical lore holds that narcissistic patients tend to be brazen and haughty in interpersonal interactions, in fact their behavior varies considerably across relationship domains, with many narcissists appearing self-confident around subordinates and peers but self-effacing when interacting with figures of authority (Morf & Rhodewalt, 2001; see also Zeigler-Hill, Myers, & Clark, 2010). When asked to describe themselves in questionnaires and interviews, dependent patients typically present themselves as being passive and timid; in fact, dependent college students compete quite aggressively to curry favor with figures of authority (Bornstein, Riggs, Hill, & Calabrese, 1996), dependent men are at significantly increased risk for perpetrating domestic violence when threatened with abandonment (Bornstein, 2006), and dependent parents (mothers and fathers alike) show elevated rates of child abuse (Bornstein, 2005).

PROCESS-FOCUSED ASSESSMENT OF PERSONALITY PATHOLOGY

There is no situation wherein complete and accurate assessment of personality pathology can be accomplished by using measures within a single modality (e.g., self-report). Accurate PD assessment in laboratory, clinical, and community settings requires that personality pathology be assessed via multiple methods (e.g., self-report and performance based), with scores obtained via different methods interpreted within the context of the psychological processes engaged by those methods. Shifting the emphasis in PD assessment from self-report to underlying process will increase understanding of the intra- and interpersonal dynamics of personality pathology. Clinicians and researchers will be better able to predict variations in PD-related responding over time and across situation, PD symptom criteria will become more precise and heuristic, and comorbidity will be reduced. Accurate assessment of personality pathology can only be accomplished by using a process-focused (PF) model of PD assessment (see Bornstein, 2002, 2009, 2011, for detailed discussions of the PF model).

The PF model of PD assessment differs from the traditional perspective in two ways. In contrast to the traditional approach, which emphasizes the convergence of scores on measures that ostensibly tap the same construct (e.g., informant report and performance-based measures of obsessiveness), the PF model highlights the value of theoretically meaningful test score divergences in delineating underlying personality dynamics. In contrast to the traditional approach, wherein correlational methods are used to quantify the relationship between test score and outcome, the PF model incorporates experimental methods to manipulate underlying PD dynamics. This enables researchers to draw more definitive conclusions regarding the nature of these hidden processes (for examples, see Bornstein, Ng, Gallagher, Kloss, & Regier, 2005; Horn, Meyer, & Mihura, 2009).

To draw clinically useful inferences regarding test score convergences and divergences and develop manipulations that shed light on the personality dynamics tapped by different tests, clinicians and clinical researchers must understand which psychological processes are engaged by different instruments. Bornstein (2009, 2011) provided preliminary process-based classifications of widely used psychological tests; these tests may be divided into five broad categories.

Self-Report Tests

When *self-report* (also called *self-attribution*) measures are used, test scores reflect the degree to which the person attributes various traits, feelings, thoughts, motives, behaviors, attitudes, or experiences to him- or herself. Because they are efficient and cost effective, self-report tests are far and away the most widely used type of PD measure in both research and clinical settings. The Millon Clinical Multiaxial Inventory (MCMI; Millon, Millon, & Davis, 1994) and the NEO Personality Inventory (NEO-PI; Costa & McCrae, 1992) are among the more widely used measures within this category.

Performance-Based Tests

In performance-based tests—traditionally called *projective tests* and more recently *stimulus attribution tests*—the person attributes meaning to ambiguous stimuli, with attributions determined in part by stimulus characteristics and in part by the person's cognitive style, emotions, motives, and need states. The Rorschach Inkblot Method (RIM; Rorschach, 1921) is the most widely used and best-known performance-based test in PD research and clinical application; others include the Thematic Apperception Test (TAT; Murray, 1943) and the Holtzman Inkblot Test (Holtzman, Thorpe, Swartz, & Herron, 1961).

Constructive Tests

In constructive tests, generation of test responses requires the person to create or construct a novel image or written description within parameters defined by the tester. The Draw a Person Test (and other projective drawings) would be classified in this category (e.g., Harris, 1963), as would various open-ended descriptions of self and significant others (e.g., Blatt's Qualitative and Structural Dimensions of Object Representations; see Blatt, Bers, & Schaffer, 1993).

Behavioral Tests

In some behavioral tests, scores are derived from indices of a person's behavior exhibited and measured in vivo, as in spot sampling (a technique wherein researchers sample respondents' behavior at randomly selected times, in multiple contexts; see Moskowitz & Sadikaj, 2012). Behavior may also be examined in a controlled setting (e.g., using joystick feedback tasks wherein moment-by-moment thoughts, behaviors, and affective reactions are rated as they occur; Lizdek, Sadler, Woody, Ethier, & Malet, 2012).

Informant-Report Tests

Scores on tests in this category are based on informants' ratings or judgments of a person's characteristic patterns of responding. Examples include the therapist version of the Shedler–Westen Assessment Procedure (Shedler & Westen, 2007) and the Informant Report version of the NEO-PI (Kurtz, Lee, & Sherker, 1999). In contrast to observational measures, which are based on direct observation of behavior, informant-report tests are based on informants' retrospective, memory-derived conclusions regarding characteristics of the target person.

OPERATIONALIZING AND IMPLEMENTING THE PF MODEL

As Bornstein (2011) noted, there are at least three ways to examine the impact of dispositional and contextual variables on test scores. First, researchers can examine naturally occurring influences (e.g., variations in mood or anxiety level); this was the approach Hirschfeld, Klerman, Clayton, and Keller (1983) used to assess the impact of changes in severity of depressive symptoms on personality traits theoretically linked with depression (e.g., dependency, self-esteem). Second, researchers can examine changes in test scores over time due to the effects of maturation (in children) or aging (in older adults). This was the approach used by Jansen and Van der Maas (1997) to detect Piagetian developmental shifts in children's reasoning and that used by Baltes (1996) to assess age-related changes in the expression of underlying dependency needs in older adults.

A third approach—least widely used but potentially most informative— is to introduce experimental manipulations that deliberately alter the processes engaged by different psychological tests. This approach allows the researcher to (a) confirm that altering these processes does in fact change test scores as expected and (b) illuminate the processes involved in tests that measure parallel constructs using contrasting methods. This was the strategy used by Bornstein and colleagues (Bornstein, Bowers, & Bonner, 1996; Bornstein, Rossner, Hill, & Stepanian, 1994) to examine the differential impact of instructional set and mood state on self-report and performance-based dependency scores; as hypothesized, deliberately inducing a negative mood state increased performance-based (but not self-report) dependency scores, whereas an instructional set that framed interpersonal dependency in positive terms increased self-report (but not performance-based) dependency. Along somewhat similar lines, Morf and Rhodewalt (2001) examined the impact of threats to self-esteem on self- and other-evaluations in narcissistic and control participants (see Besser & Priel, 2011, for evidence regarding the impact of similar manipulations on emotional responding in narcissistic and control participants).

Emphasizing this latter experimental approach to illuminating underlying process, Exhibit 11.1 summarizes in broad terms four steps involved in implementing the PF model in research and clinical settings. As Exhibit 11.1 shows, the first step in PF PD assessment involves specifying the underlying processes associated with different personality and PD measures (e.g., MCMI, RIM), and identifying variables (e.g., affect state, instructional set) that potentially alter these processes. Next, process–outcome links are operationalized and tested empirically (Step 2), and the results of these assessments are evaluated (Step 3). Finally, PF PD assessment data are contextualized by enumerating limiting conditions (e.g., flaws in experimental design) that might have influenced the results and evaluating the generalizability and ecological validity of these data by assessing the degree to which similar patterns are obtained

---

EXHIBIT 11.1
A Process-Focused Model of Personality Disorder Assessment

---

1. Identify salient personality disorder (PD) processes
    (a) Specify underlying psychological processes
    (b) Identify internal states and external variables that alter these processes
2. Operationalize and evaluate process–outcome links
    (a) Turn process-altering variables into manipulations
    (b) Delineate hypothesized outcomes
3. Interpret outcome
    (a) Process-based PD patterns
    (b) Convergences and divergences
4. Evaluate generalizability/ecological validity
    (a) Population
    (b) Context and setting

---

in different populations and settings. This latter task entails conducting replications of the initial investigation in different contexts, using new participant samples. Thus, Steps 1 through 3 will occur whenever a PF study is conducted; Step 4 represents a long-term goal that requires additional studies.

INITIAL FINDINGS USING PF METHODS

As an illustration of the breadth of approaches that have been employed in recent years and the range of PDs that has been examined with PF methods, five representative studies are described below. Some of these investigations tapped underlying PD dynamics by contrasting respondents' performance on measures that engaged different psychological processes (Bornstein, 1998; Lobbestael, Cima, & Arntz, 2013); others employed behavioral outcome measures in lieu of self-reports to illuminate cognitive and affective reactions not amenable to introspection and verbal description (Lenzenweger, Miller, Maher, & Manschreck, 2007). Still other investigations introduced experimental manipulations to deliberately alter PD-related responding (Arntz, Klokman, & Sieswerda, 2005), and one combined experimental procedures with behavioral outcome assessments (Horvath & Morf, 2009).

Implicit and Self-Attributed Dependency Needs in Dependent and Histrionic PDs

Although early models of histrionic pathology emphasized conflicts regarding sexuality as the core element of histrionic PD, later theoretical frameworks argued that issues regarding dependency are as important to histrionic dynamics as are issues regarding sexuality—perhaps more so. As the *Diagnostic and Statistical Manual of Mental Disorders* (4th ed.; *DSM–IV*; American Psychiatric Association, 1994) noted, "Without being aware of it [patients with histrionic PD] often act out a role . . . in their relationships with others. They may seem to control their partner through emotional manipulation or seductiveness on one level, whereas displaying a marked dependency on them at another level" (p. 656). Clinical writings on inter- and intrapersonal dynamics of histrionic PD have also noted that unconscious dependency strivings may play a role in histrionic pathology (see Blashfield, Reynolds, & Stennett, 2012), but until relatively recently no empirical studies had examined possible links between unacknowledged dependency strivings and histrionic PD.

To address this issue, Bornstein (1998) used self-report and performance-based measures of interpersonal dependency to contrast the underlying dynamics and expressed dependency needs of college students who scored above threshold on the Personality Diagnostic Questionnaire—Revised (PDQ–R; Hyler, Skodol, Kellman, Oldham, & Rosnick, 1990) histrionic PD and dependent PD subscales. A large sample of participants was screened to obtain a group of 28 "pure" dependent PD participants (i.e., participants who scored above threshold for dependent PD but no other PDs) and 24 pure histrionic PD participants. Separate groups of "Other PD" ($n = 77$) and "No PD" ($n = 77$) participants were included as controls. All participants completed the Interpersonal Dependency Inventory (IDI; Hirschfeld et al., 1977), a widely used measure of self-reported dependency, and the Rorschach Oral Dependency (ROD) scale (Masling, Rabie, & Blondheim, 1967), a widely used measure of performance-based dependency.

Results of this comparison were unambiguous: As expected, participants in the dependent PD group showed high levels of both implicit and self-reported dependency, and those in the histrionic PD group scored high on implicit—but not self-reported—dependency. Participants in the other two groups scored comparatively low on both dependency measures. This study provided the first direct evidence that dependent PD is associated with high levels of both underlying and expressed dependency, whereas histrionic PD is associated with high levels of underlying dependency but not self-reported (or "self-attributed") dependency. As Bornstein, Denckla, and Chung (in press) noted, these results not only enhance understanding of the intra- and interpersonal dynamics of histrionicity but also suggest that exploration of unconscious conflicts regarding dependency may be an important component of insight-oriented treatment for histrionic PD.

Induced Emotional Arousal and Schema Mode Processing in Borderline PD

Although cognitive models have proven useful in conceptualizing a number of *DSM* PDs (e.g., dependent, paranoid, avoidant, obsessive-compulsive), these models have not had as much success in explaining the intrapersonal dynamics of borderline PD. Unlike most other PDs, borderline PD is not characterized by a predictable set of dysfunctional core beliefs that are stable over time and across situation (see Linehan, 1993; Pretzer & Beck, 2005). To move beyond limitations in extant cognitive models of borderline pathology, Young, Klosko, and Weishaar (2003) proposed a schema mode model of borderline PD that shifts the focus of cognitive theory in this domain, hypothesizing that the core dysfunction underlying borderline pathology has less to do with schema content and more to do with schema instability: Under stress, people with borderline pathology "flip" more easily than other people from healthy to unhealthy schema modes. In Young et al.'s model, the patient with borderline PD is hypothesized to flip from "healthy adult" mode to "detached protector" mode under stress (detached protector mode is characterized by cognitive avoidance, denial, and dissociation, all of which serve—at least in the short term—to dampen aversive emotions).

To test this model, Arntz et al. (2005) assessed schema mode processing in 18 patients with borderline PD, 18 patients with Cluster C PD, and 18 nonpatient controls with Klokman, Arntz, and Sieswerda's (2001) Schema Mode Questionnaire (SMQ); PD diagnoses were derived from the SCID-II (First, Gibbon, Spitzer, Williams, & Benjamin, 1997). Patients were then randomly assigned to one of two conditions: (a) a negative arousal condition, wherein they viewed a 10-minute fragment of a fictional film depicting a young girl being physically, emotionally, and sexually abused by her parents, or (b) a control condition, wherein they viewed a 10-minute fragment of a travelogue. Immediately following exposure to the films, participants completed the SMQ a second time, along with a state emotion inventory.

Arntz et al. (2005) found that exposure to the abuse film increased negative emotions (i.e., anger and depression) in all participant groups. However, only participants with borderline PD showed a statistically significant increase in detached protector mode responding (i.e., increases in cognitive avoidance, denial, and dissociation) following exposure to the abuse film. Arntz et al.'s results suggest that—consistent with Young et al.'s (2003) schema mode model—a core cognitive element of borderline PD is instability in schema mode responding and susceptibility to shifts toward a syndrome-specific form of dysfunctional coping and information processing when emotionally aroused.

Abnormal Verbal Associative Patterns in Schizotypal PD

Although schizotypal PD has been included on Axis II since the multi-axial system was introduced in the *Diagnostic and Statistical Manual of Mental Disorders* (3rd ed.; *DSM–III*; American Psychiatric Association, 1980), its continued inclusion as a PD syndrome has been based more on tradition than evidence. Following Rado (1953, 1960), Meehl (1962) initially conceptualized schizotypy both as a potential precursor of schizophrenia and a dysfunctional personality style characterized by anhedonia, perceptual aberration, and odd behavior; the schizotypal person's interpersonal quirkiness ultimately leads to social rejection and increased cognitive slippage. As Lenzenweger (2006) noted, the degree to which schizotypy and schizotypal PD are physiologically and phenomenologically related to schizophrenia remains unresolved.

To address this issue, Lenzenweger, Miller, Maher, and Manschreck (2007) examined the number and quality of verbal associations spontaneously generated by 35 schizotypal undergraduates (identified with the Schizotypal

Personality Questionnaire; Raine, 1991) and 29 matched nonschizotypal controls. All of them were asked to provide open-ended descriptions of a painting: Pieter Bruegel's *The Wedding Feast*. Participants' verbalizations were analyzed with Maher, Manschreck, Linnert, and Candela's (2005) Computed Associations in Sequential Text (CAST) procedure, a software program designed to assess qualities of verbal associations by comparing target utterances to an extensive database of norms from different criterion groups (e.g., individuals with thought disorder, community adults).

Lenzenweger et al. (2007) found that schizotypal PD symptoms were associated with increases in both the number and range of verbal associations, even in undergraduates with no current evidence or prior history of thought disorder; they interpreted these results to suggest that schizotypal PD shares important information-processing features with schizophrenia spectrum syndromes. The schizotypal symptoms most strongly predictive of increased associative breadth were Odd Beliefs/Magical Thinking ($r = .31$), Unusual Perceptual Experiences ($r = .27$), and Odd Speech ($r = .35$). As Lenzenweger et al. noted, these findings suggest that schizotypal PD might be better classified as a schizophrenia-spectrum disorder (rather than as a form of personality pathology) in future versions of the *DSM*.

Sequential Activation and Suppression of Worthlessness in Narcissistic PD

Cognitive and psychodynamic models of narcissistic PD differ with respect to the processes hypothesized to drive narcissistic behavior. Most cognitive models argue that narcissistic grandiosity reflects inflated perceptions of self-worth, often traceable to early learning experiences within the family. Psychodynamic models, in contrast, view narcissism as reflecting a defense against underlying feelings of worthlessness, such that overt expressions of grandiosity are used in part to fend off awareness of one's frailty, fragility, and vulnerability (see Ronningstam, 2005, for reviews of these and other theoretical perspectives on narcissistic PD).

To test the psychodynamic "defense model" of narcissism, Horvath and Morf (2009) recruited high school and college students who obtained high versus low scores on the Narcissistic Personality Inventory (NPI; Raskin & Hall, 1979). Participants took part in a lexical decision task on a desktop computer; they were asked to distinguish a series of worthlessness-related target words (e.g., *deficient, incompetent, useless*) from nonwords as quickly as possible by pressing a button on the keyboard. Prior to each word/nonword judgment, participants were exposed to a masked subliminal prime designed to activate feelings of worthlessness (FAILURE) or to a neutral control prime (NOTE) for 35 milliseconds (ms). Stimulus onset asynchronicity (SOA) was randomized across trials, with the interval between subliminal prime and target word being 150 ms for half the trials and 2,000 ms for the remaining trials. Horvath and Morf hypothesized that narcissistic participants' reaction times for worthlessness-related words should decrease following exposure to the FAILURE prime with briefer (150 ms) SOAs, because feelings of worthlessness are still activated by the FAILURE prime at this point, facilitating word/nonword judgments. Reaction times should increase with longer (2,000 ms) SOAs, because after this interval defenses would have been activated to suppress the initial prime effect.

Results confirmed Horvath and Morf's (2009) hypothesis, such that lexical decision times for worthlessness-related words decreased significantly in the FAILURE prime condition at briefer SOAs and increased significantly at longer SOAs—but only for participants scoring high on the NPI. As Horvath and Morf (2009) noted,

> The results of this study are consistent with our hypothesis that narcissists scan for and then subsequently repress worthlessness after an ego threat. . . . Both narcissistic men and women seem to use repression as a strategy to absorb worthlessness and thereby protect their grandiose self. [These findings confirm that] narcissists are vigilant for worthlessness and are then quick and successful at avoiding it. (p. 1255)

Hostile Interpretation Bias and Aggression in Antisocial PD

Men diagnosed with antisocial PD show elevated levels of both reactive aggression (i.e., uncontrolled aggression exhibited in response to provocation or threat) and proactive aggression (i.e., goal-directed aggression that is typically more mindful and internally motivated); the processes underlying these personality–aggression links remain largely unexplored (Herve & Yuille, 2007; Stafford & Cornell, 2003). To address this issue, Lobbestael et al. (2013) assessed hostile interpretation bias (the tendency to interpret ambiguous stimuli in a hostile manner) and both forms of aggression in 37 male inpatients and outpatients diagnosed with antisocial PD and 29 community men without diagnosed personality pathology.

In an assessment of hostile interpretation bias, participants read eight brief (1–2 sentence) vignettes depicting ambiguously provocative social interactions and provided open-ended interpretations of each vignette, which were coded for level of hostile attribution (*hostile, negative, neutral,* or *positive*) on a 4-point scale. They also provided open-ended interpretations of eight TAT cards; these descriptions were coded for hostile interpretation bias on the same 4-point scale. Finally, participants completed the Reactive–Proactive Aggression Questionnaire (RPAQ; Raine et al., 2006), which yields separate scores for reactive and proactive aggression.

Results indicated that although presence and severity of antisocial PD symptoms predicted both types of aggression, only reactive aggression was mediated by hostile interpretation bias. In other words, the tendency of antisocial persons to react aggressively when provoked is due in part to their tendency to interpret this provocation as reflecting hostility on the other person's part. As Lobbestael et al. (2013) noted, these results not only illuminate the processes that underlie reactive aggression in antisocial men but also suggest promising avenues for intervention and harm reduction in patients with antisocial PD.

CONCLUSIONS AND FUTURE DIRECTIONS

As Bornstein (2003, 2007) noted, the vast majority of PD studies to date have taken a top down approach, in which PD symptoms and traits are assessed, usually via interview or questionnaire, and these data are used to derive and refine diagnostic criteria and test hypotheses regarding PD etiology, dynamics, and comorbidity. As these brief reviews of PF PD studies suggest, understanding of the intra- and interpersonal dynamics of personality pathology is enhanced if the traditional top-down approach is coupled with a bottom-up strategy wherein other types of outcome measures (e.g., behavioral, performance based) are used in addition to self-reports and experimental procedures are introduced to complement and extend the more widely used correlational procedures. Beyond illuminating the underlying dynamics of personality pathology, the PF model has some noteworthy empirical and clinical implications.

Empirical Implications

PDs differ substantially with respect to etiology and present-day dynamics, and no single theoretical model can account for all PDs. Neurological factors play a particularly strong role in certain PDs (e.g., schizotypal); for others (e.g., dependent, avoidant), cognitive elements are more pronounced (see Bornstein, 2007, 2013). For some dysfunctional personality patterns (e.g., histrionic), psychodynamic factors are particularly important (Bornstein et al., in press). Moreover, even within a given category, patients may present with multiple etiologies, varied learning histories, and contrasting present-day dynamics (e.g., paranoid PD can reflect a self-defeating cognitive style acquired within the family, underlying fears and conflicts regarding shame and vulnerability, experiences related to cultural adaptation and the challenges of assimilation, or some combination of these and other factors).

Given this etiological and dynamic diversity, it is crucial that clinicians and researchers conceptualize personality pathology from multiple theoretical frameworks (e.g., cognitive, psychodynamic, cultural, humanistic) to identify variables that mediate and moderate PD-related responding (see Bornstein, 2007). The importance of multitheoretical "nesting" of PDs is echoed in the PF framework: In contrast to traditional outcome-based PD assessment, which tends to be trait- and symptom-focused, the PF model explicitly links personality and PD assessment to constructs derived from an array of theoretical frameworks (e.g., cognitive, psychodynamic) and integrates methodologies from multiple subfields within psychology (e.g., developmental, social). By shedding light on the intrapersonal dynamics of personality pathology from multiple vantage points the PF model provides unique information regarding the antecedents and maintenance factors associated with different forms of personality pathology (e.g., schemas, defenses, attachment patterns, mental representations of self and others). Because PF methods can be used to elucidate adaptive personality dynamics as well as personality dysfunction, they may also help bridge the gap between studies of "normal" and "abnormal" personality. As several writers have pointed out, research in these two domains has diverged in recent years, to the detriment of both (see Ganellen, 2007; Markon, Krueger, & Watson, 2005; Widiger, 2011).

Clinical Implications

Although the PF model yields unique information regarding PD dynamics that traditional methods cannot, neither strategy alone yields a truly comprehensive picture of personality pathology. When the two approaches are employed in tandem, understanding of patients is enhanced: Clinicians and researchers know how patients perceive and describe themselves, as well as the intrapersonal factors—often hidden and not easily accessed via self-report—that drive their pathology. As a result, the bottom up approach inherent in the PF model enables clinical researchers to understand more fully the differences between PDs that share certain surface features but differ with respect to underlying dynamics (e.g., dependent and histrionic, paranoid and borderline). Data derived from PF studies may ultimately lead to improved symptom criteria in *DSM–6*, as well as other diagnostic systems (e.g., *International Classification of Diseases—11*, *Psychodynamic Diagnostic Manual-2*): To the extent that symptom criteria reflect patients' underlying dynamics and self-descriptions, differential diagnosis will improve.

The PF model also provides a framework within which clinicians and clinical researchers can tailor multimethod assessment batteries to assess hypothesized process features of different PDs, blending findings from nomothetic studies of PD pathology with idiographic strategies that maximize the effectiveness of assessment batteries in clinical settings. In this context, it is worth noting that PF methods may also facilitate therapeutic assessment, engaging the patient in a collaborative exploratory process in ways that traditional evaluation methods cannot (see Finn, 2007, for a detailed discussion of therapeutic assessment strategies and techniques). To the extent that PF data are used to inform patients about aspects of self- and interpersonal-functioning about which they were previously unaware (e.g., coping resources, object relations, interpersonal scripts), commitment to the therapeutic process is likely to increase, and confidence in treatment will be enhanced.

Finally, the PF framework suggests additional possibilities for intervention based on heretofore unexplored PD dynamics uncovered by PF studies. The PF model provides a framework for tracking change during the course of therapy on multiple dimensions (e.g., self-report and performance based), which enhances the assessment of treatment process and progress. It may be, for example, that change during the course of insight-oriented therapy for certain PDs is reflected in shifting underlying dynamics that set the stage for observable symptom reduction later in treatment; in this situation, PF data represent a unique intrapsychic "window" affording the clinician early indication of incipient therapeutic change.

REFERENCES

American Psychiatric Association. (1980). *Diagnostic and statistical manual of mental disorders* (3rd ed.). Washington, DC: Author.

American Psychiatric Association. (1994). *Diagnostic and statistical manual of mental disorders* (4th ed.). Washington, DC: Author.

American Psychiatric Association. (2000). *Diagnostic and statistical manual of mental disorders* (4th ed., text rev.). Washington, DC: Author.

Arntz, A., Klokman, J., & Sieswerda, S. (2005). An experimental test of the schema mode model of borderline personality disorder. *Journal of Behavior Therapy and Experimental Psychiatry, 36,* 226–239. doi:10.1016/j.jbtep.2005.05.005

Baltes, M. (1996). *The many faces of dependency in old age.* Cambridge, England: Cambridge University Press.

Besser, A., & Priel, B. (2011). Dependency, self-criticism, and negative affective responses following imaginary rejection and failure threats: Meaning-making processes as moderators or mediators. *Psychiatry: Interpersonal and Biological Processes, 74,* 31–40. doi:10.1521/psyc.2011.74.1.31

Blais, M. A., & Baity, M. R. (2006). Rorschach assessment of histrionic personality disorder. In S. K. Huprich (Ed.), *Rorschach assessment of the personality disorders* (pp. 205–221). Mahwah, NJ: Erlbaum.

Blashfield, R. K., Reynolds, S. M., & Stennett, B. (2012). The death of histrionic personality disorder. In T. A. Widiger (Ed.), *Oxford handbook of personality disorders* (pp. 603–627). New York, NY: Oxford University Press.

Blatt, S. J., Bers, S. A., & Schaffer, C. E. (1993). *The assessment of self-descriptions.* Unpublished manuscript, Yale University School of Medicine.

Bornstein, R. F. (1998). Implicit and self-attributed dependency needs in dependent and histrionic personality disorders. *Journal of Personality Assessment, 71,* 1–14. doi:10.1207/s15327752jpa7101_1

Bornstein, R. F. (2002). A process dissociation approach to objective–projective test score interrelationships. *Journal of Personality Assessment, 78,* 47–68. doi:10.1207/S15327752JPA7801_04

Bornstein, R. F. (2003). Behaviorally referenced experimentation and symptom validation: A paradigm for 21st-century personality disorder research. *Journal of Personality Disorders, 17,* 1–18. doi:10.1521/pedi.17.1.1.24056

Bornstein, R. F. (2005). Interpersonal dependency in child abuse perpetrators and victims: A meta-analytic review. *Journal of Psychopathology and Behavioral Assessment, 27,* 67–76. doi:10.1007/s10862-005-5381-1

Bornstein, R. F. (2006). The complex relationship between dependency and abuse: Converging psychological factors and social forces. *American Psychologist, 61,* 595–606. doi:10.1037/0003-066X.61.6.595

Bornstein, R. F. (2007). From surface to depth: Diagnosis and assessment in personality pathology. *Clinical Psychology: Science and Practice, 14,* 99–102. doi:10.1111/j.1468-2850.2007.00067.x

Bornstein, R. F. (2009). Heisenberg, Kandinsky, and the heteromethod convergence problem: Lessons from within and beyond psychology. *Journal of Personality Assessment, 91,* 1–8. doi:10.1080/00223890802483235

Bornstein, R. F. (2011). Toward a process-focused model of test score validity: Improving psychological assessment in science and practice. *Psychological Assessment, 23,* 532–544. doi:10.1037/a0022402

Bornstein, R. F. (2013). Combining interpersonal and intrapersonal perspectives on personality pathology. *Journal of Personality Disorders, 27,* 296–302. doi:10.1521/pedi.2013.27.3.296

Bornstein, R. F., Bowers, K. S., & Bonner, S. (1996). Effects of induced mood states on objective and projective dependency scores. *Journal of Personality Assessment, 67,* 324–340. doi:10.1207/s15327752jpa6702_8

Bornstein, R. F., Denckla, C. A., & Chung, W. J. (in press). Dependent and histrionic personality disorders. In P. H. Blaney, R. F. Krueger, & T. Millon (Eds.), *Oxford textbook of psychopathology* (3rd ed.). Oxford, England: Oxford University Press.

Bornstein, R. F., Ng, H. M., Gallagher, H. A., Kloss, D. M., & Regier, N. G. (2005). Contrasting effects of self-schema priming on lexical decisions and Interpersonal Stroop Task performance: Evidence for a cognitive/interactionist model of interpersonal dependency. *Journal of Personality, 73,* 731–762. doi:10.1111/j.1467-6494.2005.00327.x

Bornstein, R. F., Riggs, J. M., Hill, E. L., & Calabrese, C. (1996). Activity, passivity, self-denigration, and self-promotion: Toward an interactionist model of interpersonal dependency. *Journal of Personality, 64,* 637–674. doi:10.1111/j.1467-6494.1996.tb00525.x

Bornstein, R. F., Rossner, S. C., Hill, E. L., & Stepanian, M. L. (1994). Face validity and fakability of objective and projective measures of dependency. *Journal of Personality Assessment, 63,* 363–386. doi:10.1207/s15327752jpa6302_14

Cizek, G. J., Rosenberg, S. L., & Koons, H. H. (2008). Sources of validity evidence for educational and psychological tests. *Educational and Psychological Measurement, 68,* 397–412. doi:10.1177/0013164407310130

Costa, P. T., Jr., & McCrae, R. R. (1992). *Revised NEO Personality Inventory (NEO-PI–R) and NEO Five-Factor Inventory (NEO-FFI) professional manual.* Odessa, FL: Psychological Assessment Resources.

Cox, B. J., Clara, I. P., Worobec, L. M., & Grant, B. F. (2012). An empirical evaluation of the structure of *DSM–IV* personality disorders in a nationally representative sample: Results of confirmatory factor analysis in the National Epidemiologic Survey on Alcohol and Related Conditions Waves 1 and 2. *Journal of Personality Disorders, 26,* 890–901. doi:10.1521/pedi.2012.26.6.890

Crawford, M. J., Koldobsky, N., Mulder, R., & Tyrer, P. (2011). Classifying personality disorder according to severity. *Journal of Personality Disorders, 25,* 321–330. doi:10.1521/pedi.2011.25.3.321

Ekselius, L., Lindstrom, E., Knorring, L., Bodlund, O., & Kullgren, G. (1994). Comorbidity among the personality disorders in *DSM–III–R. Personality and Individual Differences, 17,* 155–160. doi:10.1016/0191-8869(94)90021-3

Fernández, J. (2013). Self-deception and self-knowledge. *Philosophical Studies, 162,* 379–400. doi:10.1007/s11098-011-9771-9

Finn, S. E. (2007). *In our clients' shoes: Theory and techniques of therapeutic assessment.* Mahwah, NJ: Erlbaum.

First, M. B., Gibbon, M., Spitzer, R. L., Williams, J. B. W., & Benjamin, L. S. (1997). *Structured Clinical Interview for DSM–IV Axis II Disorders (SCID-II).* New York, NY: Biometrics Department, New York State Psychiatric Institute.

Ganellen, R. J. (2007). Assessing normal and abnormal personality functioning: Strengths and weaknesses of self-report, observer, and performance-based methods. *Journal of Personality Assessment, 89,* 30–40. doi:10.1080/00223890701356987

Garb, H. N. (1998). *Studying the clinician: Judgment research and psychological assessment.* Washington, DC: American Psychological Association.

Harris, D. B. (1963). *Children's drawings as measures of intellectual maturity: A revision and extension of the Goodenough Draw-a-Man Test.* San Diego, CA: Harcourt Brace Jovanovich.

Herve, H., & Yuille, J. C. (Eds.). (2007). *The psychopath: Theory, research, and practice.* Mahwah, NJ: Erlbaum.

Hirschfeld, R. M. A., Klerman, G. L., Clayton, P. J., & Keller, M. B. (1983). Personality and depression: Empirical findings. *Archives of General Psychiatry, 40,* 993–998. doi:10.1001/archpsyc.1983.01790080075010

Hirschfeld, R. M. A., Klerman, G. L., Gough, H. G., Barrett, J., Korchin, S. J., & Chodoff, P. (1977). A measure of interpersonal dependency. *Journal of Personality Assessment, 41,* 610–618. doi:10.1207/s15327752jpa4106_6

Hogan, T. P., & Agnello, J. (2004). An empirical study of reporting practices concerning measurement validity. *Educational and Psychological Measurement, 64,* 802–812. doi:10.1177/0013164404264120

Holtzman, W. H., Thorpe, J. S., Swartz, J. D., & Herron, E. W. (1961). *Inkblot perception and personality.* Austin: University of Texas Press.

Horn, S. L., Meyer, G. J., & Mihura, J. L. (2009). Impact of card rotation on the frequency of Rorschach reflection responses. *Journal of Personality Assessment, 91,* 346–356. doi:10.1080/00223890902936090

Horvath, S., & Morf, C. C. (2009). Narcissistic defensiveness: Hypervigilance and avoidance of worthlessness. *Journal of Experimental Social Psychology, 45,* 1252–1258. doi:10.1016/j.jesp.2009.07.011

Huprich, S. K. (2011). Contributions from personality- and psychodynamically oriented assessment to the development of the *DSM–5* personality disorders. *Journal of Personality Assessment, 93,* 354–361. doi:10.1080/00223891.2011.577473

Huprich, S. K., Bornstein, R. F., & Schmitt, T. (2011). Self-report methodology is insufficient for improving the assessment and classification of Axis II personality disorders. *Journal of Personality Disorders, 25,* 557–570. doi:10.1521/pedi.2011.25.5.557

Hyler, S. E., Skodol, A. E., Kellman, H. D., Oldham, J. M., & Rosnick, L. (1990). Validity of the Personality Diagnostic Questionnaire—Revised: Comparison with two structured interviews. *American Journal of Psychiatry, 147,* 1043–1048.

Insel, T. R., & Wang, P. S. (2010). Rethinking mental illness. *JAMA, 303,* 1970–1971. doi:10.1001/jama.2010.555

Jansen, B. R. J., & Van der Maas, H. L. J. (1997). Statistical tests of the rule assessment methodology by latent class analysis. *Developmental Review, 17,* 321–327.

Klokman, J., Arntz, A., & Sieswerda, S. (2001). *The Schema Mode Questionnaire.* Unpublished document, Maastricht University, Maastricht, the Netherlands.

Kurtz, J. E., Lee, P. A., & Sherker, J. L. (1999). Internal and temporal reliability estimates for informant ratings of personality using the NEO-PI–R and IAS. *Assessment, 6,* 103–113. doi:10.1177/107319119900600201

Lenzenweger, M. F. (2006). Schizotaxia, schizotypy, and schizophrenia: Paul E. Meehl's blueprint for the experimental psychopathology and genetics of schizophrenia. *Journal of Abnormal Psychology, 115,* 195–200. doi:10.1037/0021-843X.115.2.195

Lenzenweger, M. F., Miller, A. B., Maher, B. A., & Manschreck, T. C. (2007). Schizotypy and individual differences in the frequency of normal associations in verbal utterances. *Schizophrenia Research, 95,* 96–102.

Linehan, M. (1993). *Cognitive behavioral treatment of borderline personality disorder*. New York, NY: Guilford Press.

Lizdek, I., Sadler, P., Woody, E., Ethier, N., & Malet, G. (2012). Capturing the stream of behavior: A computer-joystick method for coding interpersonal behavior continuously over time. *Social Science Computer Review, 30*, 512–521.

Lobbestael, J., Cima, M., & Arntz, A. (2013). The relationship between adult reactive and proactive aggression, hostile interpretation bias, and antisocial personality disorder. *Journal of Personality Disorders, 27*, 53–66. doi:10.1521/pedi.2013.27.1.53

Maher, B. A., Manschreck, T. C., Linnert, J., & Candela, S. (2005). Quantitative assessment of the frequency of normal associations in the utterances of schizophrenia patients and healthy controls. *Schizophrenia Research, 78*, 219–224. doi:10.1016/j.schres.2005.05.017

Markon, K. E., Krueger, R. F., & Watson, D. (2005). Delineating the structure of normal and abnormal personality: An integrative hierarchical approach. *Journal of Personality and Social Psychology, 88*, 139–157. doi:10.1037/0022-3514.88.1.139

Masling, J., Rabie, L., & Blondheim, S. H. (1967). Obesity, level of aspiration, and Rorschach and TAT measures of oral dependence. *Journal of Consulting Psychology, 31*, 233–239. doi:10.1037/h0020999

McWilliams, N. (2006). Some thoughts about schizoid dynamics. *Psychoanalytic Review, 93*, 1–24. doi:10.1521/prev.2006.93.1.1

Meehl, P. E. (1962). Schizotaxia, schizotypy, schizophrenia. *American Psychologist, 17*, 827–838. doi:10.1037/h0041029

Millon, T. (2011). *Disorders of personality: Introducing a DSM/ICD spectrum from normal to abnormal*. Hoboken, NJ: Wiley.

Millon, T., Millon, C., & Davis, R. (1994). *Millon Clinical Multiaxial Inventory–III*. Minneapolis, MN: National Computer Systems.

Morf, C. C., & Rhodewalt, F. (2001). Unraveling the paradoxes of narcissism: A dynamic self-regulatory processing model. *Psychological Inquiry, 12*, 177–196. doi:10.1207/S15327965PLI1204_1

Moskowitz, D. S., & Sadikaj, G. (2012). Event-contingent recording. In M. R. Mehl & T. S. Connor (Eds.), *Handbook of research methods for studying daily life* (pp. 160–175). New York, NY: Guilford Press.

Murray, H. A. (1943). *Thematic Apperception Test manual*. Cambridge, MA: Harvard University Press.

National Institute of Mental Health. (2008). *The National Institute of Mental Health Strategic Plan* (NIH Publication No. 08-6368). Retrieved from http://www.nimh.nih.gov/about/strategic-planning-reports/index.shtml

Pretzer, J. L., & Beck, A. T. (2005). A cognitive theory of personality disorders. In M. F. Lenzenweger & J. F. Clarkin (Eds.), *Major theories of personality disorder* (2nd ed., pp. 43–113). New York, NY: Guilford Press.

Rado, S. (1953). Dynamics and classification of disordered behavior. *American Journal of Psychiatry, 110,* 406–416.

Rado, S. (1960). Theory and therapy: The theory of schizotypal organization and its application to the treatment of decompensated schizotypal behavior. In S. C. Scher & H. R. Davis (Eds.), *The outpatient treatment of schizophrenia* (pp. 87–101). New York, NY: Grune & Stratton.

Raine, A. (1991). The SPQ: A scale for the assessment of schizotypal personality based on *DSM–III–R* criteria. *Schizophrenia Bulletin, 17,* 555–564. doi:10.1093/schbul/17.4.555

Raine, A., Dodge, K., Loeber, R., Gatzke-Kopp, L., Lynam, D., Reynolds, C., & Stouthamer-Loehmer, M. (2006). The Reactive–Proactive Aggression Questionnaire: Differential correlates of reactive and proactive aggression in adolescent boys. *Aggressive Behavior, 32,* 159–171. doi:10.1002/ab.20115

Raskin, R. N., & Hall, C. S. (1979). A narcissistic personality inventory. *Psychological Reports, 45,* 590. doi:10.2466/pr0.1979.45.2.590

Rogers, R. (2003). Standardizing *DSM–IV* diagnoses: The clinical applications of structured interviews. *Journal of Personality Assessment, 81,* 220–225. doi:10.1207/S15327752JPA8103_04

Ronningstam, E. (2005). *Identifying and understanding the narcissistic personality.* New York, NY: Oxford University Press.

Rorschach, H. (1921). *Psychodiagnostik.* Bern, Switzerland: Bircher.

Shedler, J., & Westen, D. (2007). The Shedler–Westen Assessment Procedure (SWAP): Making personality diagnosis clinically meaningful. *Journal of Personality Assessment, 89,* 41–55. doi:10.1080/00223890701357092

Stafford, E., & Cornell, D. (2003). Psychopathy scores predict adolescent inpatient aggression. *Assessment, 10,* 102–112. doi:10.1177/1073191102250341

von Hippel, W., & Trivers, R. (2011). The evolution and psychology of self-deception. *Behavioral and Brain Sciences, 34,* 1–16. doi:10.1017/S0140525X10001354

Widiger, T. A. (2011). Integrating normal and abnormal personality structure: A proposal for *DSM–V. Journal of Personality Disorders, 25,* 338–363. doi:10.1521/pedi.2011.25.3.338

Widiger, T. A., & Samuel, D. B. (2005). Evidence-based assessment of personality disorders. *Psychological Assessment, 17,* 278–287. doi:10.1037/1040-3590.17.3.278

Wise, E. A. (1996). Comparative validity of MMPI–2 and MCMI–II personality disorder classifications. *Journal of Personality Assessment, 66,* 569–582. doi:10.1207/s15327752jpa6603_7

Young, J. E., Klosko, J., & Weishaar, M. E. (2003). *Schema therapy: A practitioner's guide.* New York, NY: Guilford Press.

Zeigler-Hill, V., Myers, E. M., & Clark, C. B. (2010). Narcissism and self-esteem reactivity: The role of negative achievement events. *Journal of Research in Personality, 44,* 285–292. doi:10.1016/j.jrp.2010.02.005

III

MOVING TOWARD INTEGRATED AND UNIFIED MODELS OF PERSONALITY DISORDERS AND PATHOLOGY

12

AN INTEGRATIVE, PSYCHODYNAMIC FRAMEWORK OF PERSONALITY PATHOLOGY

PATRICK LUYTEN AND SIDNEY J. BLATT

This chapter presents an integrative conceptualization of personality disorders (PDs) that has emerged over the last few decades as a result of a dialogue among psychodynamic developmental psychopathology, attachment research, cognitive-behavioral theory, and, more recently, evolutionary and neuroscience approaches (Blatt, 2008; Blatt & Luyten, 2009, 2010; Luyten & Blatt, 2007, 2011, 2013). This conceptualization bridges theory-driven and descriptive multivariate models of personality pathology and reconciles variable- and person-centered approaches to classifying and treating personality pathology.

We have consistently argued, congruent with recent theoretical formulations of PD (Livesley, 2008) and proposals for the fifth edition of the *Diagnostic and Statistical Manual of Mental Disorders* (*DSM–5*; American Psychiatric Association, 2013; Skodol, 2012) about the centrality of impairments in self and relatedness (see also Chapter 8, this volume), that

http://dx.doi.org/10.1037/14549-013
Personality Disorders: Toward Theoretical and Empirical Integration in Diagnosis and Assessment,
S. K. Huprich (Editor)

personality pathology can be conceptualized, from both descriptive and theoretical points of view, as disruptions in relatedness or attachment on the one hand and in self-definition or self and identity on the other. This view provides a theoretically coherent approach to understanding processes of normal and disrupted personality development as well as therapeutic action. Well-functioning personality involves an integration (or balance) in the development of interpersonal relatedness and self-definition, with more mature levels of relatedness facilitating the development of an essentially positive and stable sense of self, identity, and autonomy that, in turn, facilitates more differentiated and integrated interpersonal relationships. By contrast, disruptive experiences throughout life, in interaction with biological predispositions, are thought to result in compensatory or defensive maneuvers in response to developmental disruptions that exaggerate one developmental line and the neglect of the other. Thus, different forms of psychopathology are not static diseases but dynamic, conflict–defense constellations that maintain a balance, however distorted and disturbed, between relatedness and self-definition (Blatt, 2008; Luyten & Blatt, 2011). Treatment, from this perspective, should thus aim at the reactivation of the dialectic interaction between relatedness and self-definition (Blatt & Shichman, 1983).

In what follows, we outline these theoretical formulations. We discuss their convergence with contemporary attachment, interpersonal, and motivational approaches to personality and discuss emerging research findings supporting the evolutionary and neurobiological foundations of relatedness and self-definition. Next, we outline the implications of these views for assessing and diagnosing personality pathology, including a discussion of the implications of these formulations for future *DSM* development and for integrating theory-driven and multivariate models of personality development such as the five-factor model. We end by outlining the implications of these formulations for clinical practice and the development of evidence-based treatments.

RELATEDNESS AND SELF-DEFINITION IN PERSONALITY DEVELOPMENT: THEORETICAL FOUNDATIONS

Basic Concepts

Relatedness and *self-definition* refer to fundamental psychological developmental processes that involve the development of (a) reciprocal, meaningful, and personally satisfying interpersonal relationships and (b) a coherent, realistic, differentiated, and essentially positive sense of self or an identity.

This emphasis on interpersonal relatedness and self-definition has been central in many theories of normal and disrupted personality development, ranging from philosophy, to evolutionary and cross-cultural psychology, to personality and social psychology and psychoanalysis (for an extensive review, see Blatt, 2008). Various personality theories have referred to these dimensions as *surrender* and *autonomy* (Angyal, 1951), *communion* and *agency* (Bakan, 1966; Pincus, 2005), *affiliation* or *intimacy* and *achievement* or *power* (McAdams, 1985; McClelland, 1985), *dependency* and *self-critical perfectionism* (Blatt, 1974, 2008), *relatedness* and *autonomy/competence* (Deci & Ryan, 2012), and, more recently, as *attachment anxiety* and *attachment avoidance* (Mikulincer & Shaver, 2007; Sibley, 2007) and *sociotropy* and *autonomy* (Beck, 1983; Clark & Beck, 1999). Similarly, Kernberg and colleagues have argued that the development of self- and other representations is intrinsically linked resulting in so-called self–object dyads that are seen as the core of personality development (Kernberg & Caligor, 2005; Yeomans & Diamond, 2010). These *two-polarities models* of personality (Luyten & Blatt, 2013) all share an emphasis on the dialectic interaction between issues of relatedness and self-definition in personality development and disruptions of this dialectic in personality pathology (Luyten & Blatt, 2011; Mikulincer & Shaver, 2007; Pincus, 2005).

From psychodynamic and cognitive developmental perspectives, Blatt and colleagues (Blatt, 2008; Blatt & Luyten, 2009; Blatt & Shichman, 1983) have argued that, throughout the life cycle, the development of the sense of self leads to increasingly mature levels of interpersonal relatedness that, in turn, facilitate further differentiation and integration in the development of the self. Beck (1983) similarly distinguished sociotropy and autonomy. Autonomy refers to an achievement-oriented personality style that is associated with attempts to maximize control over the environment. Sociotropy involves a focus on attachment to others. Beck also proposed that a balance between autonomy and sociotropy characterizes adaptive personality development. Research has provided ample evidence that consistent differences are associated with these two personality dimensions in current and early life experiences (Blatt & Homann, 1992; Blatt & Luyten, 2009; Soenens, Vansteenkiste, & Luyten, 2010), stress responsivity (Luyten et al., 2011), and interpersonal and attachment styles (Zuroff, Mongrain, & Santor, 2004).

Current interpersonal models have proposed similar dimensions underlying personality development–agency (or social dominance) and communion (or nurturance or affiliation; Benjamin, 2005; Horowitz & Strack, 2011; Horowitz et al., 2006; Kiesler, 1983; Leary, 1957; Pincus, 2005; Wiggins, 2003). These dimensions overlap both theoretically and empirically with self-definition/autonomy and relatedness/sociotropy (Luyten & Blatt, 2011).

Contemporary attachment theory also emphasizes a balance between relatedness and self-definition in normal personality development (Mikulincer & Shaver, 2007). Attachment theory essentially proposes that two dimensions—attachment avoidance and attachment anxiety (Meyer & Pilkonis, 2005; Mikulincer & Shaver, 2007; Roisman et al., 2007)—underlie attachment behavior. The dimensions are expressed in differences in internal working models (IWMs) of self and of other (Bartholomew & Horowitz, 1991), which are the expectations, beliefs, and feelings about the self and others that develop in interactions with attachment figures. Attachment avoidance is characterized by IWMs that express "discomfort with closeness" and "discomfort with depending on others" (Mikulincer & Shaver, 2007, p. 87). These IWMs overlap conceptually and empirically with the self-definition/autonomy/dominance dimension (Luyten & Blatt, 2011; Sibley, 2007). Attachment anxiety, expressed in IWMs characterized by "fear of rejection and abandonment" (Mikulincer & Shaver, 2007, p. 155), overlaps with the relatedness/sociotropy/warmth dimension. Adaptive personality functioning in contemporary attachment formulations is conceptualized, as in other two-polarities models, as a balance between relatedness and self-definition, expressed in low to moderate levels of attachment anxiety and avoidance that are typical of securely attached individuals (Mikulincer & Shaver, 2007).

Self-determination theory (Deci & Ryan, 2012), from a motivational perspective, advances very similar views about personality development. Intrinsic or autonomous motivation, characteristic of adaptive personality development, is assumed to involve a balance between autonomy and competence, on the one hand, and relatedness on the other. Autonomy and competence reflect strivings toward control over the initiation and outcome of one's activities, and relatedness refers to the need to feel related to others. Again, empirical research provides evidence for the conceptual and empirical overlap of the focus in self-determination theory on autonomy/competence and relatedness with other two-polarities models (Luyten & Blatt, 2011; Zuroff, Koestner, Moskowitz, McBride, & Bagby, 2012).

Neurobiological and Evolutionary Basis

Given the centrality of these two dimensions in human development, it is hardly surprising that relatedness and self-definition seem deeply rooted in neurobiology. The neurobiology of attachment and social cognition, for instance, demonstrates an intrinsic link, as two-polarities models assume, between the development of relatedness, affect/stress regulation, and the development of the self (Gunnar, Quevedo, De Kloet, Oitzl, & Eric, 2007; Neumann, 2008; Sbarra & Hazan, 2008).

Relatively distinct neural circuits seem to serve the development of relatedness across the life span, beginning with the earliest capacities of the child to relate to others, probably served through the so-called contingency-detection system (Fonagy, Gergely, & Target, 2007), to early bonding, mature attachment and love relationships, and parenting/caregiving behaviors. These circuits include the mesocorticolimbic, dopaminergic, and hypothalamic-midbrain-limbic-paralimbic-cortical neural circuits (Rutherford, Williams, Moy, Mayes, & Johns, 2011; Swain, Lorberbaum, Kose, & Strathearn, 2007).

Neuropeptides such as oxytocin appear to play a pivotal role in these neural circuits and thus in affiliative behavior ranging from parental care to pair bonding and sexual behavior (Insel & Young, 2001; Neumann, 2008). Their role is also important in social cognition (Feldman, Weller, Zagoory-Sharon, & Levine, 2007) and in behavioral and neuroendocrinological responses to stress (Neumann, 2008). Briefly, in the context of secure attachment, release of oxytocin appears to reinforce social experiences by its rewarding effects, foster social cognition, and lead to the down-regulation of stress. From an evolutionary perspective, the ability to relate to others may thus promote the survival of the species (and the individual) and seems to be reinforced by brain reward neurocircuitry resulting in "broaden and build" (Fredrickson, 2001) cycles typical of attachment security (Fonagy & Luyten, 2009; Mikulincer & Shaver, 2007). Attachment relationships not only lead to rewarding experiences and the down-regulation of stress but also foster positive feelings about the self and explorative behavior (Insel & Young, 2001; Neumann, 2008). Thus, they link experiences of relatedness to opportunities to develop feelings of autonomy, competence, and identity, which in turn enhance coping and affect regulation (Fonagy & Luyten, 2009; Fredrickson, 2001). Studies in this area thus provide firm neurobiological evidence for the view, central in two-polarities models of personality pathology, that disruptions in the developmental dialectic interaction between relatedness and self-definition are associated with disruptions in the neural circuits (e.g., either relative hyperactivation or hypoactivation) underlying these dimensions.

This view is further supported by findings concerning neural circuits involved in the development of the self and self-representational capacities. Research findings suggest that cortical midline structures such as the medial prefrontal cortex, posterior cingulate, precuneus, and temporal parietal junction (Lieberman, 2007; Lombardo, Chakrabarti, Bullmore, & Baron-Cohen, 2011; for a meta-analysis, see Northoff et al., 2006) not only underlie the experience of self and autonomy but are also implicated in social cognition, theory of mind, mentalizing, and, hence, social cognition with regard to others (Fonagy & Luyten, 2009; Lieberman, 2007; Lombardo et al., 2010).

The emergence of the capacity to envision and reflect upon mental states (i.e., mentalizing, the capacity to understand the self and others in terms of desires, wishes, feelings, values, and goals) probably resulted in a substantial evolutionary advantage by enabling the development of increasingly complex group and social structures, thereby laying the foundation for what is now called culture (Allen, Fonagy, & Bateman, 2008). These evolutionary processes are ongoing and may play an important role in understanding vulnerability for psychopathology, as demonstrated by research on gene–culture coevolution. It seems that several genes increase sensitivity to environmental influences and attachment experiences in particular (Ellis, Boyce, Belsky, Bakermans-Kranenburg, & van IJzendoorn, 2011). Cultures that emphasize relatedness—so-called collectivistic or interdependent cultures—may be genetically programmed to be more open to influences that are rooted in attachment relationships (Chiao & Blizinsky, 2010). For instance, Way and Lieberman (2010) found a strong correlation between the relative frequency of so-called social sensitivity genes (e.g., *5-HTTLPR, MAOA-uVNTR, OPRM1 A118G*) and the degree of individualism versus collectivism (Way & Lieberman, 2010). Moreover, collectivism mediated the negative correlation between the frequency of these alleles and depression. This emphasis on relations and social support is thus associated with reduced levels of depression in populations with a high proportion of social sensitivity alleles. Yet, the rather dramatic recent shift toward individualism in many collectivistic cultures, with rapidly disintegrating social and family structures, may result in an increase in psychopathology in these socially sensitive populations. Recent studies in Peru and Korea, for instance, do indeed report dramatically increased rates of depression and suicide (up to 90% and 280%, respectively) over the past decades (Luyten & Blatt, 2013).

The neurobiology of relatedness and self-definition once again stresses the need to move beyond the current unfruitful search for relatively unique causes and treatments for specific psychiatric disorders, as it is unlikely that specific disorders are characterized by specific psychological and neurobiological causes (Luyten, Vliegen, Van Houdenhove, & Blatt, 2008). The recent Research Domain Criteria (RDoC) initiative of the National Institute of Mental Health similarly proposed that future research should focus on the neurobiological systems that underlie basic psychological capacities (e.g., reward neurocircuitry and neural systems implicated in self-representation, theory of mind, attachment/separation fear, positive valence systems), rather than on discrete disorders. Similarly, the current efforts to identify specific effective treatments for specific disorders will probably prove less fruitful than attempts at identifying treatment principles that are effective for spectra of disorders, an issue discussed in more detail below.

IMPLICATIONS FOR ASSESSING AND DIAGNOSING PERSONALITY PATHOLOGY

Reconciling Descriptive, Empirically Derived, and Theory-Driven Approaches to Personality Development

Descriptive, empirically based, and multivariate approaches to personality (e.g., five-factor model, tripartite model) and theory-driven approaches (e.g., the two-polarities models described in this chapter) have both contributed to our understanding of personality pathology. Although descriptive diagnoses and empirically derived personality theories seem attractive from a pragmatic and psychometric perspective, purely empirically derived models tend to create a classification system that has little clinical utility in the classification and treatment of mental disorders (Spitzer, First, Shedler, Westen, & Skodol, 2008). It is therefore more productive to consider these descriptive, empirically derived, and theory-driven approaches as complementary. Descriptive diagnoses are valuable, as are multivariate personality models focusing on broad temperament features, such as neuroticism or extraversion, that are important "building blocks" of human personality. Yet, a number of contemporary theory-driven approaches have remarkable convergence with the core defining features of psychopathology, at the empirical, descriptive, and theoretical levels. Blatt and Shichman (1983) and Livesley (2008), for example, have argued persuasively that two major dysfunctions characterize PDs (i.e., problems with relatedness or attachment on the one hand and problems with autonomy or self and identity on the other). Recently, the Personality and Personality Disorders Work Group preparing for *DSM–5* advanced a similar argument (Skodol et al., 2011). Research findings indeed support the assumption that impairments in relatedness/attachment and autonomy/self-identity are the central defining descriptive features of both symptom-based and PDs. On a theoretical level, impairments in the capacity for relatedness and self-definition (and associated impairments in mental representations or cognitive affective schema of self and others) underlie these descriptive features of psychiatric disorders. These dimensions therefore provide a comprehensive theoretical framework to integrate the theory-driven and empirically derived approaches to psychopathology. Moreover, these dimensions, in theoretically meaningful ways, relate to the central dimensions underlying adaptive personality development outlined above, proposing an essential continuity between normal and disrupted personality development.

What Is Psychopathology?

From the perspective of two-polarities models, all forms of psychopathology are characterized by momentary or continuous problems in relatedness and/or self-definition. These two dimensions thus provide a parsimonious classification system of psychopathology that can inform both fundamental research and clinical practice. Two-polarities models converge to suggest that different forms of psychopathology are best conceptualized in terms of distorted modes of adaptation that derive, at different developmental levels, from variations and disruptions in the synergistic interaction between aspects of relatedness and self-definition throughout the life span. Different forms of psychopathology are thus viewed as distorted attempts to maintain a balance, however maladaptive, between relatedness and self-definition, resulting in an excessive emphasis on one developmental line to the neglect of the other (Blatt, 2008; Luyten & Blatt, 2011; Meyer & Pilkonis, 2005; Mikulincer & Shaver, 2007).

Studies indicate, congruent with these assumptions, that various PDs can indeed be organized into two configurations: one focused around issues of relatedness (an *anaclitic* configuration) and the other focused around issues of self-definition (an *introjective* configuration; see the summary in Blatt & Luyten, 2010). For instance, research has shown that individuals with features of *Diagnostic and Statistical Manual of Mental Disorders* (4th ed., *DSM–IV*; American Psychiatric Association, 1994) Dependent, Histrionic, and Borderline PDs have significantly greater concern with issues of interpersonal relatedness than with issues of self-definition. Individuals with Antisocial, Narcissistic, Paranoid, Schizoid, Schizotypal, Avoidant, and Obsessive-Compulsive features, by contrast, are more preoccupied with issues of self-definition (Blatt & Luyten, 2010; Luyten & Blatt, 2011).

Of importance, research generally indicates that there is not a one-to-one relationship between these two developmental dimensions and descriptive *DSM* categories (Ouimette & Klein, 1993). Levy, Edell, and McGlashan (2007), for example, found that patients with a *DSM–5* diagnosis of Borderline Personality Disorder (BPD) had substantial symptomatic heterogeneity. Yet, Levy et al. identified within this symptomatically heterogeneous group a more interpersonally oriented (anaclitic) type and a more self-critical (introjective) type of BPD patients, in whom issues with relatedness and self-definition, respectively, predominated.

These findings have important implications for conceptualizing, classifying, and treating psychopathology. Fundamental differences in underlying personality organization may provide a more coherent differentiation both within and between various disorders than would a symptom-based classification system, as in *DSM–5* (American Psychiatric Association, 2013). Congruent with this view, the *DSM–5* Personality and Personality Disorders Work Group recommended dropping the Dependent, Histrionic, and Schizoid PDs because of insufficient evidence supporting the distinctive nature of these disorders and, thus, their clinical utility (Skodol, 2012).

Two-polarities models can contribute substantially to this discussion by providing a rigorous and empirically supported theoretical framework for evaluating the distinctiveness of specific PDs (Horowitz et al., 2006; Meyer & Pilkonis, 2005). As detailed elsewhere (Luyten & Blatt, 2011), PDs (or clusters of PD features) that are situated near each other in a two-dimensional space defined by relatedness and self-definition probably overlap to such an extent that clinically it may no longer be useful to distinguish between them (i.e., they are characterized by similar disturbances in relatedness and self-definition, despite potential differences in their symptomatic expression). This seems likely the case for the Histrionic and Dependent PDs and for the anaclitic subgroup of BPD, because they overlap considerably in their underlying disturbances in relatedness (Kernberg & Caligor, 2005; Luyten & Blatt, 2011). At the very least, they seem to reflect similar disruptions in relatedness at different developmental levels and thus are likely to show considerable overlap and comorbidity. In contrast, PDs (or clusters of PD features) situated further apart in the two-dimensional space probably warrant consideration as separate disorders because they have different underlying features (i.e., different types of disturbances in relatedness and self-definition).

DSM–5 has also questioned the distinction between Axis I (symptom) and Axis II (personality) disorders. Again, findings derived from research based on two-polarities models can inform this discussion. Studies have shown that various symptom disorders (i.e., mood disorders, several anxiety disorders, substance abuse disorders, eating disorders, and somatoform disorders) are characterized by (temporary or chronic) impairments in the sense of self and relatedness (for reviews, see Blatt, 2008; Blatt & Luyten, 2010; Egan, Wade, & Shafran, 2011; Zuroff et al., 2004). These findings suggest that maladaptive expressions of relatedness and self-definition (e.g., dependency, self-critical perfectionism) can, therefore, best be conceptualized as *transdiagnostic vulnerability factors*, which may also partly explain the high comorbidity among "symptom" and "personality" disorders and the longitudinal relationships among both types of disorders.

For instance, two-polarities models have allowed investigators from different theoretical orientations to identify two fundamental dimensions in depression: a so-called anaclitic dimension reflecting impairments in relatedness centered on feelings of loneliness, abandonment, and neglect and an introjective dimension reflecting impairments in self-definition centering on issues of self-worth and feelings of failure and guilt (Arieti & Bemporad, 1978; Beck, 1983; Blatt, 1974, 2004; Bowlby, 1973). More than four decades of research has provided extensive evidence for differences in the early life experiences associated with these two dimensions in depression as well as differences in the clinical expression of depression, the relational and attachment style, and therapeutic response associated with these dimensions (Beck,

2009; Blatt, 2004; Blatt, Zuroff, Hawley, & Auerbach, 2010; Luyten & Blatt, 2012). Similarly, researchers working in the domain of eating disorders have identified subtypes of patients with eating disorder reflecting different levels of impairment in self and relatedness, ranging from a high-functioning/perfectionism (reflecting an excessive emphasis on self-definition) to an avoidant/depressed subtype (reflecting less emphasis on self-definition, in combination with strong avoidance of relatedness) and an emotionally dysregulated subtype (reflecting severe impairments in both relatedness and self-definition; Mascaro, Hackett, & Rilling, 2013). These subtypes have been shown to explain additional variance beyond descriptive eating disorder diagnoses in predicting clinical presentation, course, and treatment outcome (Boone, Claes, & Luyten, 2014; Luyten, Blatt, & Fonagy, 2013). Hence, in contrast to descriptive *DSM* diagnoses in the field of depression and eating disorders, research focused on impairments in levels of self and relatedness has typically yielded more meaningful relationships with vulnerability factors implicated in psychopathology, such as depression and eating disorders, their clinical presentation and course, and their treatment response. These findings suggest that it is more productive to focus on underlying personality dynamics as the basis for the classification and treatment of depression and eating disorders than on manifest symptoms alone, as in the *DSM*.

TOWARD AN INTEGRATIVE, PSYCHODYNAMIC APPROACH TO PERSONALITY PATHOLOGY

Elsewhere, we have described our attempts to reconcile various approaches and findings concerning personality pathology (Blatt & Luyten, 2009, 2010; Luyten & Blatt, 2007, 2011, 2013). Here, we summarize and update these views.

We have proposed, based on the research reviewed, that different forms of psychopathology can be situated within a hierarchical model that integrates theory-driven models that emphasize relatedness and self-definition as central coordinates in normal and disrupted personality development with empirically derived models of basic temperament and personality factors. This integration is based on three central assumptions concerning the nature of personality pathology, which are outlined below.

A Circumplex View of Normal and Disrupted Personality Development

Research indicates a growing consensus that psychopathological disorders, congruent with contemporary interpersonal approaches (Horowitz et al., 2006; Pincus, 2005), can be arranged in a two-dimensional space defined by (a) *relatedness*, ranging from high to low anxiety or warmth in relationships, and (b) *self-definition*, ranging from low to high avoidance of others. The cognitive-affective interpersonal schemas or internal working models of self and others underlying these dimensions range from relatively broad schemas to more relationship-specific working models of self and others (Blatt & Luyten, 2010; Sibley & Overall, 2010). They are part of connectionist networks that develop over the life span and that, at least in normal development, become increasingly complex, differentiated, and integrated.

This view implies that there is fundamental continuity between normal personality features and psychopathology. On this basis, research should examine the developmental pathways from more basic genetic, temperament, and personality dimensions, which, in interaction with environmental factors, lead to disruptions at different developmental levels of the structural organization of cognitive-affective schemas of self and others across the life span. The contrasting view, as promoted by the *DSM* approach, assumes that each disorder has a relatively unique (biological) cause.

Our approach also implies that correlations between different disorders situated in the two dimensional, circumplex space are expected to decrease as one moves around the circumplex, which could lead to further understanding of the vexing problem of the high comorbidity of disorders in *DSM*. Furthermore, the emphasis on cognitive-affective schemas or internal working models provides a common language across disciplines, ranging from cognitive science, cognitive-behavioral research, social and personality psychology, developmental psychopathology, and psychodynamic and neuroscience approaches.

Finally, a host of validated measures exist, from self-report questionnaires to interviews and observer-rated scales, to assess various expressions of relatedness and self-definition at different levels of abstraction (Sibley & Overall, 2007, 2010).

A Prototype Approach

The proposed model, in contrast to most descriptive approaches, assumes that psychopathological disorders are best conceptualized as prototypes in this two-dimensional space and not as categorically distinct disorders, as in the *DSM*, or as defined by arbitrary or empirically determined cutoff scores on various dimensions, as proposed by proponents of multivariate dimensional models. The approach defines different disorders in terms of *prototypical, conflict–defense constellations*, however maladaptive, that reflect attempts to establish and maintain a sense of interpersonal relatedness and self-definition at different developmental levels of organization (Blatt & Shichman, 1983; McWilliams, 1994). Hence, individual patients may resemble, to a greater or lesser extent, prototypical ways of dealing with issues of relatedness and self-definition, ranging from normal personality functioning, to subclinical psychopathology, to full-blown symptom and/or PDs.

The groundbreaking work of Drew Westen and Jonathan Shedler (Shedler & Westen, 2010; Spitzer et al., 2008) has amply demonstrated the advantages of prototypes over the *DSM* categorical approach or multivariate personality models. Clinicians indeed tend to conceptualize disorders in terms of prototypes and therefore prefer prototypical classificatory systems, which seem rooted in the human tendency to use a prototype approach for classification. Cognitive science provides further support for the notion that prototypes reflect a high time and effort ratio (Spitzer et al., 2008) that enables clinicians to consider the dynamic interactions of different dimensions, a view notably absent in the symptom-based *DSM* and multivariate personality models. Moreover, several statistical methods have been designed to investigate the nature, development, and structure of prototypes (Shedler & Westen, 2010), further emphasizing the clinical utility of the proposed model.

Furthermore, the proposed prototype approach suggests a possible underlying hierarchical organization of different disorders, thus providing a more parsimonious way of dealing with the problematic and vexing issue of comorbidity (Egan et al., 2011). For example, evidence suggests that anaclitic and introjective personality traits such as dependency and self-critical perfectionism may explain in part the high comorbidity among several Axis I disorders, as discussed previously. Similarly, the high comorbidity among depression, anxiety, and substance abuse disorders can at least be partly explained by the fact that these disorders, rather than being different "diseases," reflect different responses to and attempts to cope with issues of relatedness and self-definition (Luyten & Blatt, 2012). What are considered to be symptom-based disorders may therefore be part of a spectrum of disorders (Westen, Shedler, & Bradley, 2006). Multivariate statistical methods promise to assist in exploring such potential spectrum and/or hierarchical organizations of psychopathology.

A Dynamic, Developmental Psychopathology Perspective

A common criticism of the *DSM* is its lack of developmental sensitivity, because it typically uses the same criteria for disorders at different ages and developmental stages. Moreover, most children present with multiple problems, rendering the need for discrete diagnoses in childhood and adolescence less urgent. The *DSM* system, furthermore, insufficiently acknowledges the fundamental continuity between disorders and problems in childhood/adolescence and adulthood.

Developmental psychopathology has shown by contrast that vulnerability to psychopathology is best conceptualized on the basis of the concepts of *equifinality* and *multifinality* across the life span (Cicchetti & Rogosch, 1996). Equifinality suggests that, rather than disorders being individually distinguishable and having a relatively unique etiology, different etiological factors may in fact lead to the same developmental outcome. At the same time, particular developmental factors (e.g., temperament) may, depending on the presence other factors, lead to different developmental outcomes (multifinality). Again, this view stresses the notion that researchers and clinicians should consider the complex developmental pathways that lead to a range of end states that share common characteristics (i.e., spectra of disorders) rather than focus on specific disorders.

Empirically derived models that focus on lower level temperament factors may inform theory-driven models of personality development by studying the complex pathways of lower order, more basic, temperament and personality factors across development. Person-centered and variable-centered research may complement each other in identifying developmental trajectories of both individuals as well as specific variables implicated in the development of normal and disrupted personality development. Future research should also seek to identify the neurobiological correlates of these fundamental building blocks of personality, consistent with the RDoC initiative cited above.

These considerations can be illustrated by our consideration of two common PDs (i.e., Dependent and Avoidant PDs). Studies suggest that Dependent PD, congruent with theory-driven models, is situated in the low avoidance, high anxiety quadrant, reflecting strong desires for attachment and love in combination with strong fears of abandonment and loss of love (Luyten & Blatt, 2011; Meyer & Pilkonis, 2005). Hence, individuals with Dependent PD typically value interpersonal relationships but are constantly preoccupied with issues of rejection and abandonment. Avoidant PD, in contrast, is situated within the high anxiety, high avoidance quadrant, suggesting that these individuals are involved in an approach–avoidance conflict. On the one hand, they desire to be accepted and admired. On the other hand, they fear that will be criticized and rejected, which leads them to pull away from others. Individuals with Avoidant PD often show extremely high levels of avoidance and an almost complete denial of needs to be close to others.

Hence, these two disorders clearly reflect different ways of dealing with issues of relatedness and self-definition that can be expressed, depending on other factors, in either internalizing or externalizing symptoms. For instance, whereas young adolescents with low levels of effortful control may attempt to cope with issues of self-criticism by externalizing their struggles with these issues onto authority figures and society, expressed in antisocial behavior, other adolescents, with higher levels of effortful control (disinhibition), may express the same issues in self-critical (introjective) depression (Leadbeater,

Kuperminc, Blatt, & Hertzog, 1999). These considerations further illustrate the view that disorders are not static end-states but complex, multidetermined, dynamic, conflict–defense resolutions. For instance, individuals in the high avoidance and low anxiety quadrant may report a positive model of self, but studies clearly indicate that this results from a continuous defense against underlying feelings of insecurity and inferiority (Mikulincer & Shaver, 2007). Likewise, dependent individuals do not merely have positive models of others but also harbor feelings of jealousy and anger toward others, which they typically inhibit out of fear of abandonment and rejection (Mikulincer & Shaver, 2007).

In summary, we argue that different disorders are part of spectra of disorders (i.e., groups of disorders that share similar etiological features) that result from complex interactions between biological and psychosocial factors across the life span. Within these spectra, several disorders can be distinguished based on a prototype approach, and there might be several ways to distinguish different spectra (e.g., based on genetic, neural, and psychosocial factors).

IMPLICATIONS FOR TREATMENT

The approach proposed in this chapter argues that it may be more productive for future research to investigate the efficacy and effectiveness of broad *transdiagnostic treatments* that address basic underlying personality issues (Egan et al., 2011; Kazdin, 2011; Luyten & Blatt, 2007, 2011), rather than to continue to focus on developing specific treatments for specific disorders or symptoms in biological as well as psychosocial interventions. For instance, biological research is currently exploring the effects of the neuropeptide oxytocin in the treatment of disorders that are marked by severe problems in relatedness, such as autism, schizophrenia, social phobia, and BPD (Striepens, Kendrick, Maier, & Hurlemann, 2011). With regard to psychosocial interventions, research indicates that common features of evidence-based treatments may be primarily responsible for treatment outcome, both in "symptom" and in "personality" disorders (Bateman, 2012; Blatt et al., 2010; Wampold, Minami, Baskin, & Tierney, 2002; Westen, Novotny, & Thompson-Brenner, 2004).

The views proposed in this chapter are further supported by findings that patient features are crucial in explaining treatment outcome. Patients who are primarily preoccupied with issues of relatedness or self-definition are differentially responsive to different aspects of the treatment process, regardless of their specific diagnosis. Patients primarily preoccupied with issues of relatedness (i.e., anaclitic patients), for instance, are responsive mainly to supportive dimensions of interventions. Patients primarily preoccupied with issues of self-definition (i.e., introjective patients) have been shown to be more responsive to interpretive–exploratory dimensions (Blatt et al., 2010). Research in this context suggests a fundamental parallel between normal psychological development and the processes of therapeutic change (Luyten, Blatt, & Mayes, 2012). Just as in normal personality development, therapeutic change seems to result from a synergistic interaction of experiences of interpersonal relatedness and self-definition, of experiences of mutuality and incompatibility, of understanding and misunderstanding. Therapeutic change may thus result from the reactivation of a normal synergistic developmental process in which interpersonal experiences in the therapeutic relationship contribute to the development of the sense of self, leading to more mature expressions of interpersonal relatedness that, in turn, further foster the development of the self (Safran, Muran, & Eubanks-Carter, 2011). Therapeutic change may thus primarily result from a therapist entering the subjective world of the patient, thereby providing experiences of how one engages with others—how to think about and understand one's thoughts and feelings as well as those of others. These empathic experiences result in changes in the content and the developmental level of the cognitive structural organization of patients' representation (cognitive-affective schema) of self and other, as well as changes in their level of mentalization (reflective functioning); that is, in their ability to reflect on themselves as well as appreciate the thoughts and feelings of others (Fonagy, Luyten, & Allison, 2013).

Although further research is needed to explore more fully the factors that contribute to sustained therapeutic change, these findings demonstrate the advantages of a theoretical model that proposes a parallel between normal personality development and therapeutic change.

CONCLUSION

The findings reviewed in this chapter indicate that two-polarities models can provide researchers and clinicians with a parsimonious and theoretically encompassing model of normal and disrupted development that has immediate relevance for therapeutic intervention. These models are theoretically and empirically related to extant multivariate models of personality. This provides a fuller understanding of PDs and opens up many interesting perspectives for research and clinical practice (Luyten & Blatt, 2011).

REFERENCES

Allen, J. G., Fonagy, P., & Bateman, A. W. (2008). *Mentalizing in clinical practice*. Washington, DC: American Psychiatric Press.

American Psychiatric Association. (1994). *Diagnostic and statistical manual of mental disorders* (4th ed.). Washington, DC: Author.

American Psychiatric Association. (2013). *Diagnostic and statistical manual of mental disorders* (5th ed.). Arlington, VA: Author.

Angyal, A. (1951). *Neurosis and treatment: A holistic theory.* New York, NY: Wiley.

Arieti, S., & Bemporad, J. (1978). *Psychotherapy of severe and mild depression.* Northvale, NJ: Aronson.

Bakan, D. (1966). *The duality of human existence.* Chicago, IL: Rand McNally.

Bartholomew, K., & Horowitz, L. M. (1991). Attachment styles among young adults: A test of a four-category model. *Journal of Personality and Social Psychology, 61,* 226–244. doi:10.1037/0022-3514.61.2.226

Bateman, A. W. (2012). Treating borderline personality disorder in clinical practice [Editorial]. *The American Journal of Psychiatry, 169,* 560–563. doi:10.1176/appi.ajp.2012.12030341

Beck, A. T. (1983). Cognitive therapy of depression: New perspectives. In P. J. Clayton & J. E. Barrett (Eds.), *Treatment of depression: Old controversies and new approaches* (pp. 265–290). New York, NY: Raven Press.

Beck, A. T. (2009). Cognitive aspects of personality disorders and their relation to syndromal disorders: A psychoevolutionary approach. In C. R. Cloninger (Ed.), *Personality and psychopathology* (pp. 411–429). Washington, DC: American Psychiatric Press.

Benjamin, L. S. (2005). Interpersonal theory of personality disorders: The structural analysis of social behavior and interpersonal reconstructive therapy. In M. F. Lenzenweger & J. F. Clarkin (Eds.), *Major theories of personality disorder* (2nd ed., pp. 157–230). New York, NY: Guilford Press.

Blatt, S. J. (1974). Levels of object representation in anaclitic and introjective depression. *Psychoanalytic Study of the Child, 29,* 107–157.

Blatt, S. J. (2004). *Experiences of depression: Theoretical, clinical and research perspectives.* Washington, DC: American Psychological Association.

Blatt, S. J. (2008). *Polarities of experience: Relatedness and self-definition in personality development, psychopathology, and the therapeutic process.* Washington, DC: American Psychological Association.

Blatt, S. J., & Homann, E. (1992). Parent–child interaction in the etiology of dependent and self-critical depression. *Clinical Psychology Review, 12,* 47–91. doi:10.1016/0272-7358(92)90091-L

Blatt, S. J., & Luyten, P. (2009). A structural–developmental psychodynamic approach to psychopathology: Two polarities of experience across the life span. *Development and Psychopathology, 21,* 793–814. doi:10.1017/S0954579409000431

Blatt, S. J., & Luyten, P. (2010). Reactivating the psychodynamic approach to classify psychopathology. In T. Millon, R. F. Krueger, & E. Simonsen (Eds.), *Contemporary directions in psychopathology: Scientific foundations of the DSM–V and ICD-11* (pp. 483–514). New York, NY: Guilford Press.

Blatt, S. J., & Shichman, S. (1983). Two primary configurations of psychopathology. *Psychoanalysis and Contemporary Thought, 6,* 187–254.

Blatt, S. J., Zuroff, D. C., Hawley, L. L., & Auerbach, J. S. (2010). Predictors of sustained therapeutic change. *Psychotherapy Research, 20,* 37–54. doi:10.1080/10503300903121080

Boone, L., Claes, L., & Luyten, P. (2014). Too strict or too loose? Perfectionism and impulsivity: The relation with eating disorder symptoms using a person-centered approach. *Eating Behaviors, 15,* 17–23. doi:10.1016/j.eatbeh.2013.10.013

Bowlby, J. (1973). *Attachment and loss: Vol. 2. Separation: Anxiety and anger.* New York, NY: Basic Books.

Chiao, J. Y., & Blizinsky, K. D. (2010). Culture–gene coevolution of individualism–collectivism and the serotonin transporter gene. *Proceedings of the Royal Society B: Biological Sciences, 277,* 529–537. doi:10.1098/rspb.2009.1650

Cicchetti, D., & Rogosch, F. A. (1996). Equifinality and multifinality in developmental psychopathology. *Development and Psychopathology, 8,* 597–600. doi:10.1017/S0954579400007318

Clark, D. A., & Beck, A. T. (1999). *Scientific foundations of cognitive theory and therapy of depression.* New York, NY: Wiley.

Deci, E. L., & Ryan, R. M. (2012). Self-determination theory. In P. A. M. V. Lange, A. W. Kruglanski, & E. T. Higgins (Eds.), *Handbook of theories of social psychology* (Vol. 1, pp. 416–437). Thousand Oaks, CA: Sage.

Egan, S. J., Wade, T. D., & Shafran, R. (2011). Perfectionism as a transdiagnostic process: A clinical review. *Clinical Psychology Review, 31,* 203–212. doi:10.1016/j.cpr.2010.04.009

Ellis, B. J., Boyce, W. T., Belsky, J., Bakermans-Kranenburg, M. J., & van IJzendoorn, M. H. (2011). Differential susceptibility to the environment: An evolutionary–neurodevelopmental theory. *Development and Psychopathology, 23,* 7–28. doi:10.1017/S0954579410000611

Feldman, R., Weller, A., Zagoory-Sharon, O., & Levine, A. (2007). Evidence for a neuroendocrinological foundation of human affiliation: Plasma oxytocin levels across pregnancy and the postpartum period predict mother–infant bonding. *Psychological Science, 18,* 965–970. doi:10.1111/j.1467-9280.2007.02010.x

Fonagy, P., Gergely, G., & Target, M. (2007). The parent–infant dyad and the construction of the subjective self. *Journal of Child Psychology and Psychiatry, 48,* 288–328. doi:10.1111/j.1469-7610.2007.01727.x

Fonagy, P., & Luyten, P. (2009). A developmental, mentalization-based approach to the understanding and treatment of borderline personality disorder. *Development and Psychopathology, 21,* 1355–1381. doi:10.1017/S0954579409990198

Fonagy, P., Luyten, P., & Allison, E. (2013). *Teaching to learn from experience: Epistemic mistrust, personality, and psychotherapy.* Manuscript submitted for publication.

Fredrickson, B. L. (2001). The role of positive emotions in positive psychology: The broaden-and-build theory of positive emotions. *American Psychologist, 56,* 218–226. doi:10.1037/0003-066X.56.3.218

Gunnar, M. R., Quevedo, K., De Kloet, R. E., Oitzl, M. S., & Eric, V. (2007). Early care experiences and HPA axis regulation in children: A mechanism for later trauma vulnerability. *Progress in Brain Research, 167,* 137–149. doi:10.1016/S0079-6123(07)67010-1

Horowitz, L. M., & Strack, S. (Eds.). (2011). *Handbook of interpersonal psychology: Theory, research, assessment.* New York, NY: Wiley.

Horowitz, L. M., Wilson, K. R., Turan, B., Zolotsev, P., Constantino, M. J., & Henderson, L. (2006). How interpersonal motives clarify the meaning of interpersonal behavior: A revised circumplex model. *Personality and Social Psychology Review, 10,* 67–86. doi:10.1207/s15327957pspr1001_4

Insel, T. R., & Young, L. J. (2001). The neurobiology of attachment. *Nature Reviews Neuroscience, 2,* 129–136. doi:10.1038/35053579

Kazdin, A. E. (2011). Evidence-based treatment research: Advances, limitations, and next steps. *American Psychologist, 66,* 685–698. doi:10.1037/a0024975

Kernberg, O. F., & Caligor, E. (2005). A psychoanalytic theory of personality disorders. In M. F. Lenzenweger & J. F. Clarkin (Eds.), *Major theories of personality disorder* (2nd ed., pp. 114–156). New York, NY: Guilford Press.

Kiesler, D. J. (1983). The 1982 Interpersonal Circle: A taxonomy for complementarity in human transactions. *Psychological Review, 90,* 185–214. doi:10.1037/0033-295X.90.3.185

Leadbeater, B. J., Kuperminc, G. P., Blatt, S. J., & Hertzog, C. (1999). A multivariate mode of gender differences in adolescents' internalizing and externalizing problems. *Developmental Psychology, 35,* 1268–1282. doi:10.1037/0012-1649.35.5.1268

Leary, T. (1957). *The interpersonal diagnosis of personality.* New York, NY: Ronald Press.

Levy, K. N., Edell, W. S., & McGlashan, T. H. (2007). Depressive experiences in inpatients with borderline personality disorder. *Psychiatric Quarterly, 78,* 129–143. doi:10.1007/s11126-006-9033-8

Lieberman, M. D. (2007). Social cognitive neuroscience: A review of core processes. *Annual Review of Psychology, 58,* 259–289. doi:10.1146/annurev.psych.58.110405.085654

Livesley, J. (2008). Toward a genetically-informed model of borderline personality disorder. *Journal of Personality Disorders, 22,* 42–71. doi:10.1521/pedi.2008.22.1.42

Lombardo, M. V., Chakrabarti, B., Bullmore, E. T., & Baron-Cohen, S. (2011). Specialization of right temporo-parietal junction for mentalizing and its relation to social impairments in autism. *NeuroImage, 56,* 1832–1838. doi:10.1016/j.neuroimage.2011.02.067

Lombardo, M. V., Chakrabarti, B., Bullmore, E. T., Wheelwright, S. J., Sadek, S. A., Suckling, J., & Baron-Cohen, S. (2010). Shared neural circuits for mentalizing about the self and others. *Journal of Cognitive Neuroscience, 22,* 1623–1635. doi:10.1162/jocn.2009.21287

Luyten, P., & Blatt, S. J. (2007). Looking back towards the future: Is it time to change the *DSM* approach to psychiatric disorders? The case of depression. *Psychiatry: Interpersonal and Biological Processes, 70*, 85–99. doi:10.1521/psyc.2007.70.2.85

Luyten, P., & Blatt, S. J. (2011). Integrating theory-driven and empirically-derived models of personality development and psychopathology: A proposal for *DSM–V*. *Clinical Psychology Review, 31*, 52–68. doi:10.1016/j.cpr.2010.09.003

Luyten, P., & Blatt, S. J. (2012). Psychodynamic treatment of depression. *Psychiatric Clinics of North America, 35*, 111–129. doi:10.1016/j.psc.2012.01.001

Luyten, P., & Blatt, S. J. (2013). Interpersonal relatedness and self-definition in normal and disrupted personality development: Retrospect and prospect. *American Psychologist, 68*, 172–183. doi:10.1037/a0032243

Luyten, P., Blatt, S. J., & Fonagy, P. (2013). Impairments in self structures in depression and suicide in psychodynamic and cognitive behavioral approaches: Implications for clinical practice and research. *International Journal of Cognitive Therapy, 6*, 265–279. doi:10.1521/ijct.2013.6.3.265

Luyten, P., Blatt, S. J., & Mayes, L. C. (2012). Process and outcome in psychoanalytic psychotherapy research: The need for a (relatively) new paradigm. In R. A. Levy, J. S. Ablon, & H. Kächele (Eds.), *Psychodynamic psychotherapy research: Evidence-based practice and practice-based evidence* (2nd ed., pp. 345–360). New York, NY: Humana Press/Springer.

Luyten, P., Kempke, S., Van Wambeke, P., Claes, S. J., Blatt, S. J., & Van Houdenhove, B. (2011). Self-critical perfectionism, stress generation, and stress sensitivity in patients with chronic fatigue syndrome: Relationship with severity of depression. *Psychiatry: Interpersonal and Biological Processes, 74*, 21–30. doi:10.1521/psyc.2011.74.1.21

Luyten, P., Vliegen, N., Van Houdenhove, B., & Blatt, S. J. (2008). Equifinality, multifinality, and the rediscovery of the importance of early experiences: Pathways from early adversity to psychiatric and (functional) somatic disorders. *Psychoanalytic Study of the Child, 63*, 27–60.

Mascaro, J. S., Hackett, P. D., & Rilling, J. K. (2013). Testicular volume is inversely correlated with nurturing-related brain activity in human fathers. *Proceedings of the National Academy of Sciences, USA, 110*, 15746–15751. doi:10.1073/pnas.1305579110

McAdams, D. P. (1985). *Power, intimacy, and the life story: Personological inquiries into identity*. Homewood, IL: Dorsey.

McClelland, D. C. (1985). *Human motivation*. Cambridge, England: Cambridge University Press.

McWilliams, N. (1994). *Psychoanalytic diagnosis*. New York, NY: Guilford Press.

Meyer, B., & Pilkonis, P. A. (2005). An attachment model of personality disorder. In M. F. Lenzenweger & J. F. Clarkin (Eds.), *Major theories of personality disorder* (2nd ed., pp. 231–281). New York, NY: Guilford Press.

Mikulincer, M., & Shaver, P. R. (2007). *Attachment in adulthood: Structure, dynamics and change*. New York, NY: Guilford Press.

Neumann, I. D. (2008). Brain oxytocin: A key regulator of emotional and social behaviours in both females and males. *Journal of Neuroendocrinology, 20,* 858–865. doi:10.1111/j.1365-2826.2008.01726.x

Northoff, G., Heinzel, A., de Greck, M., Bermpohl, F., Dobrowolny, H., & Panksepp, J. (2006). Self-referential processing in our brain—A meta-analysis of imaging studies on the self. *NeuroImage, 31,* 440–457. doi:10.1016/j.neuroimage.2005.12.002

Ouimette, P. C., & Klein, D. N. (1993). Convergence of psychoanalytic and cognitive-behavioral theories of depression: An empirical review and new data on Blatt's and Beck's models. In J. M. Masling & R. F. Bornstein (Eds.), *Empirical studies of psychoanalytic theories: Vol. 4. Psychoanalytic perspectives on psychopathology* (pp. 191–223). Washington, DC: American Psychological Association.

Pincus, A. L. (2005). A contemporary integrative interpersonal theory of personality disorders. In M. F. Lenzenweger & J. F. Clarkin (Eds.), *Major theories of personality disorder* (2nd ed., pp. 282–331). New York, NY: Guilford Press.

Roisman, G. I., Holland, A., Fortuna, K., Fraley, R. C., Clausell, E., & Clarke, A. (2007). The Adult Attachment Interview and self-reports of attachment style: An empirical rapprochement. *Journal of Personality and Social Psychology, 92,* 678–697. doi:10.1037/0022-3514.92.4.678

Rutherford, H. J. V., Williams, S. K., Moy, S., Mayes, L. C., & Johns, J. M. (2011). Disruption of maternal parenting circuitry by addictive process: Rewiring of reward and stress systems. *Frontiers in Psychiatry, 2,* Article 37. doi:10.3389/fpsyt.2011.00037

Safran, J. D., Muran, J. C., & Eubanks-Carter, C. (2011). Repairing alliance ruptures. *Psychotherapy: Theory, Research, and Practice, 48,* 80–87. doi:10.1037/a0022140

Sbarra, D. A., & Hazan, C. (2008). Coregulation, dysregulation, self-regulation: An integrative analysis and empirical agenda for understanding adult attachment, separation, loss, and recovery. *Personality and Social Psychology Review, 12,* 141–167. doi:10.1177/1088868308315702

Shedler, J., & Westen, D. (2010). The Shedler–Westen Assessment Procedure: Making personality diagnosis clinically meaningful. In J. F. Clarkin, P. Fonagy, & G. O. Gabbard (Eds.), *Psychodynamic psychotherapy for personality disorders: A clinical handbook* (pp. 125–161). Washington, DC: American Psychiatric Publishing.

Sibley, C. (2007). The association between working models of attachment and personality: Toward an integrative framework operationalizing global relational models. *Journal of Research in Personality, 41,* 90–109. doi:10.1016/j.jrp.2006.03.002

Sibley, C., & Overall, N. (2007). The boundaries between attachment and personality: Associations across three levels of the attachment network. *Journal of Research in Personality, 41,* 960–967. doi:10.1177/0265407509346421

Sibley, C., & Overall, N. (2010). Modeling the hierarchical structure of personality–attachment associations: Domain diffusion versus domain differentiation. *Journal of Social and Personal Relationships, 27,* 47–70. doi:10.1177/0265407509346421

Skodol, A. E. (2012). Personality disorders in *DSM–5. Annual Review of Clinical Psychology, 8,* 317–344. doi:10.1146/annurev-clinpsy-032511-143131

Skodol, A. E., Bender, D. S., Morley, L. C., Clark, L. A., Oldham, J. M., Alarcon, R. D., . . . Siever, L. J. (2011). Personality disorder types proposed for *DSM–5. Journal of Personality Disorders, 25,* 136–169. doi:10.1521/pedi.2011.25.2.136

Soenens, B., Vansteenkiste, M., & Luyten, P. (2010). Towards a domain-specific approach to the study of parental psychological control: Distinguishing between dependency-oriented and achievement-oriented psychological control. *Journal of Personality, 78,* 217–256. doi:10.1111/j.1467-6494.2009.00614.x

Spitzer, R. L., First, M. B., Shedler, J. P., Westen, D. P., & Skodol, A. E. (2008). Clinical utility of five dimensional systems for personality diagnosis: A "consumer preference" study. *Journal of Nervous and Mental Disease, 196,* 356–374. doi:10.1097/NMD.0b013e3181710950

Striepens, N., Kendrick, K. M., Maier, W., & Hurlemann, R. (2011). Prosocial effects of oxytocin and clinical evidence for its therapeutic potential. *Frontiers in Neuroendocrinology, 32,* 426–450. doi:10.1016/j.yfrne.2011.07.001

Swain, J. E., Lorberbaum, J. P., Kose, S., & Strathearn, L. (2007). Brain basis of early parent–infant interactions: Psychology, physiology, and in vivo functional neuroimaging studies. *Journal of Child Psychology and Psychiatry, 48,* 262–287. doi:10.1111/j.1469-7610.2007.01731.x

Wampold, B. E., Minami, T., Baskin, T. W., & Tierney, S. C. (2002). A meta-(re)analysis of the effects of cognitive therapy versus "other therapies" for depression. *Journal of Affective Disorders, 68,* 159–165. doi:10.1016/S0165-0327(00)00287-1

Way, B. M., & Lieberman, M. D. (2010). Is there a genetic contribution to cultural differences? Collectivism, individualism, and genetic markers of social sensitivity. *Social Cognitive and Affective Neuroscience, 5,* 203–211. doi:10.1093/scan/nsq059

Westen, D., Novotny, C. M., & Thompson-Brenner, H. (2004). The empirical status of empirically supported psychotherapies: Assumptions, findings, and reporting in controlled clinical trials. *Psychological Bulletin, 130,* 631–663. doi:10.1037/0033-2909.130.4.631

Westen, D., Shedler, J., & Bradley, R. (2006). A prototype approach to personality disorder diagnosis. *The American Journal of Psychiatry, 163,* 846–856. doi:10.1176/appi.ajp.163.5.846

Wiggins, J. S. (Ed.). (2003). *Paradigms of personality assessment.* New York, NY: Guilford Press.

Yeomans, F., & Diamond, D. (2010). Transference-focused psychotherapy and borderline personality disorder. In J. F. Clarkin, P. Fonagy, & G. O. Gabbard (Eds.), *Psychodynamic psychotherapy for personality disorders: A clinical handbook* (pp. 209–238). Washington, DC: American Psychiatric Publishing.

Zuroff, D. C., Koestner, R., Moskowitz, D. S., McBride, C., & Bagby, R. M. (2012). Therapist's autonomy support and patient's self-criticism predict motivation during brief treatments for depression. *Journal of Social and Clinical Psychology, 31*, 903–932. doi:10.1521/jscp.2012.31.9.903

Zuroff, D. C., Mongrain, M., & Santor, D. A. (2004). Conceptualizing and measuring personality vulnerability to depression: Commentary on Coyne and Whiffen (1995). *Psychological Bulletin, 130*, 489–511. doi:10.1037/0033-2909.130.3.489

13

AN INTEGRATIVE ATTACHMENT THEORY FRAMEWORK OF PERSONALITY DISORDERS

KENNETH N. LEVY, J. WESLEY SCALA, CHRISTINA M. TEMES, AND TRACY L. CLOUTHIER

Over the last two decades, John Bowlby's attachment theory has increasingly become recognized as a clinically and theoretically useful approach for conceptualizing and understanding fundamental aspects of personality disorders (PDs). Attachment difficulties are characteristic of virtually all PDs and are often a central feature of personality pathology (Levy, 2005). For example, impoverished relationships are a cardinal feature of schizoid, avoidant, narcissistic, and antisocial PDs, whereas those with borderline personality disorder (BPD) and dependent PD struggle with feelings of aloneness and are preoccupied by fears of abandonment and the dissolution of close relationships. Furthermore, intense and stormy relationships are one of the central features of BPD (Levy, 2005), but those with dependent pathology appear incapable of functioning without the aid of others (Bornstein, 1993). A number of clinical theorists and researchers have recently begun to conceptualize these interpersonal aspects of PDs as stemming from impairments in the

http://dx.doi.org/10.1037/14549-014
Personality Disorders: Toward Theoretical and Empirical Integration in Diagnosis and Assessment,
S. K. Huprich (Editor)

underlying attachment organization (e.g., Fonagy et al., 1996; Gunderson, 1996; Levy & Blatt, 1999).

In this chapter, we articulate an attachment theoretical perspective on the development, psychopathology, and treatment of PDs. We begin with a brief review of Bowlby's theory of attachment and an overview of the evidence with respect to the major claims of attachment theory. Next, we discuss the theoretical, conceptual, and clinical links between attachment theory and PDs. We then present recent work linking attachment theory and PDs, with a focus on implications for underlying mechanisms of personality pathology. We conclude by articulating the implications of these findings for understanding PDs and noting salient issues that suggest further research.

ATTACHMENT THEORY

Attachment theory is concerned with the affective bond that emerges between child and caregiver early in development, as well as the implications of this bond for an individual's self-concept, self-regulation, and relationships throughout the life span (Bowlby, 1973, 1977). John Bowlby was a British psychiatrist and psychoanalyst who trained as a physician early last century. Although his work emerged out of an object relations tradition within psychoanalysis, he also used a combination of other scientific disciplines, including ethology, cognitive psychology, and developmental psychology, to explain affectional bonding between infants and their caregivers as well as the long-term effects these early "attachment" experiences have on the development of both personality and psychopathology. Integrating ideas from these disciplines, Bowlby postulated that the caregiver–infant attachment bond is a complex, instinctually guided behavioral system that has functioned throughout human evolution to protect the infant from danger and predators and to ensure that offspring reached sexual maturity, increasing the likelihood of reproduction. However, the survival gain of attachment lies not only in eliciting protection from caregivers but also in enhancing the infant's survival by providing comfort in times of stress and the experience of psychological containment of aversive affect states required for the development of a coherent and symbolizing self (Fonagy, 1999).

Bowlby contended that all infants become attached to their caregivers; however, he postulated that there were differences in the quality of the attachment between infants and caregivers. Bowlby hypothesized that the *felt security* provided through the attachment relationship in infancy is based on the caregiver's reliable and sensitive provision of love, comfort, and fulfillment of emotional needs, as well as food and warmth. This security is expressed in two main ways: the use of the caregiver as a safe haven to turn to in times of distress and the use of the caregiver as a secure base from which to explore one's environment. Bowlby postulated that differences in infant–caregiver relationships would lead to distinctive patterns of attachment (and therefore of safe haven and secure base behaviors). Those caregivers who provided reliable and sensitive care would produce infants characterized by secure attachment, who would turn to caregivers when scared, cold, or needing emotional support and would otherwise be able to explore the environment with a sense that the caregiver was looking out for them. Those providing less reliable and sensitive care would produce infants who would display insecure attachment patterns characterized by an inability to use the caregiver for emotional support in times of distress or to explore their environment during stress-free times.

On the basis of Bowlby's writings, a seminal study by Ainsworth, Blehar, Waters, and Wall (1978) identified three major styles of attachment in infancy—secure, avoidant, and anxious-ambivalent—and linked these styles to caregivers' parenting behavior. Later, a fourth category, disorganized-disoriented, was added (Main & Solomon, 1986, 1990). The disorganized baby displays disorganized and/or disoriented behaviors in the parent's presence, suggesting a temporary "collapse" of a behavioral strategy. The findings from Ainsworth's lab have been replicated and extended in many subsequent studies in over 10,000 infants (Bakermans-Kranenburg & van IJzendoorn, 2009), and these differences in attachment are consistently associated with differences in caretaker warmth and responsiveness (van IJzendoorn, 1995). Additionally, a number of longitudinal studies have found impressive levels of influence of infant attachment styles on subsequent functioning and adaptive potential, as well as a high degree of continuity between attachment during infancy and attachment in adulthood (Fraley, 2002).

Bowlby proposed that through repeated transactions with their attachment figures, infants form mental representations of the self and others and develop expectations about interpersonal relations, which he called *internal working models* (IWMs). This concept is central to Bowlby's theory and the idea that attachment is stable over time. These IWMs or mental representations include expectations, beliefs, emotional appraisals, and rules for processing or excluding information (i.e., defenses). IWMs can be partly conscious or partly unconscious and need not be completely consistent or coherent. According to Bowlby, they organize personality development and subsequently direct and shape future relationships by acting as a template or heuristic that contributes to shaping thoughts, feelings, and behaviors in future relationships.

The continuity of these mental models over time is rooted in the complementary nature of working models of self and other and concomitant expectations regarding one's role in interpersonal relationships. For example, an infant whose needs are typically left unmet may develop a model of others as unreliable and uncaring. Consequently, the neglected infant and child may, as an adult, believe each new person will prove to be inaccessible, uncaring, and unresponsive. Conversely, the child whose needs have been addressed in a consistent loving and supportive manner may subsequently regard others as dependable and trustworthy.

Longitudinal studies have found, consistent with Bowlby's hypothesis that attachment patterns tend to remain stable over time, that attachment classifications demonstrate considerable stability between infancy and young adulthood. Experiences in relationships during the intervening period of time contribute to the continuity or discontinuity of attachment patterns for any given individual (Fraley, 2002). Such contributions suggest that although attachment patterns are rooted in early experiences with caregivers, later relationships can influence these patterns.

Relation Between Attachment and Other Perspectives

Bowlby's IWMs are very similar to the psychoanalytic concept of mental representations proposed by other object relations theorists; however, there are two notable exceptions. First, Bowlby emphasized that IWMs were constantly being updated, whereas the psychoanalytic concept of mental representations at that time conceptualized these representations as being relatively static. Second, Bowlby stressed the realistic aspects of IWMs, writing that IWMs "are tolerably accurate reflections of the experiences those individuals actually had" (Bowlby, 1973, p. 235), whereas dominant theories of the time focused on the fantasy and distorted aspects of representations (Klein, 1948). Although Bowlby emphasized the realistic aspects of IWMs, he also understood that IWMs could be distorted in cases of severe psychopathology as seen in individuals with PD, especially those with BPD. His emphasis on the accurate aspects of IWMs was in part a reaction to Klein's emphasis on fantasy, distortion, and dismissiveness of actual experience but was also due to his focus on normative development. Accordingly, despite Bowlby's emphasis on their realistic aspects, his concept of IWMs is highly consistent with the work of Blatt (1974) on mental representations and that of Kernberg (1976) on object relations, with their focus on structural and defensive aspects of representation. Kernberg's concept of an object relation dyad (ORD) is similar to Bowlby's IWM in that both stress that representations of self and others are complementary and mutually confirming. Both concepts include unconscious aspects and affective aspects of experience and acknowledge that IMW/ORD need not be consistent, coherent, or integrated. In fact, Bowlby stressed that individuals could have multiple and inconsistent representations that could oscillate and were often dealt with through what he called *defensive exclusion*, a process remarkably similar to Kernberg's concept of splitting. These representational concepts from attachment and object relations theory are consistent with the concept of cognitive schemas as well as Mischel's (Mischel & Shoda, 1995) cognitive-affective personality system model, although representation in attachment and object relations theory includes both conscious and unconscious components and more explicitly emphasizes structural and developmental aspects of representation.

Assessment of Attachment in Adulthood

Attachment patterns are commonly assessed and described within the context of two independent research traditions: a developmental psychological tradition and a social psychological tradition. The developmental psychological tradition generally assesses attachment organization with the Adult Attachment Interview (AAI; George, Kaplan, & Main, 1985), which uses questions about experiences with childhood caregivers and how these experiences influenced one's adult personality. There are three main AAI classifications: secure, preoccupied, and dismissing. Secure individuals value attachment relationships and seem able to deal effectively with potentially invasive feelings about the past or future. Preoccupied individuals appear overwhelmed by negative emotions related to past attachment relationships. Dismissing individuals appear to defend against the awareness of painful feelings related to attachment relationships, and they often overvalue their sense of independence while devaluing close relationships. A fourth category, unresolved/disorganized, is assigned when individuals demonstrate lapses in the monitoring of speech or reasoning when discussing traumatic experiences and is thought to represent a lack of resolution of these experiences.

The social psychological tradition uses self-report measures to assess adult attachment with questions concerning an individual's attitudes about or behaviors in close relationships. Although the first self-report measures used a categorical model based on AAI classifications (Hazan & Shaver, 1987), the dimensions of anxiety and avoidance have more recently been used to define a model with four categories (Bartholomew & Horowitz, 1991): secure (low anxiety and low avoidance), preoccupied (high anxiety and low avoidance), dismissing-avoidant (low anxiety and high avoidance), and fearful-avoidant (high anxiety and high avoidance). Individuals high in attachment anxiety display intense worry in relationships, are particularly anxious about being abandoned, and use emotion regulation strategies that intensify affect related to attachment relationships. By contrast, individuals high in avoidance overvalue independence, are uncomfortable with closeness, and use emotion regulation strategies that inhibit affect related to attachment relationships. The AAI and self-report categories display poor correspondence with one another, but the dimensional scales derived from each measure are significantly related (Shaver, Belsky, & Brennan, 2000).

Regardless of how attachment patterns are assessed, attachment insecurity is associated with distress, impaired interpersonal functioning, and psychopathology (Crowell, Fraley, & Shaver, 1999). This association is consistent with Bowlby's (1977) view that attachment insecurity was central to the development of disordered personality traits and other psychopathology. This may be because attachment anxiety contributes to hypervigilance toward cues related to attachment or threat, but avoidance contributes to distancing from such cues. Given this pattern, attachment insecurity could contribute to an impaired ability to effectively invest in non-attachment-related activities, to self-regulate, and to respond to conflicts within relationships. Such contribution may be consistent with the disturbances observed in personality pathology, particularly in an interpersonal context.

AN ATTACHMENT THEORETICAL PERSPECTIVE ON PERSONALITY DISORDERS

Bowlby (1973) believed that early attachment experiences, repeatedly elaborated over time, had long-lasting effects, tended to persist across the life span, and are among the major determinants of personality. Bowlby further postulated that insecure attachment lies at the center of disordered personality traits. He believed that working models of attachment were related to "many forms of emotional distress and personality disturbance" (Bowlby, 1977, p. 201) and that attachment difficulties underlie "a whole range of adult dysfunctions," including "personality disorders" (Bowlby, 1977, p. 206). For instance, Bowlby suggested that anxious ambivalent attachment, with its "tendency to make excessive demands on others and to be anxious and clingy when they are not met," could be linked to "dependent and hysterical personalities," and that avoidant attachment—a product of caretakers' rebuffing a child's bids for comfort or protection—with a corresponding "blockage in the capacity to make deep relationships . . . may later be diagnosed a narcissistic" personality (Bowlby, 1973, p. 124) or even develop as "psychopathic personalities" (Bowlby, 1973, p. 14).

More recent work has expanded upon Bowlby's hypotheses by characterizing the links between specific attachment styles and personality in more detail. One approach, as outlined by Levy and Blatt (1999; Blatt & Levy, 2003), combines cognitive-developmental psychoanalytic theory with attachment theory to propose that more and less adaptive forms of attachment exist within both dismissing and preoccupied attachment patterns, denoting different developmental levels based upon the degrees of differentiation and integration of representational or working models that underlie these patterns. Further, these different developmental levels are believed to be associated with particular personality styles or types of personality pathology. Levy and Blatt proposed in particular that preoccupied attachment runs along a relatedness continuum from individuals without PD to those with BPD, with gregarious individuals and individuals with hysterical personality styles in the middle of the continuum. By contrast, Levy and Blatt noted that avoidant attachment runs along a self-definitional continuum: from individuals without PD who are striving for personal development to those who are more obsessive, followed respectively by those with avoidant PD, then those with narcissistic PD, and finally—at the lowest developmental levels—to those with BPD and antisocial PD. The clinical characteristics of several PDs will be discussed in terms of their predominant attachment styles based on this delineation by Levy and Blatt (1999) and later empirical research.

Although some disorders have most often been found to correspond to a preoccupied style (e.g., dependent and histrionic PDs), a dismissive style (e.g., schizoid and antisocial PDs), or a fearful style (e.g., avoidant PD), other PDs can be characterized by aspects of both preoccupied and dismissing dynamics. Or they may be sufficiently heterogeneous to be characterized by an avoidant type and a preoccupied type, as is the case with narcissistic and borderline personalities. A number of studies have found evidence for two types of narcissistic patients, those characterized by a grandiose presentation that would be more characteristic of dismissive attachment and those characterized by a vulnerable presentation that would be more characteristic of an anxious-preoccupied attachment. Following Kernberg's proposal that the grandiose and vulnerable presentations are two sides of the same coin, Levy (2012) described how narcissistic patients can vacillate between more dismissive presentations and more dependent presentations. Likewise, many clinical writers have noted that those with BPD quickly vacillate between disparate mental states. Levy and Kelly (2008) specifically noted how those with BPD can show indications of preoccupied and avoidant attachment on the AAI, as they can provide narratives that are both highly enmeshed (a preoccupied characteristic) and derogating (a dismissive characteristic) when speaking about the same situation.

RESEARCH ON ATTACHMENT AND PERSONALITY DISORDERS

In this section, we examine the growing body of research on attachment and PDs as it bears on the conceptual framework and clinical dynamics proposed by Bowlby and others. We first review clinical studies, mostly concerning the association between attachment and PDs, but also those studies that focused on basic neurocognitive and neuroscience research that either examined attachment and PD processes directly or examined constructs relevant to understanding the relationship between attachment and personality. Finally, we discuss the developmental psychopathology and psychotherapy literature relevant to attachment processes in patient groups with PD.

Association Between Attachment and Personality Disorders

Research has largely supported theoretical assertions of an overlap between PDs and insecure attachment. Much attention in the literature has been given to insecure attachment and BPD (Levy, 2005) and antisocial personality to a lesser extent. There are fewer data on attachment variables and other PDs, and what is available tends to compare dimensions of self-reported adult romantic attachment to self-reported PD symptoms (for exceptions, see Barone, 2003; Levy et al., 2006; Rosenstein & Horowitz, 1996). Within that literature, a negative relationship between attachment security and overall personality pathology has been found consistently, but the relationships between specific PDs and insecure attachment types are less consistent. Findings from both self-report and interview measures suggest that preoccupied attachment tends to be associated with histrionic, dependent, and avoidant PDs, whereas dismissing attachment tends to be associated with narcissistic, antisocial, schizoid, and paranoid PDs. Fearful attachment is associated with paranoid, schizotypal, avoidant, borderline, obsessive–compulsive, and narcissistic PDs. These findings were confirmed in a meta-analysis examining AAI distributions in clinical samples (Bakermans-Kranenburg & van IJzendoorn, 2009).

Despite some differences across studies, the findings tend to converge across both interview and self-report measures and various age groups and samples. Both preoccupied and dismissing attachment are associated with BPD, and in general preoccupied attachment is uniquely associated with the anxiety-based PDs such as dependent and Avoidant PDs; whereas dismissing attachment is associated with antisocial and narcissistic PDs and some of the Cluster A PDs (especially schizoid and paranoid PDs). Fearful avoidance has sometimes been associated with Cluster A PDs and sometimes with Cluster C PDs. However, some inconsistencies in the findings remain regarding the relationship between specific PDs and specific dimensions, or styles, of attachment. These inconsistencies suggest that other factors may be contributing to these inconsistencies. Much of this research has focused on BPD, with less attention focused on other PDs. However, the findings related to BPD may have important implications for other PDs and could guide future research.

Although the association between BPD and attachment anxiety has been fairly consistent, the association between BPD and attachment avoidance has been less so. Some studies have found no significant relationships (e.g., Meyer, Pilkonis, & Beevers, 2004), and others have found a relationship only when attachment anxiety is also high (e.g., Levy, Meehan, Weber, Reynoso, & Clarkin, 2005). In light of these inconsistencies, some researchers have suggested that the relationship between specific attachment patterns and BPD may be indirect; studies have shown that certain personality traits, such as impulsivity, aggression, and trait negative affect (Scott, Levy, & Pincus, 2009), serve as mediators that can help to explain the relationship between adult attachment and BPD. Rejection sensitivity and negative views of self have also been shown to mediate the attachment–BPD relationship (Boldero et al., 2009). Other findings suggest that fearful forms of attachment (i.e., the combination of attachment anxiety and avoidance) are associated with reactive aggression, attachment avoidance is associated with self-harm, and attachment anxiety is associated with anger and irritability in patients with BPD (Critchfield, Levy, Clarkin, & Kernberg, 2008). Additionally, there is evidence that preoccupied attachment interacts with anger and social dysfunction to predict BPD (Morse et al., 2009).

Taken together, these findings suggest the presence of a significant but indirect relationship between adult attachment and BPD that is consistent with the main tenets of attachment theory. In times of distress, securely attached adults tend to seek support from attachment figures in the form of physical contact, supportive comments, and emotional support, all of which are behaviors analogous to the secure base and safe haven behavior observed in children by Bowlby (1988). However, in insecurely attached adults, these distress-reducing behaviors are disrupted. As a result, such individuals are more vulnerable to experiencing intense feelings of anger, aggression, and impulsivity, all of which are primary characteristics of BPD (Levy et al., 2006). Thus, one's attachment style appears to be related to aspects of personality and personality traits, which are in turn related to personality pathology such as BPD. Additionally, the hypersensitivity to rejection and negative views of self observed in BPD can be understood in the context of Bowlby's conceptualization of internal working models of the self and other in relationships (Bowlby, 1973). It appears that some of the attachment-related difficulties experienced by individuals with BPD may be due in part to the presence of internal working models of others that are characterized by an expectation that others will be rejecting and by an internal working model of the self that is negative.

Another possible reason for the inconsistent findings with regard to BPD is the heterogeneity of the disorder (Johansen, Karterud, Pedersen, Gude, & Falkum, 2004). Because BPD is a polythetic disorder in which five of nine criteria are needed for the diagnosis, there are 256 different ways to meet criteria for BPD. Given the heterogeneity of BPD, we would suggest that different attachment processes may be prominent in some patients with BPD having a particular clinical presentation, whereas other attachment processes may be prominent in other patients with BPD characterized by a different clinical presentation. Levy (2005; Levy et al., 2005) noted that those with BPD are characterized by aspects of both preoccupied and dismissing attachment processes.

Psychophysiological and Neurobiological Correlates of Attachment and Personality Disorders

Consistent with Bowlby's notion of attachment as a biologically based behavioral system, a line of research has developed that focuses on understanding the biological correlates of attachment through the use of psychophysiology measures such as electrodermal activity (skin conductance) and heart rate. Beginning in the late 1970s, Sroufe and Waters (1977) demonstrated that both secure and insecurely attached children experienced an increase in heart rate during the separation phase of the Strange Situation. During the reunion phase, securely attached children's heart rate returned to baseline quickly, whereas avoidantly attached children's heart rate continued at an elevated rate. This finding provided some of the first evidence that avoidant children, who appear calm and indifferent, are actually stressed by the situation and employ behavioral strategies (e.g., ignoring the parent, engaging a toy) aimed at reducing or defending against distress, albeit ineffectively.

More recently, researchers have studied similar processes in adults by collecting psychophysiology data during attachment-relevant tasks designed to activate the attachment system, such as the AAI. Dismissing adults who minimize negative emotions related to attachment experiences through the use of deactivating strategies experience higher levels of conflict and inhibition, as evidenced by an increased skin conductance response, particularly on AAI questions that ask about separation (or threatened separation) from and rejection by parents (Dozier & Kobak, 1992). Across multiple studies, dismissing attachment appears to be related to skin conductance increases in response to attachment-related stressors, whereas preoccupied attachment tends to be unrelated to such increases (e.g., Diamond, Hicks, & Otter-Henderson, 2006). There is also evidence that both dismissing and preoccupied adults demonstrate a greater divergence between their self-reported reactivity and their psychophysiological reactivity (Diamond et al., 2006), supporting the notion that the defensive strategies employed by insecurely attached individuals may effectively help to regulate behavioral responses to attachment-related stressors but do not seem to aid in the regulation of physiological arousal.

Although little research has directly examined attachment-related differences in psychophysiological reactivity among individuals with PD, there is some evidence to suggest that these individuals may be particularly vulnerable to experiencing breakdowns in defensive behavioral strategies aimed at reducing distress in response to attachment-related stressors, as evidenced by physiological reactivity. For example, high levels of life stress and high symptom load have been shown to moderate the relationship between attachment avoidance and vagal withdrawal (Ehrenthal, Irgang, & Schauenburg, in press). High life stress and high symptom load predicted a larger vagal withdrawal, which is indicative of less adaptive self-regulation. Given that individuals with PDs tend to experience high levels of life stress and a multitude of other symptoms (Zanarini et al., 1998), it seems likely that these individuals may be at particular risk for breakdowns in adaptive processes that help minimize distress in the face of attachment-related stressors.

Oxytocin, Attachment, and Personality Disorders

Oxytocin is a neuropeptide that has a primary function in facilitating labor and contractions during childbirth, as well as lactation after childbirth. Additionally, human and animal research suggests that oxytocin plays an important role in affiliative behaviors and in the development and maintenance of close attachments (Heinrichs & Domes, 2008). Intranasally administered oxytocin has been shown to increase accuracy in the recognition of emotions in faces, particularly for more complex emotions (Domes, Heinrichs, Michel, Berger, & Herpetz, 2007); to increase judgments of the trustworthiness and attractiveness of faces (Theodoridou, Rowe, Penton-Voak, & Rogers, 2009); and to increase trust in a social trust game (Kosfeld, Heinrichs, Zak, Fischbacher, & Fehr, 2005). Additionally, among insecurely attached but healthy populations, oxytocin may help to increase feelings of secure attachment and decrease feelings of insecure attachment (Buchheim et al., 2009).

However, when insecure attachment exists simultaneously with certain types of psychopathology, as is often the case in BPD and other PDs, the generally positive effects of oxytocin do not seem to persist. In contrast, it appears that oxytocin may actually have an opposite effect on individuals with BPD in that it decreases, rather than increases, feelings of trust and cooperation (Bartz et al., 2011). These findings raise the important question of why oxytocin appears to function differently in individuals with BPD than in healthy populations. One possible explanation is that oxytocin actually functions differently at a biological level. However, given that the response of biological systems (e.g., the hypothalamic–pituitary–adrenal axis) following oxytocin administration is similar in individuals with BPD and healthy controls (Simeon et al., 2011), this explanation is unlikely.

It is more plausible and consistent with an attachment theoretical perspective that individuals with BPD respond differently than healthy individuals to the feelings elicited by oxytocin because they experience and interpret the feelings of closeness elicited by oxytocin differently. Whereas these feelings are typically experienced as positive and comforting and responded to with increased prosocial behaviors such as trust and cooperation, those with BPD experience the feelings of closeness as dangerous. They respond with fear, anxiety, and increased vulnerability and thus become less trusting and cooperative and more antagonistic. This interpretation is consistent with and sheds light on psychotherapy findings indicating that supportive interventions, particularly validations, which are typically experienced positively in patients without PD, result in increased disorganization in individuals with BPD (Prunetti et al., 2008).

Neuroscience Research

In the context of the experimental psychopathology and psychophysiological research reviewed above, the growing area of research using functional magnetic resonance imaging (fMRI) technology can help us to begin to understand the relationship between PDs and attachment at yet another level of analysis. There is a vast neuroscience literature relevant for understanding the neurological basis of PDs. However, rather than providing a comprehensive review of this literature, the following section focuses on select literature that has direct implications for understanding the neural correlates of attachment and PDs. As is the case with the previously reviewed literature, much of the research on PDs and attachment using fMRI technology has focused on BPD; however, some research also exists on antisocial, narcissistic, and schizotypal PDs. We begin by examining research relevant for understanding the neural basis of attachment-related constructs in healthy populations, then discuss the implications of attachment-related neuroscience research in the context of BPD, and follow with a brief review of relevant literature on other PDs.

Attachment and fMRI in Healthy Populations

According to Bowlby, the attachment system is automatically activated in response to real or imagined physical or psychological threats and motivates individuals to seek or maintain support and proximity from their attachment figures (that is, other individuals who are trusted to provide support and safety in times of distress). Experimental studies have supported this assumption among healthy populations by showing that individuals are able to more quickly identify proximity-related words (Mikulincer, Birnbaum, Woddis, & Nachmias, 2000), as well as the names of their attachment figures

(Mikulincer, Gillath, & Shaver, 2002), in a lexical decision-making task when primed with threat-related words. Additionally, there are important attachment style differences such that attachment anxiety is associated with heightened accessibility of attachment figure representations, and attachment avoidance is associated with decreased accessibility when the threat-related prime is *separation*. These findings can be interpreted as evidence that in the context of threat, proximity-related thoughts, as well as thoughts of one's attachment figures, become activated and are readily accessible, but that one's attachment style may influence the degree to which these representations are accessible.

More recent research using fMRI has taken these findings a step further and identified attachment style differences in specific brain regions that are associated with attachment security. Canterberry and Gillath (2013) found that when anxiously attached participants were primed with security words (e.g., comfort, embrace, love, support), compared to insecure words (e.g., loss, lonely, rejected, abandon), they had increased activation in areas of the brain (e.g., posterior cingulate, paracentral, inferior parietal, orbitofrontal cortex, superior frontal) that would suggest they experienced the secure primes with more emotional intensity and at the same time had difficulty regulating the emotions. Among avoidantly attached participants, increased activation was observed in areas of the brain associated with memory (e.g., parahippocampal gyrus), suggesting the possibility that these individuals may be making repeated memory retrieval attempts due to a lack of easily accessible secure representations. Additionally, these individuals showed increased activations in the amygdala and insula, areas that are associated with processing of salient or aversive emotional stimuli. Thus, not only are differences in activation of the attachment system evident at the behavioral level, but there is evidence from neural imaging studies to suggest that these differences are reflected at the level of the brain.

Also relevant for understanding individual differences in attachment styles is research on the ways in which attachment style may influence one's reactions to emotionally salient social cues, such as facial expressions. According to Bowlby, IWMs, or mental representations of the self and others, include expectations, beliefs, emotional appraisals, and rules for processing or excluding information that direct and shape thoughts, feelings, and behaviors in future relationships. Thus, when one is confronted with emotionally salient information, the structure of one's IWM of the self and other may influence the ways in which that information is evaluated and responded to, and these differences should be evident at the neural level. It appears in particular that anxiously attached individuals are particularly sensitive to cues of social punishment, as reflected by increased activation in the left amygdala in response to negative feedback in the form of angry faces during social game, whereas avoidantly attached individuals show decreased responsiveness to social reward, as evidenced by reduced activation in the striatum and ventral tegmental areas in response to positive feedback in the form of smiling faces (Vrtička, Andersson, Grandjean, Sander, & Vuilleumier, 2008). These findings are consistent with theoretical assertions of attachment theory and behavioral observations showing that anxiously attached individuals tend to show a hypervigilance for emotionally salient social cues (Dozier & Kobak, 1992; Mikulincer & Shaver, 2007; Rom & Mikulincer, 2003; Zeijlmans van Emmichoven, van IJzendoorn, de Ruiter, & Brosschot, 2003), whereas individuals with avoidant attachment styles tend to downplay the importance of emotionally relevant information (Dozier & Kobak, 1992). There is some evidence that purposefully distancing oneself, or downregulating one's response to emotional stimuli, may help to regulate emotional response to social situations (Koenigsberg et al., 2010).

Attachment and fMRI in Populations With Personality Disorder

There are a few perspectives, using fMRI, that are relevant for thinking about the relationship between attachment and PDs. One such perspective views *mentalization*, or the ability to understand oneself and others in terms of mental states, as an important capacity that contributes to one's ability to function in close relationships (Fonagy & Bateman, 2008). These authors view failures in the capacity to mentalize as a core feature of BPD. From this perspective, mentalization emerges from the attachment relationship and fully develops in the context of a secure attachment. However, when the attachment relationship is not secure, particularly in the context of malevolence or traumatic experiences that are common in BPD, the attachment system can become disorganized. Fonagy, Luyten, and Strathearn (2011) argued that "the disorganization of attachment relationships . . . disorganizes the self-structure, creating incoherence and splitting, which makes stress particularly hard to manage" (p. 49). As a result, they argued, the attachment system can become hyperreactive and generate intense emotional states. In the context of these intense emotional states, the capacity to reflect and assess the intentions of the self and others becomes impossible and may contribute to some of the interpersonal difficulties experienced by individuals with BPD.

These theoretical assertions are consistent with our knowledge of emotional arousal and stress regulation. Fonagy et al. (2011) argued that as arousal and stress increase, a switch occurs in which processing goes from cortical systems important for the use of executive function and controlled processing (i.e., mentalizing) to subcortical systems related to automatic responding (i.e., nonmentalizing). Neuroimaging evidence suggests that when individuals try to suppress negative thoughts, attachment anxiety may be associated with a reliance on brain areas relevant for memory and emotion processing (e.g., hippocampus, anterior temporal pole, dorsal anterior cingulate) and with less reliance on areas of the brain related to emotion regulation (e.g., orbitofrontal cortex; Gillath, Bunge, Shaver, Wendelken, & Mikulincer, 2005). In patients with BPD, behavioral inhibition appears to be limited in the context of negative emotion, as evidenced by decreased activation in prefrontal brain regions and increased amygdala activity in these individuals compared with controls (Silbersweig et al., 2007).

Thus, individuals with BPD, who tend to have insecure attachment styles and are prone to intense emotional states and a hyperreactivity of the attachment system, may have a lower set point for switching from cortical to subcortical neural systems and therefore from controlled to automatic, or non-mentalizing, modes. Given the proneness to switch to nonmentalizing modes and therefore to experience failures in mentalization, it follows that at the behavioral level, this may be manifested by a decreased ability to understand the emotional states of others and to respond in an emotionally and behaviorally appropriate manner. There is evidence from numerous fMRI studies that individuals with BPD tend to respond to emotional stimuli with increased activation, compared with controls, in subcortical areas of the brain (e.g., amygdala; New et al., 2012). Hazlett et al. (2012), contrasting patients with BPD with patients who had schizotypal PD and healthy controls, found that patients with BPD had a slower return to baseline activity in the amygdala following the onset of pleasant and unpleasant (but not neutral) photographs. This finding suggests that individuals with BPD have long-lasting reactions to emotional cues. Further, patients with BPD reported low levels of self-reported affect suggesting a lack of understanding of their own emotional state.

Other Personality Disorders

There is little neuroscience literature directly relevant for understanding the relationship between attachment and other PDs. However, a few studies providing evidence for neural correlates consistent with key features of each PD have implications for understanding the ways in which individuals may function in attachment relationships. For example, Narcissistic PD has been shown to be associated with structural and functional abnormalities in areas of the brain associated with empathy: Individuals with Narcissistic PD have decreased gray matter and activation during an empathy task (Fan et al., 2011; Schulze et al., 2013).

Developmental Psychopathology Research

Much developmental psychopathology research has examined how attachment influences the development of PDs. Most of this research has focused on BPD. In general, these studies have examined how attachment experiences interact with other dispositional factors (e.g., genetics, temperament) to influence the development of PD features. Some studies also examine this topic by looking at a range of psychological outcomes in the children of parents with PDs.

Prospective longitudinal studies on BPD symptomatology illustrate how early attachment experiences, particularly when examined along with other dispositional traits, appear to be powerful predictors of later borderline personality pathology and likely influence personality development via their influence on the elaboration and consolidation of mental representations over the life span (or, rather, through disturbances in this process). Carlson, Egeland, and Sroufe (2009) followed a group of individuals from infancy to adulthood and found that—in addition to infant temperament and disposition—a number of early relationship and representational factors predicted adult BPD symptoms. In particular, disorganized infant attachment (18 months), maltreatment (12–18 months), maternal hostility and boundary confusion (18–42 months), family disruption related to father presence (12–64 months), and overall family stress (3–42 months) were predictive of later BPD symptoms. Disturbance in emotion regulation, behavior, attention, relationship functioning, and self-representation in adolescence were also predictive of adult borderline symptoms. Using a similar design, Crawford, Cohen, Chen, Anglin, and Ehrensaft (2009) examined the trajectory of BPD symptoms over time with a particular focus on the effect of maternal separations prior to age 5. Extended early separations (i.e., those lasting 1 month or more) were predictive of more BPD symptoms in adolescence and early adulthood as well as slower developmental declines in symptoms. Difficult temperament in middle childhood, child abuse, and attachment anxiety and avoidance in adolescence were also predictive of adult BPD symptoms, with only temperament acting as a partial mediator between early separations and later symptoms.

Additional studies have further explored the relationship between attachment and the development of BPD in adolescence and early adulthood; these studies have generally found that attachment anxiety is particularly related to negative outcomes during this period. For example, measured in early adolescence, preoccupied attachment predicts increased risky sexual behavior and aggression (both features of BPD) over the course of adolescence, as well as steeper rates of growth in these behaviors (Kobak, Zajac, & Smith, 2009). Further, one investigation of potential pathways between attachment, personality features, and borderline symptoms (Scott et al., 2009) found that trait impulsivity and negative affect fully mediate the relationship between attachment anxiety and BPD symptoms in young adults, suggesting that these temperamental traits may contribute to the development of BPD when they occur in the context of high levels of attachment anxiety.

Other studies have examined how attachment and early relationship experiences more generally interact with genes and underlying biological systems to contribute to the development of personality pathology. Research on a polymorphism in the serotonin transporter gene (5-HTTLPR), wherein a short allele (either homozygous or heterozygous) has been implicated in different areas of behavioral dysregulation, has been one fruitful area of study. Kochanska, Philibert, and Barry (2009) found a strong interaction between infant attachment organization and alleles of this gene with regard to self-regulation in early childhood, with security of attachment a strong predictor of good regulatory capacities for those with the short 5-HTTLPR allele. Zimmerman, Mohr, and Spangler (2009) found a similar pattern in adolescents with regard to regulation of autonomy and aggression. Both of these studies suggest that attachment may affect the expression of genes related to dysregulation. Taken together, these studies reflect how constitutional factors may combine with attachment-related experiences to influence how an individual is affected by external stressors and perturbations. That is, individuals with high constitutional disadvantage likely have a lower threshold for environmental perturbations to overwhelm their capacity to assimilate and accommodate to their environment, whereas those with a lower constitutional load may be resilient to greater perturbations and require greater disruption to develop personality pathology.

To better understand the development and transmission of personality pathology, researchers have focused on the offspring of parents with PDs. Findings from these studies suggest that child–parent interactions are often atypical and disturbed among these parents, affecting later attachment and functioning, particularly in the areas of psychosocial function and emotion regulation.

In a Still Face paradigm study, Crandell, Patrick, and Hobson (2003) found that mothers with BPD were more likely to act insensitively, vacillating between intrusive and disengaged behaviors. In turn, their infants showed more dazed looks and looking away during the Still Face portion of the protocol and also showed lowered affect and continued dazed looks during the play after the Still Face. On follow-up, 80% of the infants of the mothers with BPD showed signs of disorganized attachment, including frightened and disoriented behavior during attachment bids, further illustrating the continuing nature of this style of interaction as well as its impact (Hobson, Patrick, Crandell, García-Pérez, & Lee, 2005). Newman, Stevenson, Bergman, and Boyce (2007) showed that infants of mothers with BPD were similarly detached and lacked attentiveness toward their mothers, also suggesting that these ways of relating were reflective of disturbances in attachment between mother and child.

Other studies (e.g., Macfie & Swan, 2009) have found that children of mothers with BPD provided narratives about parent figures with significantly more role reversal, fear of abandonment, and more negative parent–child relationship expectations than did children of mothers without BPD. In terms of emotion regulation, children of mothers with BPD displayed significantly more reality/fantasy confusion, self/fantasy boundary confusion, fantasy proneness, intrusion of traumatic material, and lower narrative coherence than did controls.

Psychotherapy Research

Bowlby conceptualized attachment theory as having relevance for psychotherapy, particularly as manifested in the relationship between therapist and patient. He described the therapist's function as "provid[ing] the patient with a secure base from which to explore both himself and also his relations with all those with whom he has made or might make, an affectional bond" (Bowlby, 1977, p. 421). In other words, Bowlby theorized that the role of the therapist was "to provide the patient with a temporary attachment figure" and that this role would serve several therapeutic goals. That is, the therapist would help the patient explore past and present attachments, as well as how these attachments inform the patient's IWMs and how they affect the patient's relationships both inside and outside of therapy. This kind of exploration would allow patients to revise IWMs and to internalize the relationship with the therapist as a safe haven they can return to internally during times of distress. Many existing psychotherapies employ techniques or principles that are concordant with these tenets of attachment theory, and interventions that are more explicitly based on attachment theory are increasingly being developed. In the realm of PD treatment, some existing empirically supported interventions are either explicitly or implicitly based on attachment theory, and the techniques employed in these treatments echo the therapeutic roles proposed by Bowlby. In addition, a growing body of research has focused on how patient attachment affects the process and outcome of psychotherapy for PDs as well as how patient attachment may change over the course of treatment.

Attachment-Based Treatments for Personality Disorders

As noted earlier, attachment theory acts as an underlying theoretical basis for multiple treatments for PDs. Most of these treatments are designed for BPD. One such treatment, mentalization-based therapy (Fonagy & Bateman, 2008), is explicitly based upon attachment theory. Fonagy and Bateman (2008) proposed that those with BPD are not able to develop the capacity to reflect on the intentional behavior in the self and others by reflecting on mental states within the context of an early attachment relationship. The primary goal of treatment is to foster the development of this capacity, with the idea that doing so in turn leads to more stability in terms of one's sense of self and in relationships with others. Mentalization-based therapy has demonstrated efficacy over short-term and long-term follow-up with regard to reduction of depressive symptoms, suicidality, parasuicidality, and length of inpatient stays as well as improvement in social functioning (see Fonagy & Bateman, 2008, for a review).

Otto Kernberg's (1976) theory of BPD, upon which transference-focused psychotherapy (TFP; Clarkin, Yeomans, & Kernberg, 2006) is based, is not explicitly grounded in attachment theory, but much of it is consistent with the central tenets of this theory. In particular, Kernberg theorized that BPD is characterized by unintegrated and undifferentiated representations of self and others (i.e., identity diffusion), as well as the use of immature defenses and poor reality testing. In terms of development, Kernberg has noted, the representational difficulties at the core of BPD result from disturbances in the internalization of early attachment relationships. Accordingly, a primary goal of TFP is for the patient to develop more integrated and differentiated representations of self and others, largely through analysis of the transference that emerges between therapist and patient. The efficacy of TFP in contributing to symptomatic change in patients with BPD has been demonstrated in two randomized controlled trials (Clarkin, Levy, Lenzenweger, & Kernberg, 2007; Doering et al., 2010), and Levy et al. (2006) showed its efficacy with regard to changes in attachment representations and security.

Attachment and the Process and Outcome of Psychotherapy
for Personality Disorders

A number of researchers and theorists have examined how client attachment affects psychotherapy process and outcome for clients with PDs and how client attachment patterns can change as a result of treatment. These studies typically assess client attachment prior to treatment and examine how it relates to later outcomes. Unsurprisingly, a general finding has been that secure attachment prior to treatment predicts better treatment outcomes across treatments for patients with PDs (Meyer, Pilkonis, Proietti, Heape, & Egan, 2001; Strauss et al., 2006). However, many clients with PDs present with more insecure or disorganized attachment classifications, and research suggests that different attachment patterns (e.g., anxious vs. avoidant) may differentially predict trajectories of treatment engagement, process, and outcome. Therefore, understanding how these different attachment styles may impact treatment is important in making predictions about the course of treatment for these individuals.

Clinical and theoretical writers have suggested that clients with PDs who are more anxiously attached (particularly those with preoccupied attachment) may initially present as very engaged and interested in pursuing treatment (Levy & Blatt, 1999). Empirical studies have indicated that individuals with high levels of attachment anxiety are more likely to report their distress and seek help for emotional difficulties (Vogel & Wei, 2005). Additionally, preoccupied individuals appear to use medical services more frequently; for instance, preoccupied individuals with Cluster B PDs report longer medical hospitalizations than do matched individuals of other attachment classifications (Hoermann, Clarkin, Hull, & Fertuck, 2004). Although preoccupied clients may appear more disclosing and dependent on clinicians, they are not more compliant with treatment recommendations (Riggs, Jacobvitz, & Hazen, 2002). Additionally, there is evidence that anxious attachment may be especially predictive of poorer treatment outcomes among both preoccupied and fearful-avoidant clients with a variety of PDs (Fonagy et al., 1996; Strauss et al., 2006). By contrast, more avoidantly attached individuals tend to report less distress and are reluctant to seek help (Vogel & Wei, 2005), and they tend to be less compliant with treatment recommendations and to develop weaker therapeutic alliances than do individuals of other attachment classifications (Mallinckrodt, Porter, & Kivlighan, 2005). In spite of this, some evidence suggests that dismissing attachment at the onset of treatment may predict better outcomes than will more anxious attachment patterns, at least in a sample of patients with mixed diagnoses (Fonagy et al., 1996). Additional work with samples with PD is needed to determine whether these findings generalize to such samples.

Researchers have begun to investigate how client attachment may change during the course of treatment for PDs. Levy et al. (2006) examined changes in attachment status in 90 patients with BPD who were randomized to one of three treatments: TFP, dialectical behavior therapy, or a modified psychodynamic supportive psychotherapy. After a year of treatment, 31.8% (seven of 22) of patients who received TFP changed from insecure to secure with regard to attachment, and this change was not observed in the other treatments. Additionally, this finding was replicated in a randomized controlled trial of TFP (Doering et al., 2010) by Buchheim, Hörz, Rentrop, Doering, and Fischer-Kern (2012).

Another recent study examined shifts in attachment as a result of short-term inpatient treatment in a sample of women diagnosed with BPD, avoidant PD, or both disorders. Strauss, Mestel, and Kirchmann (2011) found that although patients experienced symptom reduction, there was little evidence of a shift in attachment security, suggesting that shifts from insecure to secure attachment are less likely in short-term treatment than in long-term treatment. Taken together, these findings suggest that psychotherapy may indeed impact client attachment in clients with BPD, but that this impact may differ depending on treatment length or other characteristics.

In addition to considering attachment as a moderator or outcome of treatment, some preliminary work has indicated that attachment-related constructs may also be used to examine psychotherapy process. Samstag, Muran, Wachtel, Slade, and Safran (2008) used the narrative coherence coding system from the AAI on sessions that were randomly selected from the first third of treatment to examine psychotherapy process as a predictor of treatment outcome in a sample of clients who were primarily diagnosed with Cluster C PDs (with comorbid depression and/or anxiety). Coherence ratings were significantly higher in clients who experienced better outcomes than in those who experienced poor outcomes or dropped out of treatment. These findings suggest that more coherent narratives in psychotherapy sessions may indicate particularly fruitful collaboration within the client–therapist dyad. It is also possible that client characteristics, including attachment, may influence the level of narrative coherency, which may in turn influence the course of psychotherapy.

CONCLUSION

Attachment theory provides a cogent and empirically based model for PDs that has both parsimony and breadth. It can explain both the intrapsychic and interpersonal aspects in ways that are consistent with research findings from a host of studies across multiple domains of knowledge, such as evolutionary biology, ethology/comparative psychology, developmental psychology, experimental social-personality psychology, and neuroscience (Levy, Beeney, & Temes, 2011).

Additionally, attachment theory not only is consistent with but also has broadly influenced and enhanced a number of theoretical orientations including psychodynamic (Eagle & Wolitzky, 2009), interpersonal (Klerman, Weissman, Rounsaville, & Chevron, 1984), cognitive (McBride & Atkinson, 2009), and behavioral (Sterkenburg, Janssen, & Schuengel, 2008). Moreover, attachment theory provides a framework for thinking integratively across these different clinical orientations.

The advantage of an attachment theory perspective, compared with that of psychoanalysis, object relations theory, and interpersonal theory, is its strong developmental evidence base. Although it is conceptually rich, is very nuanced, and is developing an increasing evidence base, psychoanalysis is particularly weak in terms of direct tests of developmental concepts. Attachment theory provides a crisp and testable framework for which much evidence exists. Similarly, although research on interpersonal theory has established a solid psychometric base and revealed important findings regarding person perception and interpersonal dynamics in individuals with PD, it does not have the broad evidence base of attachment theory, particularly with regard to development, non-self-reported outcomes, and longitudinal continuity and discontinuity. For these reasons we feel that attachment theory offers a parsimonious, broad, and integrative framework for conceptualizing normative personality development as well as PDs. Attachment theory is a rich theoretical model with a strong evidence base and thus is a promising approach for conceptualizing and studying PDs in the 21st century.

REFERENCES

Ainsworth, M., Blehar, M., Waters, E., & Wall, S. (1978). *Patterns of attachment: A psychological study of the strange situation*. Oxford, England: Erlbaum.

Bakermans-Kranenburg, M. J., & van IJzendoorn, M. H. (2009). The first 10,000 adult attachment interviews: Distributions of adult attachment representations in non-clinical and clinical groups. *Attachment & Human Development, 11*, 223–263. doi:10.1080/14616730902814762

Barone, L. (2003). Developmental protective and risk factors in borderline personality disorder: A study using the Adult Attachment Interview. *Attachment & Human Development, 5*, 64–77. doi:10.1080/1461673031000078634

Bartholomew, K., & Horowitz, L. M. (1991). Attachment styles among young adults: A test of a four-category model. *Journal of Personality and Social Psychology, 61*, 226–244. doi:10.1037/0022-3514.61.2.226

Bartz, J., Simeon, D., Hamilton, H., Kim, S., Crystal, S., Braun, A., . . . Hollander, E. (2011). Oxytocin can hinder trust and cooperation in borderline personality disorder. *Social Cognitive and Affective Neuroscience, 6*, 556–563. doi:10.1093/scan/nsq085

Blatt, S. J. (1974). Levels of object representation in anaclitic and introjective depression. *Psychoanalytic study of the child, 29*(10), 7–157.

Blatt, S. J., & Levy, K. N. (2003). Attachment theory, psychoanalysis, personality development, and psychopathology. *Psychoanalytic Inquiry, 23*, 102–150. doi:10.1080/07351692309349028

Boldero, J. M., Hulbert, C. A., Bloom, L., Cooper, J., Gilbert, F., Mooney, J. L., & Salinger, J. (2009). Rejection sensitivity and negative self-beliefs as mediators of associations between the number of borderline personality disorder features and self-reported adult attachment. *Personality and Mental Health, 3*, 248–262. doi:10.1002/pmh.93

Bornstein, R. F. (1993). *The dependent personality*. New York, NY: Guilford Press.

Bowlby, J. (1973). *Attachment and loss: Vol. 2. Separation*. New York, NY: Basic Books.

Bowlby, J. (1977). The making and breaking of affectional bonds: I. Aetiology and psychopathology in the light of attachment theory. *British Journal of Psychiatry, 130*, 201–210. doi:10.1192/bjp.130.3.201

Bowlby, J. (1988). *A secure base: Parent–child attachment and healthy human development*. New York, NY: Basic Books.

Buchheim, A., Heinrichs, M., George, C., Pokorny, D., Koops, E., Henningsen, P., . . . Gündel, H. (2009). Oxytocin enhances the experience of attachment security. *Psychoneuroendocrinology*, *34*, 1417–1422. doi:10.1016/j.psyneuen.2009.04.002

Buchheim, A., Hörz, S., Rentrop, M., Doering, S., & Fischer-Kern, M. (2012, September). *Attachment status before and after one year of transference focused psychotherapy (TFP) versus therapy as usual (TAU) in patients with borderline personality disorder.* Paper presented at the meeting of the International Congress on Borderline Personality Disorder and Allied Disorders, Amsterdam, the Netherlands.

Canterberry, M., & Gillath, O. (2013). Neural evidence for a multifaceted model of attachment security. *International Journal of Psychophysiology*, *88*, 232–240. doi:10.1016/j.ijpsycho.2012.08.013

Carlson, E. A., Egeland, B., & Sroufe, L. A. (2009). A prospective investigation of the development of borderline personality symptoms. *Development and Psychopathology*, *21*, 1311–1334. doi:10.1017/S0954579409990174

Clarkin, J. F., Levy, K. N., Lenzenweger, M. F., & Kernberg, O. F. (2007). Evaluating three treatments for borderline personality disorder: A multiwave study. *The American Journal of Psychiatry*, *164*, 922–928. doi:10.1176/appi.ajp.164.6.922

Clarkin, J. F., Yeomans, F., & Kernberg, O. F. (2006). *Psychotherapy for borderline personality disorder: Focusing on object relations.* Arlington, VA: American Psychiatric Publishing.

Crandell, L. E., Patrick, M. P. H., & Hobson, R. P. (2003). "Still-face" interactions between mothers with borderline personality disorder and their 2-month-old infants. *British Journal of Psychiatry*, *183*, 239–247. doi:10.1192/bjp.183.3.239

Crawford, T. N., Cohen, P. R., Chen, H., Anglin, D. M., & Ehrensaft, M. (2009). Early maternal separation and the trajectory of borderline personality disorder symptoms. *Development and Psychopathology*, *21*, 1013–1030. doi:10.1017/S0954579409000546

Critchfield, K. L., Levy, K. N., Clarkin, J. F., & Kernberg, O. F. (2008). The relational context of aggression in borderline personality disorder: Using adult attachment style to predict forms of hostility. *Journal of Clinical Psychology*, *64*, 67–82. doi:10.1002/jclp.20434

Crowell, J. A., Fraley, R. C., & Shaver, P. R. (1999). Measurement of individual differences in adolescent and adult attachment. In J. Cassidy & P. R. Shaver (Eds.), *Handbook of attachment: Theory, research, and clinical applications* (pp. 434–465). New York, NY: Guilford Press.

Diamond, L. M., Hicks, A. M., & Otter-Henderson, K. (2006). Physiological evidence for repressive coping among avoidantly attached adults. *Journal of Social and Personal Relationships*, *23*, 205–229. doi:10.1177/0265407506062470

Doering, S., Hörz, S., Rentrop, M., Fischer-Kern, M., Schuster, P., Benecke, C., . . . Buchheim, P. (2010). Transference-focused psychotherapy v. treatment by community psychotherapists for borderline personality disorder: Randomized controlled trial. *British Journal of Psychiatry, 196,* 389–395. doi:10.1192/bjp.bp.109.070177

Domes, G., Heinrichs, M., Michel, A., Berger, C., & Herpertz, S. C. (2007). Oxytocin improves "mind reading" in humans. *Biological Psychiatry, 61,* 731–733. doi:10.1016/j.biopsych.2006.07.015

Dozier, M., & Kobak, R. R. (1992). Psychophysiology in attachment interviews: Converging evidence for deactivating strategies. *Child Development, 63,* 1473–1480. doi:10.2307/1131569

Eagle, M. N., & Wolitzky, D. L. (2009). Adult psychotherapy from the perspectives of attachment theory and psychoanalysis. In J. H. Obegi & E. Berant (Eds.), *Attachment theory and research in clinical work with adults* (pp. 351–378). New York, NY: Guilford Press.

Ehrenthal, J. C., Irgang, M., & Schauenburg, H. (in press). Insecure attachment and the breakdown of regulatory defenses under high life stress: Psychophysiological evidence. *Journal of Social and Clinical Psychology.*

Fan, Y., Wonneberger, C., Enzi, B., de Greck, M., Ulrich, C., Tempelmann, C., . . . Northoff, G. (2011). The narcissistic self and its psychological and neural correlates: An exploratory fMRI study. *Psychological Medicine, 41,* 1641–1650. doi:10.1017/S003329171000228X

Fonagy, P. (1999). Psychoanalysis and attachment theory. In J. Cassidy & P. R. Shaver (Eds.), *Handbook of attachment: Theory, research, and clinical applications* (pp. 595–624). New York, NY: Guilford Press.

Fonagy, P., & Bateman, A. W. (2008). The development of borderline personality disorder—A mentalizing model. *Journal of Personality Disorders, 22,* 4–21. doi:10.1521/pedi.2008.22.1.4

Fonagy, P., Leigh, T., Steele, M., Howard, S., Kennedy, R., Mattoon, G., . . . Gerber, A. (1996). The relation of attachment status, psychiatric classification, and response to psychotherapy. *Journal of Consulting and Clinical Psychology, 64,* 22–31. doi:10.1037/0022-006X.64.1.22

Fonagy, P., Luyten, P., & Strathearn, L. (2011). Borderline personality disorder, mentalization, and the neurobiology of attachment. *Infant Mental Health Journal, 32,* 47–69. doi:10.1002/imhj.20283

Fraley, R. C. (2002). Attachment stability from infancy to adulthood: Meta-analysis and dynamic modeling of developmental mechanisms. *Personality and Social Psychology Review, 6,* 123–151. doi:10.1207/S15327957PSPR0602_03

George, C., Kaplan, N., & Main, M. (1985). *The Adult Attachment Interview.* Unpublished manuscript, University of California at Berkeley.

Gillath, O., Bunge, S. A., Shaver, P. R., Wendelken, C., & Mikulincer, M. (2005). Attachment-style differences in the ability to suppress negative thoughts: Exploring the neural correlates. *NeuroImage, 28,* 835–847. doi:10.1016/j.neuroimage.2005.06.048

Gunderson, J. G. (1996). The borderline patient's intolerance of aloneness: Insecure attachments and therapist availability. *The American Journal of Psychiatry, 153*, 752–758.

Hazan, C., & Shaver, P. (1987). Romantic love conceptualized as an attachment process. *Journal of Personality and Social Psychology, 52*, 511–524. doi:10.1037/0022-3514.52.3.511

Hazlett, E. A., Zhang, J., New, A. S., Zelmanova, Y., Goldstein, K. E., Haznedar, M. M., . . . Chu, K. W. (2012). Potentiated amygdala response to repeated emotional pictures in borderline personality disorder. *Biological Psychiatry, 72*, 448–456. doi:10.1016/j.biopsych.2012.03.027

Heinrichs, M., & Domes, G. (2008). Neuropeptides and social behaviour: Effects of oxytocin and vasopressin in humans. *Progress in Brain Research, 170*, 337–50. doi:10.1016/S0079-6123(08)00428-7

Hobson, R. P., Patrick, M., Crandell, L., García-Pérez, R., & Lee, A. (2005). Personal relatedness and attachment in infants of mothers with borderline personality disorder. *Development and Psychopathology, 17*, 329–347. doi:10.1017/S0954579405050169

Hoermann, S., Clarkin, J. F., Hull, J. W., & Fertuck, E. A. (2004). Attachment dimensions as predictors of medical hospitalizations in individuals with *DSM–IV* Cluster B personality disorders. *Journal of Personality Disorders, 18*, 595–603. doi:10.1521/pedi.18.6.595.54791

Johansen, M., Karterud, S., Pedersen, G., Gude, T., & Falkum, E. (2004). An investigation of the prototype validity of the borderline *DSM–IV* construct. *Acta Psychiatrica Scandinavica, 109*, 289–298. doi:10.1046/j.1600-0447.2003.00268.x

Kernberg, O. F. (1976). *Object relations theory and clinical psychoanalysis*. New York, NY: Aronson.

Klein, M. (1948). *Contributions to psycho-analysis, 1921–1945*. London, England: Hogarth Press.

Klerman, G. L., Weissman, M. M., Rounsaville, B. J., & Chevron, E. S. (1984). *Interpersonal psychotherapy of depression*. New York, NY: Basic Books.

Kobak, R., Zajac, K., & Smith, C. (2009). Adolescent attachment and trajectories of hostile-impulsive behavior: Implications for the development of personality disorders. *Development and Psychopathology, 21*, 839–851. doi:10.1017/S0954579409000455

Kochanska, G., Philibert, R. A., & Barry, R. A. (2009). Interplay of genes and early mother–child relationship in the development of self-regulation from toddler to preschool age. *Journal of Child Psychology and Psychiatry, 50*, 1331–1338. doi:10.1111/j.1469-7610.2008.02050.x

Koenigsberg, H. W., Fan, J., Ochsner, K. N., Liu, X., Guise, K., Pizzarello, S., . . . Siever, L. J. (2010). Neural correlates of using distancing to regulate emotional responses to social situations. *Neuropsychologia, 48*, 1813–1822. doi:10.1016/j.neuropsychologia.2010.03.002

Kosfeld, M., Heinrichs, M., Zak, P. J., Fischbacher, U., & Fehr, E. (2005, June 2). Oxytocin increases trust in humans. *Nature, 435,* 673–676. doi:10.1038/nature03701

Levy, K. N. (2005). The implications of attachment theory and research for understanding borderline personality disorder. *Development and Psychopathology, 17,* 959–986. doi:10.1017/S0954579405050455

Levy, K. N. (2012). Subtypes, dimensions, levels, and mental states in narcissism and narcissistic personality disorder. *Journal of Clinical Psychology, 68,* 886–897. doi:10.1002/jclp.21893

Levy, K. N., Beeney, J. E., & Temes, C. M. (2011). Attachment and its vicissitudes in borderline personality disorders. *Current Psychiatry Reports, 13,* 50–59. doi:10.1007/s11920-010-0169-8

Levy, K. N., & Blatt, S. J. (1999). Attachment theory and psychoanalysis: Further differentiation within insecure attachment patterns. *Psychoanalytic Inquiry, 19,* 541–575. doi:10.1080/07351699909534266

Levy, K. N., & Kelly, K. M. (2008). Using interviews to assess adult attachment. In J. H. Obegi & E. Berant (Eds.), *Attachment theory and research in clinical work with adults* (pp. 121–151). New York, NY: Guilford Press.

Levy, K. N., Meehan, K. B., Kelly, K. M., Reynoso, J., Clarkin, J. F., & Kernberg, O. F. (2006). Change in attachment patterns and reflective function in a randomized control trial of transference-focused psychotherapy for borderline personality disorder. *Journal of Consulting and Clinical Psychology, 74,* 1027–1040. doi:10.1037/0022-006X.74.6.1027

Levy, K. N., Meehan, K. B., Weber, M., Reynoso, J., & Clarkin, J. F. (2005). Attachment and borderline personality disorder: Implications for psychotherapy. *Psychopathology, 38,* 64–74. doi:10.1159/000084813

Macfie, J., & Swan, S. A. (2009). Representations of the caregiver–child relationship and of the self, and emotion regulation in the narratives of young children whose mothers have borderline personality disorder. *Development and Psychopathology, 21,* 993–1011. doi:10.1017/S0954579409000534

Main, M., & Solomon, J. (1986). Discovery of a new, insecure-disorganized-disoriented attachment pattern. In T. B. Brazelton & M. Yogman (Eds.), *Affective development in infancy* (pp. 95–124). Norwood, NJ: Ablex.

Main, M., & Solomon, J. (1990). Procedures for identifying infants as disorganized/disoriented during the Ainsworth Strange Situation. In M. T. Greenberg, D. Cicchetti, & E. M. Cummings (Eds.), *Attachment in the preschool years: Theory, research and intervention* (pp. 95–124). Chicago, IL: University of Chicago Press.

Mallinckrodt, B., Porter, M. J., & Kivlighan, D. M., Jr. (2005). Client attachment to therapist, depth of in-session exploration, and object relations in brief psychotherapy. *Psychotherapy: Theory, Research, Practice, Training, 42,* 85–100. doi:10.1037/0033-3204.42.1.85

McBride, C., & Atkinson, L. (2009). Attachment theory and cognitive-behavioral therapy. In J. H. Obegi & E. Berant (Eds.), *Attachment theory and research in clinical work with adults* (pp. 434–458). New York, NY: Guilford Press.

Meyer, B., Pilkonis, P. A., & Beevers, C. G. (2004). What's in a (neutral) face? Personality disorders, attachment styles, and the appraisal of ambiguous social cues. *Journal of Personality Disorders, 18,* 320–336.

Meyer, B., Pilkonis, P. A., Proietti, J. M., Heape, C. L., & Egan, M. (2001). Attachment styles and personality disorders as predictors of symptoms course. *Journal of Personality Disorders, 15,* 371–389. doi:10.1521/pedi.15.5.371.19200

Mikulincer, M., Birnbaum, G., Woddis, D., & Nachmias, O. (2000). Stress and accessibility of proximity-related thoughts: Exploring the normative and intra-individual components of attachment theory. *Journal of Personality and Social Psychology, 78,* 509–523. doi:10.1037/0022-3514.78.3.509

Mikulincer, M., Gillath, O., & Shaver, P. R. (2002). Activation of the attachment system in adulthood: Threat-related primes increase the accessibility of mental representations of attachment figures. *Journal of Personality and Social Psychology, 83,* 881–895. doi:10.1037/0022-3514.83.4.881

Mikulincer, M., & Shaver, P. R. (2007). *Attachment in adulthood: Structure, dynamics, and change.* New York, NY: Guilford Press.

Mischel, W., & Shoda, Y. (1995). A cognitive-affective system theory of personality: Reconceptualizing situations, dispositions, dynamics, and invariance in personality structure. *Psychological Review, 102,* 246–268. doi:10.1037/0033-295X.102.2.246

Morse, J. Q., Hill, J., Pilkonis, P. A., Yaggi, K., Broyden, N., Stepp, S., . . . Feske, U. (2009). Anger, preoccupied attachment, and domain disorganization in borderline personality disorder. *Journal of Personality Disorders, 23,* 240–257. doi:10.1521/pedi.2009.23.3.240

New, A. S., aan het Rot, M., Ripoll, L. H., Perez-Rodriguez, M. M., Lazarus, S., Zipursky, E., . . . Siever, L. J. (2012). Empathy and alexithymia in borderline personality disorder: Clinical and laboratory measures. *Journal of Personality Disorders, 26,* 660–675. doi:10.1521/pedi.2012.26.5.660

Newman, L. K., Stevenson, C. S., Bergman, L. R., & Boyce, P. (2007). Borderline personality disorder, mother–infant interaction, and parenting perceptions: Preliminary findings. *Australian and New Zealand Journal of Psychiatry, 41,* 598–605. doi:10.1080/00048670701392833

Prunetti, E., Framba, R., Barone, L., Fiore, D., Sera, F., & Liotti, G. (2008). Attachment disorganization and borderline patients' metacognitive responses to therapists' expressed understanding of their states of mind: A pilot study. *Psychotherapy Research, 18,* 28–36. doi:10.1080/10503300701320645

Riggs, S. A., Jacobvitz, D., & Hazen, N. (2002). Adult attachment and history of psychotherapy in a normative sample. *Psychotherapy: Theory, Research, Practice, Training, 39,* 344–353. doi:10.1037/0033-3204.39.4.344

Rom, E., & Mikulincer, M. (2003). Attachment theory and group processes: The association between attachment style and group-related representations, goals, memories, and functioning. *Journal of Personality and Social Psychology, 84,* 1220–1235. doi:10.1037/0022-3514.84.6.1220

Rosenstein, D. S., & Horowitz, H. A. (1996). Adolescent attachment and psychopathology. *Journal of Consulting and Clinical Psychology, 64*, 244–253. doi:10.1037/0022-006X.64.2.244

Samstag, L. W., Muran, J. C., Wachtel, P. L., Slade, A., & Safran, J. D. (2008). Evaluating negative process: A comparison of working alliance, interpersonal behavior, and narrative coherency among three psychotherapy outcome conditions. *American Journal of Psychotherapy, 62*, 165–194.

Schulze, L., Dziobek, I., Vater, A., Heekeren, H. R., Bajbouj, M., Renneberg, B., . . . Roepke, S. (2013). Gray matter abnormalities in patients with narcissistic personality disorder. *Journal of Psychiatric Research, 47*, 1363–1369. doi:10.1016/j.jpsychires.2013.05.017

Scott, L. N., Levy, K. N., & Pincus, A. L. (2009). Adult attachment, personality traits, and borderline personality disorder features in young adults. *Journal of Personality Disorders, 23*, 258–280. doi:10.1521/pedi.2009.23.3.258

Shaver, P. R., Belsky, J., & Brennan, K. A. (2000). The adult attachment interview and self-reports of romantic attachment: Associations across domains and methods. *Personal Relationships, 7*, 25–43. doi:10.1111/j.1475-6811.2000.tb00002.x

Silbersweig, D., Clarkin, J. F., Goldstein, M., Kernberg, O. F., Tuescher, O., Levy, K. N., . . . Stern, E. (2007). Failure of frontolimbic inhibitory function in the context of negative emotion in borderline personality disorder. *The American Journal of Psychiatry, 164*, 1832–1841. doi:10.1176/appi.ajp.2007.06010126

Simeon, D., Bartz, J. A., Hamilton, H., Crystal, S., Braun, A., Ketay, S., & Hollander, E. (2011). Oxytocin administration attenuates stress reactivity in borderline personality disorder: A pilot study. *Psychoneuroendocrinology, 36*, 1418–1421. doi:10.1016/j.psyneuen.2011.03.013

Sroufe, L. A., & Waters, E. (1977). Heart rate as a convergent measure in clinical and developmental research. *Merrill-Palmer Quarterly, 23*, 3–27.

Sterkenburg, P. S., Janssen, C. G. C., & Schuengel, C. (2008). The effect of an attachment-based behavior therapy for children with visual and severe intellectual disabilities. *Journal of Applied Research in Intellectual Disabilities, 21*, 126–135. doi:10.1111/j.1468-3148.2007.00374.x

Strauss, B., Kirchmann, H., Eckert, J., Lobo-Drost, A., Marquet, A., Papenhausen, R., . . . Höger, D. (2006). Attachment characteristics and treatment outcome following inpatient psychotherapy: Results of a multisite study. *Psychotherapy Research, 16*, 579–594. doi:10.1080/10503300600608322

Strauss, B. M., Mestel, R., & Kirchmann, H. A. (2011). Changes of attachment status among women with personality disorders undergoing inpatient treatment. *Counselling and Psychotherapy Research, 11*, 275–283. doi:10.1080/14733145.2010.548563

Theodoridou, A., Rowe, A. C., Penton-Voak, I. S., & Rogers, P. J. (2009). Oxytocin and social perception: Oxytocin increases perceived facial trustworthiness and attractiveness. *Hormones and Behavior, 56*, 128–132. doi:10.1016/j.yhbeh.2009.03.019

van IJzendoorn, M. H. (1995). Adult attachment representations, parental responsiveness, and infant attachment: A meta-analysis on the predictive validity of the adult attachment interview. *Psychological Bulletin, 117*, 387–403. doi:10.1037/0033-2909.117.3.387

Vogel, D. L., & Wei, M. (2005). Adult attachment and help-seeking intent: The mediating roles of psychological distress and perceived social support. *Journal of Counseling Psychology, 52*, 347–357. doi:10.1037/0022-0167.52.3.347

Vrtička, P., Andersson, F., Grandjean, D., Sander, D., & Vuilleumier, P. (2008). Individual attachment style modulates human amygdala and striatum activation during social appraisal. *PLoS ONE, 3*(8), e2868. doi:10.1371/journal.pone.0002868

Zanarini, M. C., Frankenburg, F. R., Dubo, E. D., Sickel, M. A., Trikha, A., Levin, A., & Reynolds, V. (1998). Axis I comorbidity of borderline personality disorder. *The American Journal of Psychiatry, 155*, 1733–1739.

Zeijlmans van Emmichoven, I. A., van IJzendoorn, M. H., de Ruiter, C., & Brosschot, J. F. (2003). Selective processing of threatening information: Effects of attachment representation and anxiety disorder on attention and memory. *Development and Psychopathology, 15*, 219–237. doi:10.1017/S0954579403000129

Zimmerman, P., Mohr, C., & Spangler, G. (2009). Genetic and attachment influences on adolescents' regulation of autonomy and aggressiveness. *Journal of Child Psychology and Psychiatry, 50*, 1339–1347. doi:10.1111/j.1469-7610.2009.02158.x

14

AN INTEGRATIVE INTERPERSONAL FRAMEWORK FOR UNDERSTANDING PERSONALITY PATHOLOGY

NICOLE M. CAIN AND EMILY B. ANSELL

Patients with personality disorders (PDs) often present for psychotherapy due to difficulties in their relationships with others. They are likely to view others as a source of frustration and to report significant interpersonal problems and distress. Quite often, their interpersonal behavior exacerbates their other presenting problems, such as mood disorders, anxiety disorders, and substance use. Symptom criteria reflect the salience of interpersonal dysfunction within PD diagnoses. Clinicians of all theoretical orientations who treat personality pathology are inevitably faced with threats to the therapeutic alliance, dissolution of important relations, and damage to the patient's life caused by entrenched maladaptive interpersonal behaviors. Given the centrality of self–other difficulties associated with personality pathology, it is not surprising that many PD theorists (e.g., Benjamin, 2003; Clarkin, Yeomans, & Kernberg, 2006; Linehan, 1993) emphasize, at least in part, the primacy of interpersonal dysfunction.

http://dx.doi.org/10.1037/14549-015
Personality Disorders: Toward Theoretical and Empirical Integration in Diagnosis and Assessment,
S. K. Huprich (Editor)

In this chapter, we present the contemporary integrative interpersonal theory framework (Pincus, 2005; Pincus & Ansell, 2013) and its associated treatment strategies (Anchin & Pincus, 2010; Benjamin, 2003) for personality pathology. Interpersonal theory offers tools to make predictions about interpersonal behavior, distinguishes varying effects of social behavior on the expression of psychopathology, and measures clinically significant variability in social behavior over time. These tools cut across theoretical orientations, offering an integrative platform by which to discuss the commonalities and unique attributes underlying personality pathology. Conceiving of personality pathology as fundamentally interpersonal in its expression (Hopwood, Wright, Ansell, & Pincus, 2013) allows clinicians and researchers to integrate across psychodynamic, social learning, dialectical, and cognitive-behavioral treatments to assess, intervene, but also mutually understand issues at the level of problematic social behaviors.

In this chapter, we review the basic tenets of interpersonal theory; the primacy of agency and communion in understanding self–other relational difficulties; the processes by which interpersonal interactions promote, maintain, or mitigate pathology; and the ways in which interpersonal theory informs our understanding of both adaptive and maladaptive interpersonal behavior. We also focus on current research supporting this framework for understanding personality pathology. Finally, we describe how to apply an integrative interpersonal framework to the treatment of personality pathology.

CONTEMPORARY INTEGRATIVE INTERPERSONAL THEORY

The interpersonal tradition offers a nomological network (Cronbach & Meehl, 1955; Pincus & Wright, 2010) that is well suited for and explicitly interested in pantheoretical integration. In other words, the interpersonal tradition offers an integrative theoretical and empirical model designed to describe and test the observable manifestations of interpersonal behavior as well as the relationship between interpersonal theory and other models of personality pathology. The integrative underpinnings of interpersonal theory were best described by Horowitz et al. (2006):

> Because the interpersonal approach harmonizes so well with all of these theoretical approaches, it is integrative: It draws from the wisdom of all major approaches to systematize our understanding of interpersonal phenomena. Although it is integrative, however, it is also unique, posing characteristic questions of its own. (p. 82)

Here we present a review of the main assumptions that underlie contemporary interpersonal theory, which both facilitate its integrative nature and define its unique characteristics.

The Interpersonal Situation

One of the main assumptions of contemporary interpersonal theory is that the most important expressions of personality and psychopathology occur in phenomena involving more than one person, described by Sullivan (1953) as the *interpersonal situation*. Pincus and Ansell (2013) noted that the interpersonal situation is the experience of a pattern of relating self with other, associated with varying levels of anxiety (or security), in which learning takes place that significantly influences the development of self-concept and social behavior. The interpersonal situation is intimately tied to the genesis, development, maintenance, and mutability of personality and PD through the continuous patterning and repatterning of interpersonal experience (social learning) in an effort to satisfy fundamental human motives (e.g., attachment and communion, autonomy and agency) in ways that increase security and self-esteem (positively reinforcing) and avoid anxiety (negatively reinforcing). Over time, this social learning leads to the development of mental representations of self and others (Blatt, Auerbach, & Levy, 1997) as well as enduring patterns of adaptive or maladaptive interpersonal behavior (Benjamin, 2003; Pincus, 2005).

A potential misinterpretation of the term *interpersonal* is to assume that it refers to a limited class of phenomena that can be observed only in the immediate interaction between two proximal people. In contemporary interpersonal theory, the term is not a geographic indicator of locale. It is not meant to generate a dichotomy between what is inside the person and what is outside the person (Pincus & Ansell, 2013). Interpersonal functioning occurs not only between people but also inside people's minds via the capacity for mental representation of self and others (e.g., Blatt et al., 1997). At the core of these different conceptions of covert interpersonally related structures and processes—variously referred to as cognitive interpersonal schemas (Safran, 1990a, 1990b), internal working models (Benjamin, 2003), object relations (Clarkin et al., 2006), or personifications (Sullivan, 1953)—is the view that developmental experiences within family and peer relationships, in dynamic interaction with biological temperament, ingrain certain sensitivities, expectancies, and motives that give rise to the disturbed interpersonal relations of patients with PD. These representational structures, elaborated over the life span by one's interpersonal experiences and metacognitive processes (e.g., self-reflection), act as templates reflexively guiding and organizing one's network of perceptions, thoughts, feelings, and motivations in significant relationships (Pincus & Hopwood, 2012).

Agency and Communion

Another main assumption of contemporary interpersonal theory is that agency and communion, core domains of human existence (Wiggins, 2003), provide an integrative metastructure for conceptualizing interpersonal situations and their mental representations (Pincus, 2005). *Agency* refers to the condition of being a differentiated individual, and it is manifested in strivings for power and mastery, which can protect and enhance one's differentiation. *Communion* refers to the condition of being part of a larger social entity, and it is manifested in strivings for intimacy, union, and solidarity with the larger entity. These metaconcepts form a superordinate structure, and this structure may take on different forms.

One form that has been used across instruments, referred to as the *interpersonal circumplex* (IPC; Leary, 1957; Wiggins, 2003), has been used to describe both adaptive and maladaptive interpersonal behavior. Wiggins (2003) noted that agency and communion encompass the fundamental interpersonal motives, strivings, and values of human relations. Thus, when seeking to understand essential motivations in interpersonal situations, it is important to consider both the agentic and communal nature of the individual's interpersonal goals (e.g., to be in control; to be close—or their opposites) and the specific behaviors enacted to achieve those goals. Agentic and communal traits imply enduring patterns of perceiving, thinking, feeling, and behaving that describe an individual's relational tendencies aggregated across interpersonal situations (i.e., one's interpersonal style). The IPC classifies the nature and intensity of distinct interpersonal acts.

The Interpersonal Circumplex

Empirical research into diverse interpersonal taxa, such as traits (Wiggins, 2003), problems (Alden, Wiggins, & Pincus, 1990), sensitivities (Hopwood et al., 2011), values (Locke, 2000), and strengths (Hatcher & Rogers, 2009), converges in suggesting that the structure of interpersonal functioning takes the form of a circle (or circumplex) with the two underlying dimensions of dominance–submission (agency) on the vertical axis and nurturance–coldness (communion) on the horizontal axis (Pincus & Hopwood, 2012). The geometric properties of circumplex models give rise to unique computational methods for assessment and research (Wright, Pincus, Conroy, & Hilsenroth, 2009) that will not be reviewed here. Rather, in this chapter, we use the IPC to anchor description of theoretical concepts. Blends of dominance and nurturance can be located along the 360° perimeter of the circle. Interpersonal qualities close to one another on the perimeter are conceptually and statistically similar, qualities at 90° are conceptually and statistically independent, and qualities 180° apart are conceptual and statistical opposites. Thus, we can use circumplex models to describe a person's typical ways of relating to others and refer to that person's interpersonal style or theme.

Using IPC models to classify individuals in terms of their agentic and communal characteristics is often referred to as *interpersonal diagnosis*

(Pincus & Wright, 2010). Of importance, however, traits and behaviors are not isomorphic, rendering the interpersonal meaning of a given behavior ambiguous without consideration of the person's interpersonal motives or goals (Horowitz et al., 2006). Thus, a certain trait or behavior (whether adaptive or maladaptive) may not necessarily be expressed in a particular interpersonal situation or relationship, or dictate a particular emergent process. For this level of specificity, contemporary interpersonal theory moves past static individual differences and uses other conceptualizations of psychopathology.

Interpersonal Pathoplasticity

The contemporary interpersonal tradition assumes a *pathoplastic* relationship between interpersonal functioning and many forms of psychopathology. Pathoplasticity is characterized by a mutually influencing, non-etiological relationship between psychopathology and another psychological system (Widiger & Smith, 2008). It was initially conceptualized as a model identifying personality-based subtypes of depression—dependent/sociotropic/anaclitic versus self-critical/autonomous/introjective (e.g., Beck, Freeman, Davis, & Associates, 2004; Blatt, 2004)—but its scope has been broadened to personality and psychopathology in general. Pathoplasticity assumes that the expression of certain maladaptive behaviors, symptoms, and mental disorders tends to occur in the larger context of an individual's personality. Likewise, it is assumed that personality has the potential for influencing the content and focus of symptoms and will likely shape the responses and coping strategies individuals employ when presented with psychological and social stressors.

Interpersonal pathoplasticity can describe the observed heterogeneity in the phenotypic expression of psychopathology (e.g., Cain et al., 2012), predict variability in response to psychotherapy within a disorder (e.g., Alden & Capreol, 1993), and account for a lack of uniformity in regulatory strategies displayed by those who otherwise are struggling with similar symptoms (e.g., Wright, Pincus, Conroy, & Elliot, 2009). The identification of interpersonal subtypes within a singular psychiatric diagnosis allows clinicians to anticipate and understand differences in patients' expressions of distress and their typical patterns in the interpersonal situation needed to regulate their self, affect, and relationships. Empirical investigations have found that interpersonal problems exhibit pathoplastic relationships with symptoms and mental disorders, in patients with generalized anxiety disorder (Przeworski et al., 2011) and major depression (Cain et al., 2012).

Recent research suggests that some *Diagnostic and Statistical Manual of Mental Disorders* (DSM) PDs may also exhibit interpersonal pathoplasticity, although research in this area is quite new. For example, Alden and Capreol (1993) found two interpersonal subtypes of avoidant PD, a warm-submissive type and a cold-submissive type, which exhibited differential responses to treatment interventions emphasizing exposure and skills training respectively. In addition, recent conceptualizations of narcissistic PD that include both grandiosity and vulnerability (Pincus & Lukowitsky, 2010) suggest that pathological narcissism may also exhibit interpersonal pathoplasticity. While narcissistic grandiosity involves arrogance, exploitativeness, and inflated self-importance, narcissistic vulnerability is characterized by self- and affect dysregulation in response to self-enhancement failures and lack of needed recognition and admiration (e.g., Zeigler-Hill & Besser, 2013; Zeigler-Hill, Clark, & Pickard, 2008). Despite sharing the core narcissistic pathology, these two presentations of pathological narcissism exhibit very different interpersonal expressions (one domineering, the other avoidant; Pincus & Lukowitsky, 2010). Finally, Wright et al. (2013) explored interpersonal pathoplasticity in borderline PD (BPD) and found six interpersonal subtypes: intrusive, vindictive, avoidant, nonassertive, moderate exploitable, and severe exploitable. These interpersonal subtypes differ in terms of clinically relevant features, such as antisocial features, self-injury, and past suicide attempts, leading Wright et al. to conclude that assessing interpersonal pathoplasticity adds incremental clinical utility above PD diagnosis.

Interpersonal Variability

The addition of pathoplasticity greatly extends the empirical and practical utility of interpersonal diagnosis. However, describing psychopathology with relationally based, dispositional personality concepts implying marked consistency of relational functioning is still insufficient and does not exhaust contemporary interpersonal diagnostic approaches (Pincus & Wright, 2010). Even patients described by a particular interpersonal style do not robotically emit the same behaviors without variation. Recent advances in the measurement and analysis of intraindividual variability (e.g., Ram & Gerstorf, 2009) converge to suggest that dynamic aspects of interpersonal behavior warrant further investigation and clinical assessment. This accumulating body of research indicates that individuals are characterized not only by their stable individual differences in mean levels of behavior but also by stable differences in their variability in psychological states (Fleeson, 2001), behaviors (Moskowitz, Russell, Sadikaj, & Sutton, 2009), affect (Kuppens, Van Mechelen, Nezlek, Dossche, & Timmermans, 2007), and even personality traits themselves (Hopwood et al., 2009) across time and situations.

Moskowitz and Zuroff (2004) introduced the terms *flux*, *pulse*, and *spin* to describe the stable levels of intraindividual variability in interpersonal behaviors sampled from the IPC. *Flux* refers to variability about an individual's mean behavioral score on agentic or communal dimensions (e.g., dominant flux, submissive flux, friendly flux, hostile flux). *Spin* refers to variability of the angular coordinates about the individual's mean interpersonal theme on the interpersonal circle. *Pulse* refers to variability of the overall extremity of the emitted behavior. Low spin would thus reflect a narrow repertoire of interpersonal behaviors enacted over time. Low pulse reflects little variability in behavioral intensity, and if it were associated with a high mean intensity generally, it would be consistent with the enactment of consistently extreme interpersonal behaviors. This dynamic lexicon has important implications for the assessment of normal and abnormal behavior. Theory and research suggest that the assessment of intraindividual variability offers unique and important new methods for the description of personality pathology.

For example, Russell, Moskowitz, Zuroff, Sookman, and Paris (2007) differentiated individuals with BPD from nonclinical control participants on the basis of intraindividual variability of interpersonal behavior over a 20-day period. Individuals with BPD reported a similar mean level of agreeable (communal) behavior more than did their nonclinical counterparts, but participants with BPD displayed greater flux in their agreeable behaviors. This suggests that nonclinical control participants demonstrated consistent agreeable behavior across situations but individuals with BPD varied greatly in their agreeable behaviors, vacillating between high and low levels. Results also showed that individuals with BPD endorsed higher mean levels of quarrelsome behavior and higher levels of flux in quarrelsome behavior than did controls. Individuals with BPD also demonstrated greater spin, suggesting greater behavioral lability, than did their nonclinical counterparts. The contemporary interpersonal framework includes flux, pulse, and spin as constructs of behavioral variability that can differentiate the phenomenological expression of personality pathology.

Interpersonal Signatures

One final assumption of interpersonal theory is that interpersonal behavior is reciprocally influential in ongoing human transaction. Using the agency and communion metaframework allows researchers and clinicians to model both stability and variability in self–other social processes. These self–other patterns, described by their agentic and communal qualities, are referred to as *interpersonal signatures* (Fournier, Moskowitz, & Zuroff, 2009). Research on interpersonal signatures is based on the seminal work of Mischel and Shoda (1995) on the cognitive-affective processing system, or CAPS. The CAPS framework argues that individuals encode the psychological features of a given situation through a complex configuration of within-person structures and processes (i.e., cognitive-affective units) that include competencies ("I feel capable of performing behavior X"), expectancies

("If I perform behavior X, then outcome Y will follow"), values ("Outcome Y is important to me"), and goals. This complex system of interrelated structures and processes gives rise to stable but situation-contingent *if-then* dispositions or behavioral signatures, such that each individual demonstrates stable levels of behavior within situations and stable patterns of behavior across situations. Within interpersonal theory, the situations in which cognitive and affective processing are primarily observed are interpersonal in nature along dimensions of agency and communion. Thus Fournier et al. (2009) coined the term *interpersonal signatures* to signify the integration of the CAPS framework with interpersonal theory.

Using the IPC to investigate interpersonal signatures has been referred to as adaptive and maladaptive transaction cycles (Kiesler, 1991) and self-fulfilling prophecies (Carson, 1969). Reciprocal relational patterns are socially reinforced through various transactional influences impacting self and other as they resolve, negotiate, or disintegrate the interpersonal situation. Interpersonal behaviors tend to pull, elicit, invite, or evoke "restricted classes" of responses from the other in a continual, dynamic transactional process. Carson (1991) referred to this as an *interbehavioral contingency process*, where "there is a tendency for a given individual's interpersonal behavior to be constrained or controlled in more or less predictable ways by the behavior received from an interaction partner" (p. 191). Thus, interpersonal signatures are the consistent agentic and communal behavioral responses to the perceived agentic and communal characteristics of others in an interpersonal situation (Pincus & Wright, 2010).

The IPC provides conceptual anchors and a lexicon to systematically describe interpersonal signatures. The most basic of these processes is referred to as *interpersonal complementarity* (Carson, 1969; Kiesler, 1983). Interpersonal complementarity occurs when there is a match between the interpersonal goals of each person. That is, reciprocal patterns of activity evolve where the agentic and communal needs of both persons are met in the interpersonal situation, leading to stability and the likely recurrence of the pattern. Carson (1969) first proposed that complementarity could be defined via the IPC based on the social exchange of status (agency) and love (communion), as reflected in reciprocity for the vertical dimension (i.e., dominance pulls for submission; submission pulls for dominance) and correspondence for the horizontal dimension (friendliness pulls for friendliness; hostility pulls for hostility). Kiesler (1983) extended the principles of reciprocity and correspondence to complementary points along the entire IPC perimeter (e.g., hostile dominance pulls for hostile submission, friendly dominance pulls for friendly submission). Although complementarity is neither the only reciprocal interpersonal pattern that can be described by the IPC nor a proposed universal law of interaction, empirical studies consistently find support for its probabilistic predictions (Sadler, Ethier, & Woody, 2011). Complementarity is considered a common baseline for the reciprocal influence of interpersonal behavior in healthy social relations. Deviations from complementarity are likely to disrupt interpersonal relations and may be indicative of pathological functioning (Fournier et al., 2009; Pincus et al., 2009). Common non-complementary interpersonal signatures in psychotherapy with patients with PD include responding to therapist warmth with fear, suspicion, anger, or indifference; engaging in power struggles with the therapist for control; and chronic passivity in the face of all therapeutic efforts to mobilize the patient.

Interpersonal Signatures and Personality Disorders

Complementarity should not be conceived of as simply a behavioral stimulus–response chain of events. Rather, mediating internal psychological processes (e.g., each interactant's self–other schemas, the motives and needs embedded in these schemas, and their effects on subjective experience) influence the likelihood of complementary interpersonal signatures. An individual's chronic deviations from complementary reciprocal patterns of social behavior may be indicative of personality pathology, as these deviations suggest impairments in (a) recognizing the consensual understanding of interpersonal situations (e.g., psychotherapy), (b) adaptively communicating one's own interpersonal needs and motives, and (c) comprehending the needs of others and the intent of their interpersonal behavior (Anchin & Pincus, 2010). In such cases, the individual pulls consistently and rigidly for responses that complement his or her own interpersonal behavior but has significant difficulty reciprocating with responses that are complementary to the other's behavior. This reduces the likelihood that the agentic and communal motives of both persons will be satisfied in the interpersonal situation, creating disturbed interpersonal relations (Pincus 2005; Pincus & Hopwood, 2012; Sullivan, 1953).

Normality, then, reflects the tendency or capacity to perceive self and other in generally undistorted forms. That is, healthy individuals are generally able to accurately encode the agentic and communal behaviors of others, and the relationship is stable. However, this is not always the case in psychotherapy with patients with PD. Therapists generally attempt to work in their patients' best interest and promote a positive therapeutic relationship. Patients who are generally free of PD typically enter therapy hoping for relief of their symptoms and are capable of experiencing the therapist as potentially helpful and benign. With complementary goals of seeking help and giving help, the therapist and patient are likely to develop a complementary interpersonal signature (i.e., a therapeutic alliance). Despite psychotherapists taking a similar stance with patients with PD, the beginning of therapy is often quite rocky, as the patients tend to view the therapists with fear, idealization, contempt, and so on. Thus treatment often starts with noncomplementary interpersonal signatures, difficulties establishing a therapeutic alliance, and ongoing negotiation of the therapeutic relationship and frame.

What leads to patients' distorted perceptions of interpersonal situations and, subsequently, maladaptive interpersonal signatures? Psychodynamic, attachment, cognitive, and interpersonal theories converge in suggesting that dyadic mental representations are key influences on the perception and subjective elaboration of interpersonal input (Pincus, 2005). Individuals exhibit tendencies to organize their experience in certain ways (i.e., they have particular interpersonal schemas, expectancies, sensitivities, memories, fantasies, etc.). Interpersonal theory posits two main pathways by which one's schemas, expectancies, sensitivities, memories, and fantasies can distort the organization of interpersonal experience, one that is outside of awareness and one that is experienced consciously.

Parataxic Distortions

Sullivan (1953) proposed the concept of *parataxic distortion* to describe the mediation of social behavior by internal psychological processes. He suggested that this occurs "when, beside the interpersonal situation as defined within the awareness of the speaker, there is a concomitant interpersonal situation quite different as to its principle integrating tendencies, of which the speaker is more or less completely unaware" (p. 92). The effects of unreflective, schema-driven distortions on interpersonal relations can occur in several forms, including chronic distortions of new interpersonal experiences (input), generation of rigid, extreme, and/or chronically nonnormative interpersonal behavior (output), and dominance of self-protective motives (Horowitz et al., 2006) leading to the disconnection of interpersonal input and output.

Healthy interpersonal relations are generally promoted by the capacity to organize and elaborate incoming interpersonal input in generally undistorted ways, allowing for the agentic and communal needs of self and other to be mutually satisfied within the contextual norms of the situation. In contrast, maladaptive interpersonal functioning is promoted when the perception of the interpersonal situation is, without apparent awareness, encoded in distorted or biased ways, leading to increased interpersonal insecurity and maladaptive interpersonal signatures (output) that disrupt interpersonal relations. In psychotherapy, this can be identified by a preponderance of noncomplementary interpersonal signatures between therapist and patient, as well as in patients' reports of their relationships with others. To account for the development and frequency of such distortions in personality pathology, interpersonal theory also outlines key maturational, motivational, and regulatory principles (see Benjamin, 2003; Pincus, 2005).

Self-Protective Motives

Beyond agency and communion, contemporary interpersonal theory identifies another class of interpersonal motives referred to as *self-protective motives*. Such motives can be described as arising "as a way of defending oneself from feelings of vulnerability that are related to relational schemas" that often take the form of "strategies people use to reassure themselves that they possess desired communal (e.g., likable) and agentic (e.g., competent) self-qualities" (Horowitz et al., 2006, pp. 75–76). To the extent that a patient's early social learning occurred in a toxic developmental environment, the more likely the patient is to exhibit parataxic distortions of interpersonal situations, feel threatened and vulnerable due to his or her characteristic ways of organizing interpersonal experience, and engage in self-protective interpersonal behavior that is noncontingent with the behavior of others or the normative situational press (Pincus & Hopwood, 2012). The severity of personality pathology can be evaluated in terms of the pervasiveness of parataxic distortions and self-protective motives across time and situations. Severe personality pathology is often reflected in pervasive rigid or chaotic parataxic distortions. The former render the experience of most interpersonal situations functionally equivalent (and typically anxiety provoking and threatening to the self); the latter render the experience of interpersonal situations highly inconsistent and unpredictable (commonly oscillating between secure and threatening organizations of experience).

Treatment Implications

Pincus and Hopwood (2012) noted that there is no single interpersonal psychotherapy; rather, intervention techniques are drawn from a variety of therapeutic approaches that view interpersonal processes as central to the development of pathology and to the patient's experience of distress. Based on the contemporary interpersonal tradition, the treatment of maladaptive interpersonal patterns aims to promote new interpersonal awareness and learning, which in turn leads to improved relational capacity and a subsequent reduction in symptoms. Appropriate intervention strategies are selected on the basis of the core interpersonal processes that define a patient's pathology as well as how that pathology is expressed within the interpersonal situation, the stage of therapy, the quality of the therapeutic relationship, and other relevant patient and therapist characteristics (Anchin & Pincus, 2010; Pincus & Hopwood, 2012).

Central to interpersonal theory is the therapeutic relationship, which provides a proximal interpersonal situation through which to explore the patient's core interpersonal processes. The therapeutic relationship is both a vehicle for change and a context through which all intervention techniques are employed. This requires the therapist to be actively engaged in the therapeutic relationship as a *participant observer* (Anchin & Pincus, 2010). As a *participant*, the therapist is reflective on his or her reactions to the patient, which often reflect the predominant interpersonal impacts of the patient's behavior on others. Of importance, the therapist is also an *observer* who is acutely attuned to interpersonal communication occurring in the patient's behavior, tone of voice, gestures, and symptoms. The therapist observes and reflects on what is occurring in the therapeutic relationship and begins to identify parataxic distortions that give rise to disturbed, noncomplementary interpersonal relations between patient and therapist.

Pincus (2005) articulated a treatment framework for personality pathology that integrates contemporary interpersonal theory with Kernberg's (1975) object-relations-based understanding of personality structure. In this approach, the therapist utilizes a sequence of clarifications, confrontations, and well-timed interpretations to identify and explore parataxic distortions that may be occurring in the therapeutic relationship as well as the relevant regulatory goal (Pincus, 2005). For example, in the initial stages of treatment, the therapist may be curious with the patient about how he or she perceives the therapist and ask to hear more about the patient's perceptions and distortions, thus clarifying how the patient views the therapist at any given point in session. As the therapy progresses, the therapist begins to gently point out and confront the discrepancies between the proximal interpersonal situation (e.g., the therapeutic relationship) and the internal interpersonal situation (e.g., the patient's parataxic distortions), understanding that this will stress the therapeutic relationship and evoke anxiety in the patient. Finally, in the later stages of therapy, the therapist begins to link the patient's distorted view of self and other in the therapeutic relationship to internal representations via interpretation. The timing of the interpretation phase is important. Depending on the type and severity of PD pathology, it may take the therapist quite some time to begin interpreting the links between the patient's views of self and other, their early relationships, and their symptoms and functional impairments.

Developmental Antecedents, Toxic Learning Environments, and Past Social Learning

Once the therapist identifies and articulates the patient's maladaptive interpersonal patterns through clarifications and confrontations, these patterns are linked via interpretation to developmental antecedents, toxic early environments, and past social learning in an effort to understand the etiology and maintenance of these characteristic patterns of relating to others. Benjamin's (2003) developmental learning and loving theory (DLL) argued that attachment itself is the fundamental motivation that catalyzes social learning processes. Benjamin proposed three developmental "copy processes" that describe the ways in which early interpersonal experiences are internalized as a function of achieving either secure or insecure attachment. The first is *identification*, which is defined as "treating others as one has been treated." To the extent that individuals strongly identify with early caretakers, there will be a tendency to act toward others in ways that copy how important others have acted toward the developing person. This tendency mediates the selection of interpersonal output and may lead to repetition of such behavior regardless of agentic and communal goals and behaviors of actual others (i.e., noncomplementary patterns). The second is *recapitulation*, which is defined as "maintaining a position complementary to an internalized other." This process can be described as reacting "as if the internalized other is still there and in control." In this case, new interpersonal input is likely to be distorted such that the proximal other is experienced as similar to the internalized other, or new interpersonal input from the proximal other may simply be ignored and behavior recapitulates old patterns with the dominant internalized other. The third is *introjection*, which is defined as "treating the self as one has been treated." Treating the self in introjected ways maintains security and esteem despite noncomplementary behavior in relations with others.

Pincus and Ansell (2013) extended the catalysts of social learning beyond the attachment motivation by proposing that reciprocal interpersonal patterns develop in concert with emerging motives that take developmental priority. These developmentally emergent motives may begin with the formation of early attachment bonds and felt security, but separation–individuation and the experiences of self-esteem and additional unfolding motives may then become priorities. Interpersonal patterns can also be associated with traumatic learning that leads to self-protective motives as well as coping strategies for impinging events such as early loss of an attachment figure, childhood illness or injury, and neglect or abuse. Identifying the developmental and traumatic catalysts for internalization and social learning allows for greater understanding of current interpersonal behaviors. For example, in terms of achieving adult attachment relationships, some individuals have developed hostile strategies (e.g., verbally or physically fighting) in order to elicit some form of interpersonal connection, and others have developed submissive strategies (e.g., avoiding conflict and deferring to the wishes of the other) in order to be liked and elicit gratitude. A person's social learning history will significantly influence that person's ability to accurately organize new interpersonal experiences.

As noted earlier, depending on the type and severity of the PD, the process of linking maladaptive interpersonal patterns to developmental antecedents may progress quite slowly. It is possible that the therapist may not get to the developmental antecedents at all. For example, the patient may end treatment before the developmental and traumatic catalysts for internalization and social learning are fully identified. However, if the therapist focuses on linking present symptoms and impairments to past social learning, the patient's will to change may be evoked and new social learning can occur both inside and outside of treatment. As for Benjamin's (2003) interpersonal reconstructive therapy, the goal of this treatment approach is to support the part of the patient that is ready, willing, and able to change his or her maladaptive interpersonal patterns. It is often the case that, with a PD patient, the more regressive part of the patient is dominant early on in the therapy. It then becomes the primary task of the therapist to form an alliance with the growth-oriented part of the patient from the very beginning of the therapy and to engage that part of the patient in the process of new social learning within the context of the therapeutic relationship. This new social learning can evoke the patient's will to change and allow the patient to develop new and more adaptive interpersonal patterns (Benjamin, 2003; Pincus & Hopwood, 2012).

Integrating Contemporary Integrative Interpersonal Theory With Other Models of Personality Pathology

Many theorists agree that personality pathology contains within it a core theme of interpersonal dysfunction (Benjamin, 2003; Clarkin et al., 2006; Hopwood et al., 2013; Linehan, 1993; Luyten & Blatt, 2013; Pincus, 2005). Proposed changes to *DSM* PDs have been put on hold for the fifth edition of the *DSM*, awaiting further research and revisions. However, one such proposal, the Level of Personality Functioning Scale (Bender, Morey, & Skodol, 2011; Morey et al., 2011), conceptualizes personality pathology severity along a continuum of self–other functioning and aligns with one of the basic tenets of contemporary integrative interpersonal theory: that the core of personality pathology pertains to dysfunction in understanding the self in relation to other and that differences may be understood along the dimensions of communion, empathy, or interpersonal relatedness and agency, self-direction, or self-esteem, depending on preferred model or theoretical orientation (Bender, 2013; Hopwood et al., 2013). In this way, interpersonal theory serves to unite, along common themes, many of the existing and diverse models of personality theory and pathology.

In particular, many of the commonly identified symptoms of personality pathology across theories can be thought of as manifestations within the interpersonal situation and these commonalities suggest target areas for integration between models. For example, Safran (1990a, 1990b) synthesized cognitive therapy with key principles from the interpersonal tradition. The central goal of Safran's cognitive-interpersonal therapy (CIT) is to identify and modify dysfunctional cognitive structures and interpersonal patterns in a patient's life. Safran noted the development of cognitive interpersonal schemas, or representations of self–other interactions, that hold the goals and if-then contingencies that regulate current and future interpersonal functioning, similar to interpersonal signatures. In CIT, awareness of interpersonal schemas increases as the therapist continually draws the patient's attention to relevant interpersonal behaviors occurring at different points in the therapeutic relationship. In this regard, the CIT therapist acts as a participant observer and helps the patient to recognize his or her interpersonal schemas as they are occurring in the here and now in the therapeutic relationship. To monitor the appearance of interpersonal schemas between sessions, the therapist assigns homework and the patient begins to identify and change his or her automatic relational style both inside and outside of sessions. Contemporary integrative interpersonal theory expands upon CIT's approach by quantifying and characterizing the interpersonal signature of a given client along the dimensions of agency and communion. This allows for diagnostic assessment based on interpersonal patterns and provides the therapist with a specific focus for treatment, which is to provide new interpersonal experiences for the patient with PD. This may be accomplished by responding to the patient in a new and therapeutic manner that counteracts typical interpersonal patterns (aka signatures) and helps to disconfirm dysfunctional interpersonal schemas.

There are also many points of overlap between contemporary integrative interpersonal theory and object-relations-based approaches to personality pathology, such as transference-focused psychotherapy (TFP) developed for the treatment of BPD (Clarkin et al., 2006). An object relation is a representation of self linked to a representation of other via affect (i.e., a scared, victimized self linked to a sadistic, abusive other via fear), most often learned in infancy and childhood through interactions with caregivers. Within contemporary interpersonal theory, the interpersonal patterns of these object relations may be understood as reflecting the internal interpersonal world that may in turn motivate and influence changes in external interpersonal behavior. Treatment models such as TFP emphasize observing how the patient relates to the therapist in order to gradually define the dominant object relation that the patient is exhibiting in the here-and-now interaction in the therapy session. To do this, the therapist must pay close attention to the patient's interpersonal communications, both verbal and nonverbal. Object-relations-based approaches note the importance of transference and countertransference in helping the therapist to understand the patient's dominant object relation in session, similar to Sullivan's use of parataxic distortion to understand disturbed interpersonal relations. As noted earlier, Pincus (2005) articulated an integrated treatment framework that combines key interpersonal principles with the treatment strategies of TFP (clarification, confrontation, and interpretation). This integrated model aims to help patients with personality pathology link their maladaptive interpersonal patterns to developmental antecedents through a series of well-timed clarifications, confrontations, and interpretations, thus leading to more adaptive interpersonal patterns.

From an attachment-based perspective, Benjamin (2003) noted the interpersonal chaos that dominates the developmental history and attachment system of the patient with BPD. This chaos often leads to abandonment fears, which subsequently lead to variability in daily social behaviors. This variability often involves compensatory interpersonal strategies aimed to reduce abandonment by others; it can be thought of as a unique interpersonal signature associated with BPD. In this way, idealization might be viewed as an expression of overly communal behavior while devaluation may be understood as a hostile (low communion) and aggressive (high dominance) social behavior. The oscillation between these two interpersonal stances (variability, or spin) is just as important as the mean level behavior (communal versus hostile). With this interpersonal understanding in mind, therapies may then seek to mitigate this social behavior variability while decreasing hostile social behaviors.

Linehan (1993) also noted interpersonal developmental antecedents that maintain the symptoms of BPD. In particular, the biosocial theory describes how the combination of biological vulnerability and an invalidating social environment leads to the emotion regulation difficulties central to BPD. For example, if a child expresses the need for affection (a communal need) more intensely than a caregiver is able to tolerate, the caregiver may respond with frustration or scorn (invalidation). The child eventually learns to blunt, mask, or distort interpersonal experiences, thereby developing maladaptive interpersonal signatures that lead to subsequent interpersonal problems and emotion dysregulation. Linehan's dialectical behavior therapy (DBT) includes treatment strategies that emphasize interpersonal validation and acceptance. For example, the DBT therapist aims to accurately reflect the patent's interpersonal communications; articulate unverbalized emotions, thoughts, or behavior patterns; and communicate how current interpersonal behavior makes sense in terms of past social learning in the invalidating environment. An awareness of the principles of contemporary interpersonal theory would allow a clinician using DBT to understand and characterize the interpersonal signatures of patients along the dimensions of agency and communion.

Finally, mentalization-based conceptualizations have also been suggested as an integrative point across therapies for PDs (Fonagy & Bateman, 2006). *Mentalizing*, or the ability of an individual to attend to the mental states of self and other, articulates the importance of both attachment (communion) and agency. Disruptions occur when perceptions of self and other behavior become dysregulated. Contemporary integrative interpersonal theory may offer a useful way to explore these disruptions in mentalizing ability by addressing the discrepancies between perception and behavior in relation to others.

It is important to note that we are not arguing that these theories and treatments of personality pathology can or should be reduced to the two dimensions of agency and communion. However, interpersonal theory offers a common fixed point to focus on disruptions in self–other relatedness along the dimensions of agency and communion and thus may be a translational bridge across theoretical models. Therefore, assessment that focuses on agentic and communal difficulties may be useful across treatment approaches, and intervention techniques may be more effectively compared when examined for changes within the interpersonal framework.

CONCLUSION

In summary, we argue that contemporary interpersonal theory can play a central role in advancing the treatment of personality pathology because of its particular focus on agentic and communal aspects of relational functioning, the reciprocal nature of relational behavior, the identification of maladaptive interpersonal signatures associated with distorted perceptions of self and other and the self-protective motives they evoke, and the role of interpersonal copy processes in healthy and abnormal personality development. Contemporary interpersonal theory provides a framework that translates across theories to aid in the measurement and description of complex interpersonal problems that signify personality pathology. It is important to note that contemporary interpersonal theory is broader than simple semantics may suggest. This theory reflects the external and internal social learning, beliefs, and emotions an individual may have in relation to others. In this sense it measures implicit and explicit, perceptions and behavior, and internal and external dimensions of social dysfunction. Future research should continue to investigate this integrative interpersonal framework for identifying, describing, and treating the disturbed interpersonal relations of personality pathology (Pincus, 2011). More research is needed to understand how revised models of personality pathology (e.g., proposals for future editions of *DSM*) may integrate with existing models of agency and communion and how difficulties on these dimensions may underlie the severity and type of personality pathology.

REFERENCES

Alden, L. E., & Capreol, M. J. (1993). Avoidant personality disorder: Interpersonal problems as predictors of treatment response. *Behavior Therapy, 24,* 357–376. doi:10.1016/S0005-7894(05)80211-4

Alden, L. E., Wiggins, J. S., & Pincus, A. L. (1990). Construction of circumplex scales for the Inventory of Interpersonal Problems. *Journal of Personality Assessment, 55,* 521–536. doi:10.1207/s15327752jpa5503&4_10

Anchin, J. C., & Pincus, A. L. (2010). Evidence-based interpersonal psychotherapy with personality disorders: Theory, components, and strategies. In J. J. Magnavita (Ed.), *Evidence-based treatment of personality dysfunction: Principles, methods, and processes* (pp. 113–166). Washington, DC: American Psychological Association.

Beck, A. T., Freeman, A., Davis, D. D., & Associates. (2004). *Cognitive therapy for personality disorders* (2nd ed.). New York, NY: Guilford Press.

Bender, D. S. (2013). An ecumenical approach to conceptualizing and studying the core of personality psychopathology: A commentary on Hopwood et al. *Journal of Personality Disorders, 27,* 311–319. doi:10.1521/pedi.2013.27.3.311

Bender, D. S., Morey, L. C., & Skodol, A. E. (2011). Toward a model for assessing level of personality functioning in *DSM–5,* Part I: A review of theory and methods. *Journal of Personality Assessment, 93,* 332–346. doi:10.1080/00223891.2011.583808

Benjamin, L. S. (2003). *Interpersonal reconstructive therapy: Promoting change in nonresponders.* New York, NY: Guilford Press.

Blatt, S. J. (2004). *Experiences of depression: Theoretical, clinical, and research perspectives.* Washington, DC: American Psychological Association.

Blatt, S. J., Auerbach, J. S., & Levy, K. N. (1997). Mental representations in personality development, psychopathology, and the therapeutic process. *Review of General Psychology, 1,* 351–374. doi:10.1037/1089-2680.1.4.351

Cain, N. M., Ansell, E. B., Wright, A. G., Hopwood, C. J., Thomas, K. M., Pinto, A., . . . Grilo, C. M. (2012). Interpersonal pathoplasticity in the course of major depression. *Journal of Consulting and Clinical Psychology, 80,* 78–86. doi:10.1037/a0026433

Carson, R. C. (1969). *Interaction concepts of personality.* Chicago, IL: Aldine.

Carson, R. C. (1991). The social-interactional viewpoint. In M. Hersen, A. Kazdin, & A. Bellack (Eds.), *The clinical psychology handbook* (2nd ed., pp. 185–199). New York, NY: Pergamon Press.

Clarkin, J. F., Yeomans, F. E., & Kernberg, O. F. (2006). *Psychotherapy for borderline personality: Focusing on object relations.* Washington, DC: American Psychiatric Publishing.

Cronbach, L. J., & Meehl, P. E. (1955). Construct validity in psychological tests. *Psychological Bulletin, 52*, 281–302. doi:10.1037/h0040957

Fleeson, W. (2001). Toward a structure- and process-integrated view of personality: Traits as density distributions of states. *Journal of Personality and Social Psychology, 80*, 1011–1027. doi:10.1037/0022-3514.80.6.1011

Fonagy, P., & Bateman, A. (2006). Mechanism of change in mentalization-based treatment of borderline personality disorder. *Journal of Clinical Psychology, 62*, 411–430. doi:10.1002/jclp.20241

Fournier, M., Moskowitz, D. S., & Zuroff, D. (2009). The interpersonal signature. *Journal of Research in Personality, 43*, 155–162. doi:10.1016/j.jrp.2009.01.023

Hatcher, R. L., & Rogers, D. T. (2009). Development and validation of a measure of interpersonal strengths: The Inventory of Interpersonal Strengths. *Psychological Assessment, 21*, 554–569. doi:10.1037/a0017269

Hopwood, C. J., Ansell, E. B., Pincus, A. L., Wright, A. G. C., Lukowitsky, M. R., & Roche, M. J. (2011). The circumplex structure of interpersonal sensitivities. *Journal of Personality, 79*, 707–740. doi:10.1111/j.1467-6494.2011.00696.x

Hopwood, C. J., Newman, D. A., Donnellan, B. M., Markowitz, J. C., Grilo, C. M., Sanislow, C. A., . . . Morey, L. C. (2009). The stability of personality traits in individuals with borderline personality disorder. *Journal of Abnormal Psychology, 118*, 806–815. doi:10.1037/a0016954

Hopwood, C. J., Wright, A. G. C., Ansell, E. B., & Pincus, A. P. (2013). The interpersonal core of personality pathology. *Journal of Personality Disorders, 27*, 270–295. doi:10.1521/pedi.2013.27.3.270

Horowitz, L. M., Wilson, K. R., Turan, B., Zolotsev, P., Constantino, M. J., & Henderson, L. (2006). How interpersonal motives clarify the meaning of interpersonal behavior: A revised circumplex model. *Personality and Social Psychology Review, 10*, 67–86. doi:10.1207/s15327957pspr1001_4

Kernberg, O. F. (1975). *Borderline conditions and pathological narcissism.* New York, NY: Aronson.

Kiesler, D. J. (1983). The 1982 Interpersonal Circle: A taxonomy for complementarity in human transactions. *Psychological Review, 90*, 185–214. doi:10.1037/0033-295X.90.3.185

Kiesler, D. J. (1991). Interpersonal methods of assessment and diagnosis. In C. R. Snyder & D. R. Forsyth (Eds.), *Handbook of social and clinical psychology* (pp. 438–468). New York, NY: Pergamon Press.

Kuppens, P., Van Mechelen, I., Nezlek, J. B., Dossche, D., & Timmermans, T. (2007). Individual differences in core affect variability and their relationship to personality and psychological adjustment. *Emotion, 7*, 262–274. doi:10.1037/1528-3542.7.2.262

Leary, T. (1957). *Interpersonal diagnosis of personality.* New York, NY: Ronald Press.

Linehan, M. M. (1993). *Cognitive-behavioral treatment for borderline personality disorder.* New York, NY: Guilford Press.

Locke, K. D. (2000). Circumplex scales of interpersonal values: Reliability, validity, and applicability to interpersonal problems and personality disorders. *Journal of Personality Assessment, 75,* 249–267. doi:10.1207/S15327752JPA7502_6

Luyten, P., & Blatt, S. J. (2013). Interpersonal relatedness and self-definition in normal and disrupted personality development: Retrospect and prospect. *American Psychologist, 68,* 172–183. doi:10.1037/a0032243

Mischel, W., & Shoda, Y. (1995). A cognitive-affective system theory of personality: Reconceptualizing situations, dispositions, dynamics, and invariance in personality structure. *Psychological Review, 102,* 246–268. doi:10.1037/0033-295X.102.2.246

Morey, L. C., Berghuis, H., Bender, D. S., Verheul, R., Krueger, R. F., & Skodol, A. E. (2011). Toward a model for assessing level of personality functioning in *DSM–5,* Part II: Empirical articulation of a core dimension of personality pathology. *Journal of Personality Assessment, 93,* 347–353. doi:10.1080/00223891.2011.577853

Moskowitz, D. S., Russell, J. J., Sadikaj, G., & Sutton, R. (2009). Measure people intensively. *Canadian Psychology/Psychologie Canadienne, 50,* 131–140.

Moskowitz, D. S., & Zuroff, D. C. (2004). Flux, pulse, and spin: Dynamic additions to the personality lexicon. *Journal of Personality and Social Psychology, 86,* 880–893. doi:10.1037/0022-3514.86.6.880

Pincus, A. L. (2005). A contemporary integrative interpersonal theory of personality disorders. In J. Clarkin & M. Lenzenweger (Eds.), *Major theories of personality disorder* (2nd ed., pp. 282–331). New York, NY: Guilford Press.

Pincus, A. L. (2011). Some comments on nomology, diagnostic process, and narcissistic personality disorder in the *DSM–5* proposal for personality and personality disorder disorders. *Personality Disorders: Theory, Research, and Treatment, 2,* 41–53. doi:10.1037/a0021191

Pincus, A. L., & Ansell, E. B. (2013). Interpersonal theory of personality. In J. Suls & H. Tennen (Eds.), *Handbook of psychology: Vol. 5. Personality and social psychology* (2nd ed., pp. 141–159). Hoboken, NJ: Wiley.

Pincus, A. L., Ansell, E. B., Pimentel, C. A., Cain, N. M., Wright, A. G., & Levy, K. N. (2009). Initial construction and validation of the Pathological Narcissism Inventory. *Psychological Assessment, 21,* 365–379. doi:10.1037/a0016530

Pincus, A. L., & Hopwood, C. J. (2012). A contemporary interpersonal model of personality pathology and personality disorder. In T. A. Widiger (Ed.), *Oxford handbook of personality disorders* (pp. 372–398). Oxford, United Kingdom: Oxford University Press.

Pincus, A. L., & Lukowitsky, M. R. (2010). Pathological narcissism and narcissistic personality disorder. *Annual Review of Clinical Psychology, 6,* 421–446. doi:10.1146/annurev.clinpsy.121208.131215

Pincus, A. L., & Wright, A. G. C. (2010). Interpersonal diagnosis of psychopathology. In L. M. Horowitz & S. Strack (Eds.), *Handbook of interpersonal psychology* (pp. 359–381). Hoboken, NJ: Wiley.

Przeworski, A., Newman, M. G., Pincus, A. L., Kasoff, M. B., Yamasaki, A. S., Castonguay, L. G., & Berlin, K. S. (2011). Interpersonal pathoplasticity in individuals with generalized anxiety disorder. *Journal of Abnormal Psychology, 120,* 286–298. doi:10.1037/a0023334

Ram, N., & Gerstorf, D. (2009). Time-structured and net intraindividual variability: Tools for examining the development of dynamic characteristics and processes. *Psychology and Aging, 24,* 778–791. doi:10.1037/a0017915

Russell, J. J., Moskowitz, D. S., Zuroff, D. C., Sookman, D., & Paris, J. (2007). Stability and variability of affective experience and interpersonal behavior in borderline personality disorder. *Journal of Abnormal Psychology, 116,* 578–588. doi:10.1037/0021-843X.116.3.578

Sadler, P., Ethier, N., & Woody, E. (2011). Interpersonal complementarity. In L. M. Horowitz & S. Strack (Eds.), *Handbook of interpersonal psychology* (pp. 123–142). Hoboken, NJ: Wiley.

Safran, J. D. (1990a). Towards a refinement in cognitive therapy in light of interpersonal theory: I. Theory. *Clinical Psychology Review, 10,* 87–105. doi:10.1016/0272-7358(90)90108-M

Safran, J. D. (1990b). Towards a refinement in cognitive therapy in light of interpersonal theory: II. Practice. *Clinical Psychology Review, 10,* 107–121. doi:10.1016/0272-7358(90)90109-N

Sullivan, H. S. (1953). *The interpersonal theory of psychiatry.* New York, NY: Norton.

Widiger, T. A., & Smith, G. T. (2008). Personality and psychopathology. In O. P. John, R. Robins, & L. A. Pervin (Eds.), *Handbook of personality: Theory and research* (3rd ed., pp. 743–769). New York, NY: Guilford Press.

Wiggins, J. S. (2003). *Paradigms of personality assessment.* New York, NY: Guilford Press.

Wright, A. G. C., Hallquist, M. N., Scott, L. N., Stepp, S. D., Nolf, K. A., & Pilkonis, P. A. (2013). Clarifying interpersonal heterogeneity in borderline personality disorder using latent mixture modeling. *Journal of Personality Disorders, 27,* 125–143. doi:10.1521/pedi.2013.27.2.125

Wright, A. G. C., Pincus, A. L., Conroy, D. E., & Elliot, A. J. (2009). The pathoplastic relationship between interpersonal problems and fear of failure. *Journal of Personality, 77,* 997–1024. doi:10.1111/j.1467-6494.2009.00572.x

Wright, A. G. C., Pincus, A. L., Conroy, D. E., & Hilsenroth, M. J. (2009). Integrating methods to optimize circumplex description and comparison of groups. *Journal of Personality Assessment, 91,* 311–322. doi:10.1080/00223890902935696

Zeigler-Hill, V., & Besser, A. (2013). A glimpse behind the mask: Facets of narcissism and feelings of self-worth. *Journal of Personality Assessment, 95,* 249–260. doi:10.1080/00223891.2012.717150

Zeigler-Hill, V., Clark, C. B., & Pickard, J. D. (2008). Narcissistic subtypes and contingent self-esteem: Do all narcissists base their self-esteem on the same domains? *Journal of Personality, 76,* 753–774. doi:10.1111/j.1467-6494.2008.00503.x

15

AN INTEGRATING AND COMPREHENSIVE MODEL OF PERSONALITY PATHOLOGY BASED ON EVOLUTIONARY THEORY

THEODORE MILLON AND STEPHEN STRACK

As an idea, personality is many thousands of years old. Historically, the word *personality* derives from the Greek term *persona*, originally representing the theatrical mask used by dramatic players. Its meaning has changed through history. As a mask assumed by an actor, it suggested pretense of appearance; that is, the possession of traits other than those that actually characterized the individual behind the mask. In time, the term *persona* lost its connotation of pretense and illusion and began to represent not the mask but the apparent, explicit, or manifest features of the person. The third and most recent meaning that the term *personality* has acquired delves beneath surface impressions and turns the spotlight on the inner, less revealed, and hidden psychological qualities of the individual. Thus, through history the meaning of the term has shifted from external illusion to surface reality and, finally, to opaque or veiled inner characteristics.

http://dx.doi.org/10.1037/14549-016
Personality Disorders: Toward Theoretical and Empirical Integration in Diagnosis and Assessment,
S. K. Huprich (Editor)

Personality is seen today as a complex pattern of deeply embedded psychological characteristics that are often nonconscious and not easily altered, and which express themselves insidiously in almost every facet of functioning. Intrinsic and pervasive, these traits emerge from the complicated matrix of biological dispositions and learning experiences that ultimately constitute the individual's complex and distinctive pattern of perceiving, feeling, thinking, coping, and behaving. Personality thus cannot be characterized by a single aspect of functioning. Instead, it is best defined as the patterning of multiple dispositional styles and traits across the entire matrix of the person.

To elaborate, in the first years of life each child displays a wide variety of behaviors. Although exhibiting a measure of consistency consonant with the child's constitutional disposition, the ways in which the child responds to and copes with the environment tend to be largely spontaneous, changeable, and unpredictable. These seemingly random and capricious behaviors serve an important exploratory function. The child is "trying out" a variety of behavioral alternatives for managing his or her environment. Over time, the child begins to discern which of these actions enable him or her to achieve his or her desires and avoid discomfort. Endowed with certain capacities, energies, and temperaments, and through experience with parents, siblings, and peers, the child learns to discriminate which activities are both permissible and rewarding and which are not.

When this sequence is traced over time, it can be seen that a shaping process has taken place in which the child's initial range of diverse behaviors gradually becomes narrowed, selective, and finally crystallized into preferred ways of relating to others and coping with the world. These learned behaviors not only persist but are accentuated as a result of being repetitively reinforced by a limited social environment. Given continuity in biological makeup and a narrow band of experiences for learning behavioral alternatives, the child acquires a pattern of psychological traits that are deeply etched and difficult to modify. This pattern of traits constitutes the child's personality; that is, ingrained and habitual ways of psychological functioning that emerge from the individual's entire developmental history and that, over time, come to characterize the child's unique identity.

The many characteristics of which personality is composed are not a potpourri of unrelated perceptions, feelings, thoughts, and behaviors but a tightly knit organization of attitudes, habits, and emotions. One may start in life with more or less random and diverse feelings and reactions, but the repetitive sequences of reinforcing experiences to which the individual is exposed narrow his or her repertoire to particular emotions, beliefs, and behavioral strategies that become prepotent and characterize the individual's personally distinctive way of dealing with others and relating to the self.

DIFFERENTIATING NORMALITY FROM
PATHOLOGY OF PERSONALITY

Numerous attempts have been made to develop definitive criteria for distinguishing psychological normality from abnormality. Some of these criteria focus on features that characterize the so-called normal, or ideal, state of mental health, as illustrated in the writings of Offer and Sabshin (1974, 1991; Strack, 2006); others have sought to specify criteria for concepts such as abnormality or psychopathology. The most common criterion employed is a statistical one in which normality is determined by those behaviors that are found most frequently in a social group, and pathology (or abnormality) is determined by features that are uncommon in that population. Some of the more diverse criteria used to signify normality are a capacity to function autonomously and competently, a tendency to adjust to one's social environment effectively and efficiently, a subjective sense of contentment and satisfaction, and the ability to self-actualize or to fulfill one's potentials. Psychopathology would be noted by deficits among the preceding (e.g., Maslow, 1968).

Central to our understanding of these terms is the recognition that normality and pathology are relative concepts; they represent arbitrary points on a continuum or gradient, because no sharp line divides normal from pathological behavior. Not only is personality so complex that certain areas of psychological functioning operate normally while others do not, but environmental circumstances change such that behaviors and strategies that prove adaptive at one time in life fail to do so at another. Moreover, the features that differentiate normal from abnormal functioning must be extracted from a complex of signs that not only wax and wane but often develop in an insidious and unpredictable manner.

Pathology results from the same forces as those involved in the development of normal functioning. Important differences in the character, timing, and intensity of these influences will lead some individuals to acquire pathological features and others to develop adaptive ones. When an individual displays an ability to cope with the environment in a flexible manner, and when his or her typical perceptions and behaviors foster increments in personal satisfaction, he or she may be said to possess a normal or healthy personality. Conversely, when average or everyday responsibilities are responded to inflexibly or defectively, or when the individual's perceptions and behaviors result in increments in personal discomfort or curtail opportunities to learn and to grow, we may speak of a pathological or maladaptive pattern.

Despite the tenuous and fluctuating nature of the normality–pathology distinction, three features may be abstracted from the flow of behavioral characteristics may serve as differentiating criteria: an adaptive inflexibility, a tendency to foster vicious or self-defeating circles (Horney, 1945), and a tenuous emotional stability under conditions of stress (Millon, 1969, 1981). Each is elaborated briefly next.

Adaptive Inflexibility

The alternative strategies the individual employs for relating to others, for achieving goals, and for coping with stress are not only few in number but appear to be practiced rigidly; that is, they are imposed upon conditions for which they are ill suited. The individual not only is unable to adapt effectively to the circumstances of his or her life but arranges the environment to avoid objectively neutral events that are perceived as stressful. As a consequence, the individual's opportunities for learning new, more adaptive behaviors are reduced and his or her life experiences become ever more narrowly circumscribed.

Vicious Circles

All of us manipulate our environments to suit our needs. What distinguishes pathological from normal patterns is not only their rigidity and inflexibility but also their tendency to foster vicious circles. What this means is that the person's habitual perceptions, needs, and behaviors perpetuate and intensify preexisting difficulties. Maneuvers such as protective constriction, cognitive distortion, and behavior generalization are processes by which individuals restrict their opportunities for new learning, misconstrue essentially benign events, and provoke reactions from others that reactivate earlier problems. In effect, then, pathological personality patterns are themselves pathogenic; that is, they generate and perpetuate existent dilemmas, provoke new predicaments, and set into motion self-defeating sequences with others, which cause their already established difficulties to not only persist but to be aggravated further.

Tenuous Stability

The third feature that distinguishes abnormal from normal personalities is a fragility or lack of resilience under conditions of subjective stress. Given the ease with which the already troubled are vulnerable to events that reactivate the past, and given their inflexibility and paucity of effective coping mechanisms, they are now extremely susceptible to new difficulties and disruptions. Faced with recurrent failures, anxious lest old and unresolved conflicts reemerge, and unable to recruit new adaptive strategies, these persons are likely to revert to pathological ways of coping. As a consequence, they display less adequate control over their emotions and ultimately experience increasingly subjective and distorted perceptions of reality.

TOWARD A SCIENCE OF PERSONALITY DISORDERS

It is necessary to go beyond current conceptual boundaries in understanding personality disorders (PDs); more specifically, we need to explore carefully reasoned, as well as intuitive, hypotheses that draw their principles, if not their substance, from more established, "adjacent" sciences. Such steps may bear new conceptual fruits and may provide a foundation that can undergird and guide our discipline's currently primitive explorations. Much of personality, no less psychology as a whole, remains adrift, divorced from broader spheres of scientific knowledge, isolated from firmly grounded, if not universal principles, leading one to continue building the patchwork of concepts and data domains that characterizes our field. Preoccupied with but a small part of the larger puzzle or fearing accusations of reductionism, many fail to draw on the rich possibilities to be found in other realms of scholarly pursuit. With few exceptions, cohering concepts that would connect our subject to those of its sister sciences have not been developed.

Despite the shortcomings of historic and contemporary theoretical schemas in the human sciences, systematizing principles and abstract concepts may be able to "facilitate a deeper seeing, a more penetrating vision that goes beyond superficial appearances to the order underlying them" (Bowers, 1977). For example, pre-Darwinian taxonomists, such as Linnaeus, limited themselves to "apparent" similarities and differences among animals as a means of constructing their classification categories. Darwin was not seduced by appearances. Rather, he sought to understand the principles by which overt features came about. His classifications were based not only on descriptive qualities but also on explanatory ones.

Efforts to construct a personality disorder science cannot be undertaken successfully if approached as an isolated classification task. It should be seen as but one intermediary step in building a truly mature clinical science, an interconnected element, a singular quest that derives its logic and rationale as but one of several interrelated components, namely:

1. *Universal scientific principles*—principles grounded in the ubiquitous laws of nature, which, despite varied forms of expression (e.g., physics, psychology) may provide an undergirding framework for guiding and constructing relatively delimited or focused subject-oriented theories.
2. *Subject-oriented theories*—explanatory and heuristic conceptual schemas that are consistent with established knowledge in both their own and related sciences and from which reasonably accurate propositions concerning pathological personality conditions can be both deduced and understood, facilitating the development of a formal classification schema.

3. *Classification of a normal-to-abnormal personality spectra*—a taxonomic schema of adaptive and maladaptive taxa that can be derived logically from the theory and arranged to provide a cohesive framework within which its major categories, domains, and traits can readily be grouped and differentiated, permitting the development of coordinated assessment tools.
4. *Clinical personality assessment instruments*—tools that are empirically grounded and sufficiently sensitive quantitatively to enable the theory's propositions and hypotheses to be adequately investigated and evaluated and the domains and traits constituting its spectrum categories to be readily identified (diagnosed) and measured (dimensionalized), specifying target areas for therapeutic intervention.
5. *Integrated treatment interventions*—strategies and techniques of therapy, designed in accord with the theory and oriented to modify problematic clinical traits and symptoms consonant with professional standards and social responsibilities.

ON THE IMPORTANCE OF THEORY TO A PERSONALITY DISORDERS TAXONOMY

Science cannot exist merely as a descriptive venture that consists in observing, categorizing, and cross-correlating various phenomena. Instead, it proceeds by establishing superordinate theoretical principles that unify the various manifestations of its subject domain. Even if reliable observations of great or even perfect positive predictive power could be made through some infallible methodology, these indicators would stand simply as isolated facts unassimilated as scientific knowledge, at least until they are unified on some theoretical basis. Predictive power alone will not make a science. Scientific explanations derive from theoretical principles that operate above the level of empirical observations. Empirical findings are of value when they predict, but theoretical principles are necessary because they explain.

In a clinical science, one is required to utilize the fecundity of theory to deal with the inevitable contradictions of a morass of empirical data in order to develop a coherent picture of the person, guiding the diverse data in ways that make sense. As noted, superordinate theory lies at a higher explanatory level than do the individual measures that constitute the "raw data." Theory reintegrates the full individual who has been fractionated among a variety of data scales and observations. A successful and coherent personality picture does not come into being of its own accord but is constructed theoretically.

Philosophers of science agree, further, that it is theory which provides the conceptual glue that binds the elements of a classification together. Moreover, a good theory not only summarizes and incorporates extant realms of knowledge but also possesses what Hempel (1965) called its "systematic import"; that is, it originates and develops new observations and new methods. In setting out a theory of PDs, what is desired is not merely a list of descriptive categories and their correlated attributes but an explanatory schema based on theoretical principles.

A fully developed taxonomy must seek a schema that "carves nature at its joints," so to speak. In this regard, it was Hempel (1965) again who distinguished between natural and artificial classification systems. The biological sexes, male and female, and the periodic table of elements are both examples of classifications schemes that can be viewed as possessing "objective" existence in nature. Of course, we seek to classify not genders or chemical elements but persons. In so doing, we seek the ideal of a classification taxonomy that is "natural"; that is, one that inheres in the larger subjects of science and is not arbitrarily imposed on it. Not only is it consonant with respect to its own subject domain, but it is also consonant with other realms of science. The notion that the validity of a scientific subject can be established only by utilizing the valid principles of an external subject was confirmed by the distinguished mathematical philosopher Kurt Godel (1931).

The purpose of a clinical science in PD is to develop a theory of the person. That scientists would want to develop a theory of the person without a corresponding theory of explanatory constructs of the person is somewhat puzzling. When classification theory is ignored in favor of exclusively empirical inductions or factor analytically derived orthogonal dimensions, that essentially is what has been done (Widiger, 2003). A theoretically grounded perspective embodies well-ordered and codified links between constructs and provides a generative basis for making clinical inferences from a small number of fundamental principles. Our fellow theorists in other chapters (e.g., South, Chapter 7; Luyten & Blatt, Chapter 12; Cain & Ansell, Chapter 14) have provided a solid ground for their models, albeit each less comprehensive and less theoretically generative than we judge ideal.

As noted, it is our strong conviction that a PD science will never be adduced satisfactorily simply by observation alone, nor by statistical analyses of numerous separate pieces of evidence. We believe we must move beyond the boundaries of piecemeal research. Only in this way can a modern opaque and complexly interrelated classificatory system of personality styles, types, and disorders be satisfactorily constructed (Millon, 2011). Anything short of such a transcendent context of guiding principles will deter us from advancing the devilishly complicated task of building a scientifically valid and clinically useful set of personality constructs.

It is unfortunate that the number of theories that have been advanced to "explain" PDs is directly proportional to the internecine squabbling found in the literature. Ostensibly toward the end of pragmatic sobriety, those of an empirically based and inductive-statistical orientation have sought to persuade our profession of the failings of premature theoretical formalization, warning that one cannot arrive at the desired future by lifting science by its own bootstraps. No one argues against the view that theories that float, so to speak, on their own, unconcerned with the empirical domain, should be seen as the fatuous achievements they are and the travesty they make of the virtues of a truly coherent conceptual system. Formal theory should not be pushed far beyond the data, and its derivations should be linked at all points to established observations and research. However, a theoretical framework can be a compelling instrument for coordinating and giving consonance to a complex of diverse data. Progress does not advance by "brute empiricism" alone; that is, by merely piling up more descriptive and more experimental data (i.e., evidence). What is elaborated and refined in theory is understanding, an ability to see relations more plainly, to conceptualize categories more accurately, and to create greater overall coherence in a subject; that is, to integrate its elements in a more logical, consistent, and intelligible fashion.

An example from the fields of engineering and physics may be helpful. Engineers have provided superb products and solutions in every sphere of life, from constructing bridges to decoding the aerodynamics of space flight. But none of the field's achievements could have been attained without the thoughtful use of the principles of physics, its undergirding laws, their application, measures, and interactions. So, too, must our progress in understanding the processes of personality functioning be undergirded by the principles of biology; specifically, the application of evolutionary laws.

EVOLUTIONARY THEORY OF PERSONALITY POLARITIES

The propositions of theory are formed when certain attributes that have been categorized have been shown or have been hypothesized to be logically or causally related to other attributes or categories. The latent taxa that undergird a scientific schema are not mere collections of overtly similar attributes or categories but are a linked or unified pattern of known or presumed relations among them. This theoretically grounded pattern of relations provides the foundation of a clinical science.

Before we elaborate where "disorders" arise within the human species, a few more words must be said concerning analogies between evolution and ecology, on the one hand, and personality, on the other. During its life history an organism develops an assemblage of traits that contribute to its individual survival and reproductive success, the two essential components of "fitness" formulated by Darwin. Such assemblages, termed *complex adaptations* and *strategies* in the literature of evolutionary ecology, are close biological equivalents to what psychologists have conceptualized as personality styles and structures. In biology, explanations of a life history strategy of adaptations refer primarily to biogenic variations among constituent traits, their overall covariance structure, and the nature and ratio of favorable to unfavorable ecologic resources that have been available for purposes of extending longevity and optimizing reproduction. Such explanations are not appreciably different from those used to account for the development of personality styles or functions.

Bypassing the usual complications of analogies, a relevant and intriguing parallel may be drawn between the phylogenic evolution of the genetic composition of a species and the ontogenic development of an individual organism's adaptive strategies (i.e., its personality style). At any point in time, a species will possess a limited set of genes that serve as trait potentials. Over succeeding generations the frequency distributions of these genes will likely change in their relative proportions depending on how well the traits they undergird contribute to the species' "fittedness" within its varying ecological habitats. In a similar fashion, individual organisms begin life with a limited subset of their species' genes and the trait potentials they subserve. Over time, the salience of these trait potentials—not the proportion of the genes themselves—will become differentially prominent as the organism interacts with its environments. It "learns" from these experiences which of its traits fit best (i.e., are most optimally suited to its ecosystem). In phylogenesis, then, actual gene frequencies change during the generation-to-generation adaptive process, whereas in ontogenesis it is the salience, or prominence, of gene-based traits that changes as adaptive learning takes place. Parallel evolutionary processes occur, one within the life of a species, the other within the life of an organism. What is seen in the individual organism is a shaping of latent potentials into adaptive and manifest styles of perceiving, feeling, thinking, and acting; these distinctive ways of adaptation, engendered by the interaction of biologic endowment and social experience, comprise the elements of what is termed *personality styles*. It is a formative process in a single lifetime that parallels gene redistributions among species during their evolutionary history.

Lest the reader assume that those seeking to wed the sciences of evolution and ecology find themselves fully welcome in their respective fraternities, there are those who assert that, "despite pious hopes and intellectual convictions, [these two disciplines] have so far been without issue" (Lewontin, 1979). This judgment is now both dated and overly severe, but numerous conceptual and methodological impediments do face those who wish to bring these fields of biologic inquiry into fruitful synthesis—no less employ them to construe the styles and disorders of personality. Nevertheless, recent developments bridging ecological and evolutionary theory are well under way and hence do offer some justification for extending their principles to human styles of adaptation.

PHYLOGENETIC STAGES OF EVOLUTION

The theoretical model that follows derives explicitly from evolutionary theory (Millon, 1990). In essence, it seeks to explicate the structure and styles of personality with reference to deficient, imbalanced, or conflicted modes of ecological survival, adaptation, and reproductive strategy.

Four phylogenetic stages in which evolutionary principles are significant are herein labeled *Existence, Adaptation, Replication,* and *Abstraction.* The first relates the serendipitous transformation of random or less organized states into those possessing distinct structures of greater organization; the second refers to homeostatic processes employed to sustain survival in open ecosystems; the third pertains to reproductive styles that maximize the diversification and selection of ecologically effective attributes; and the fourth concerns the emergence of competencies that foster anticipatory planning and reasoned decision making. Polarities derived from the first three stages (pleasure–pain, passive–active, other–self) are used to construct a theoretically embedded scientific system of PDs (Millon, 1990, 1996, 2011).

1. The first component of the theory, *existence,* concerns the maintenance of integrative phenomena, whether nuclear particle, virus, or human being, against the background of entropic decompensation. Evolutionary mechanisms derived from this stage encompass acts of both *life-enhancement* and *life-preservation.* The former are concerned with orienting individuals toward improvement in the quality of life; the latter with orienting individuals away from actions or environments that decrease the quality of life or even jeopardize existence itself. These are called *existential aims* in the theory. At the highest level of abstraction such mechanisms form, phenomenologically or metaphorically, as a "pleasure–pain polarity." Some individuals possess deficits in these crucial polar substrates (e.g., the schizoid). In terms of ontogenetic growth stages, the pleasure–pain polarity is recapitulated in a *sensory-attachment* phase, a major purpose of which is the learned discrimination of pain and pleasure signals.

2. Existence, however, is but an initial phase. Once an integrative structure exists, it must maintain its existence through exchanges of energy and information with its environment. The second evolutionary stage relates to what is termed the *modes of adaptation*; it is also framed as a two-part polarity, a *passive* orientation (i.e., a tendency to accommodate to one's ecological niche) versus an *active* orientation (i.e., a tendency to modify or intervene in one's surrounds). These modes of adaptation differ from the first phase of evolution, that of *being*, in that they regard how that which is, endures. In terms of ontogenetic growth stages, these modes are recapitulated in a *sensorimotor-autonomy* phase, during which the child either progresses in assuming an active disposition toward his or her physical and social context or perpetuates the passive dependent mode of prenatal and infantile existence.
3. Although organisms may exist well adapted to their environments, the existence of any life-form is time limited. To circumvent this limitation, organisms progress through a *replicatory phase* by which they are prepared to create progeny. This phase relates to what evolutionary scientists (Prigogine, 1972; Rushton, 1985) have referred to as an *r-* or *self-propagating* strategy (political individualism), at one polar extreme, and a *K-* or *other-nurturing* strategy (political community), at the second extreme. Psychologically, the former strategy is disposed toward actions that are egotistic and uncaring; the latter is disposed toward actions that are affiliative and solicitous (Bakan, 1966; Blatt, 2008; Millon, 1969).

What will be proposed in the following paragraphs is clearly conjectural, perhaps overly extended in its speculative reach. In essence, it seeks to deduce the structure and styles of personality with reference to the processes of ontogenetic natural selection, more specifically to deficient, imbalanced, or conflicted survival objectives; alternate modes of ecologic adaptation; and contrasting methods of reproductive strategy (Millon, 1990, 2010).

In line with the concept of natural selection, each complex species, from insects, to fish, to birds, to mammals, displays distinctive commonalities in its adaptive or survival style. Within each species, however, there are differences in style and differences in the success with which its various members adapt to the diverse and changing environments they face. It is these differences in adaptive and maladaptive styles that constitute what we would term *personality*, its spectra, normal and abnormal, and their trait domains.

According to Theodore Millon, evolutionary theory's most vigorous supporter, evolution is the logical choice as a scaffold upon which to develop a science of PDs (Millon, 1990). In creating a taxonomy of personality styles and disorders based on evolutionary principles, one faces a number of tasks: How can its multitrait components and their processes best be organized so that their relevance to personality composites and their disorders be clearly seen? It will be necessary to start in answering this question by utilizing the evolutionary constructs we called *polarities* in prior paragraphs.

DERIVING THE PERSONALITY DISORDERS FROM THE POLARITY MODEL

Some personalities exhibit a reasonable balance on one or other of the polarity pairs. Not all individuals fall at the center, of course. Individual differences in both personality features and overall style will reflect the relative positions and strengths of each polarity component. Personalities we have termed *deficient* lack the capacity to experience or to enact certain aspects of the three polarities (e.g., the schizoid has a faulty substrate for both pleasure and pain); those spoken of as *imbalanced* lean strongly toward one or another extreme of a polarity (e.g., the dependent is oriented to receiving support from others); and those we judge *conflicted* struggle with ambivalences toward opposing ends of a bipolarity (e.g., the passive-aggressive vacillates between adhering to the expectancies of others and enacting what is wished for one's self). Consistent with integrative logic, the polarity foundation is central to our personality characterizations. The following brief descriptions illustrate the connection between the theoretical polarities and the various personalities that comprise the evolutionary model:

1. *Schizoid personality.* Schizoid persons are those in whom both pleasure and pain polarity systems are deficient; that is, they lack the capacity, relatively speaking, to experience life's events as either painful or pleasurable.
2A. *Avoidant personality.* The second clinically meaningful combination based on problems in the pleasure–pain polarity comprises individuals with a diminished ability to experience pleasure but with a hyperactive sensitivity and responsiveness to pain.
2B. *Depressive personality.* Both avoidant and depressive personalities have a diminished ability to experience pleasure and a comparable tendency to be overly sensitive to pain (i.e., events of a foreboding, disquieting, and anguishing character). However, avoidants have learned to anticipate these troublesome

events. Depressives are notably more passive than the anxiously proactive avoidant.

3. *Dependent personality*. Following the polarity model, one must ask whether particular clinical consequences occur among individuals who are markedly imbalanced interpersonally by virtue of turning almost exclusively toward others or toward themselves. Dependents have learned not only to turn to others as their source of nurturance and security but to wait passively for their leadership in providing them.

4A. *Histrionic personality*. Also turning to others as their primary strategy are a group of personalities that take an active dependency stance. They achieve their goal of maximizing protection, nurturance, and reproductive success by engaging busily in a series of seductive, gregarious, and attention-getting maneuvers.

4B. *Exuberant personality*. This group of individuals is unusual by virtue of the central role they give to the active pursuit of the pleasurable side of the pain–pleasure polarity. Typically energetic and buoyant in manner, they may become overly animated, scattered, and manic.

5. *Narcissistic personality*. Persons falling into the "independent" personality pattern also exhibit an imbalance in their replication strategy; in this case, however, there is a primary reliance on self rather than others. These individuals are noted by their egotistic self-involvement; they experience primary pleasure simply by passively being or focusing on themselves.

6A. *Antisocial personality*. Those whom we characterize as exhibiting the active-independent orientation resemble the outlook, temperament, and socially unacceptable behaviors of the *Diagnostic and Statistical Manual of Mental Disorders* (DSM) Antisocial Personality. These individuals act to counter the expectation of pain and depredation by engaging in duplicitous and often illegal behaviors.

6B. *Sadistic personality*. In some, the usual properties associated with pain and pleasure are conflicted or reversed. These individuals not only seek or create objectively "painful" events but experience them as "pleasurable." Both the sadistic and self-defeating patterns are labeled as discordant patterns.

7. *Compulsive personality*. The compulsive personality represents a pattern conflicted on the self–other polarity but with a passive bent. Such individuals display a picture of distinct other directedness, consistency in social compliance, and interpersonal respect.

8A. *Negativistic (passive-aggressive) personality.* This pattern is also conflicted on the self–other polarity but instead assumes a more active orientation toward this reversal than does the compulsive. Although their struggle represents an inability to resolve conflicts similar to those of the passive-ambivalent (compulsives), such individuals behave obediently one time and defiantly the next.

8B. *Masochistic (self-defeating) personality.* Like the sadistic personality, these clients are conflicted on the pleasure–pain polarity. These individuals interpret events and engage in relationships in a manner that is at variance with this deeply rooted polarity, and they relate to others in an obsequious and self-sacrificing manner.

9. *Schizotypal personality.* This PD represents a cognitively dysfunctional and maladaptively detached orientation in multiple polarity domains. Schizotypal personalities experience minimal pleasure; they have difficulty consistently differentiating between self and other strategies and between active and passive modes of adaptation.

10. *Borderline personality.* This PD corresponds to the theory's emotionally dysfunctional and maladaptively ambivalent polarity orientation. Conflicts exist across the board, between pleasure and pain, active and passive, and self and other.

11. *Paranoid personality.* These individuals have a vigilant mistrust of others and an edgy defensiveness against anticipated criticism and deception. Driven by a high sensitivity to pain (rejection-humiliation) and oriented strongly to the self polarity, these persons exhibit a touchy irritability, a need to assert themselves but not necessarily in action.

Numerous combinations of these preceding personalities exist and demonstrate the rich diversity of styles and disorders that clinicians must come to understand; many of these combinations are illustrated and discussed in Millon (2011).

OTHER SYSTEMATIC APPROACHES ILLUSTRATE PART–WHOLE FALLACIES AND LACK OF AN INTEGRATING THEORY

A problem with some approaches to understanding and classifying the PDs is that they assert that the part domain to which they give priority is key to the whole personality. Hence, they are inclined either to locate other components of a person's makeup in a repetitively secondary position or to assign them a place of irrelevance. No matter how brilliant their formulations may be (and we may want here to recognize the illuminating work of some of these theorists; e.g., Beck, Benjamin, Blatt, Gunderson, Kernberg, Kiesler, Livesley, Stone, Widiger, and Wiggins), their restricted focus on one methodology or one facet of personality constrains the potential richness of their ideas, their potential scope, and their ultimate power and clinical utility. Nevertheless, it behooves the serious reader to reflect on the views stated by authors in the previous chapters in this book, and also in a recent issue of the *Journal of Personality Disorders* (Bender, 2013; Bornstein, 2013; Clarkin, 2013; Hopwood, Wright, Ansell, & Pincus, 2013). Thus, the key role of interpersonal models can be subsumed by more extensive perspectives and vice versa.

Our evolutionary approach seeks to build a structural edifice that utilizes all components of the entire personologic domain from the start. The emphasis is on the simultaneous explication and interplay of all "latent entities"; that is, all the multiple and diverse clinical domains that account for the personologic subject. The distinguishing orientation of the evolutionary approach is that it seeks to encompass and display the interactions among all domains of the entire personologic realm at once on the basis of a small number of theoretical principles (Millon, 1984, 1990, 2011).

A question that must be asked is, "What domain categories and distinctive trait clusters should PDs be composed of and thereby organized?" Although some consider personality as being primarily psychodynamic or primarily interpersonal, we regard such positions as overly narrow and restrictive. The integrative perspective encouraged by our evolutionary model views personality as a multidetermined and multireferential construct that should be studied across a variety of content areas. The term *multireferential* is an important one. We have noted that one way of dealing with the subject is simply to assess personality in accord with a single focus, effectively eliminating the eclecticism of divergent perspectives through a dismissive dogmatism. A truly comprehensive science, however, one that is logically consonant with the integrative nature of personality as a construct, requires that personality be assessed systematically across multiple personologic domains (Millon, 1984). Scientific approaches that do not address these multiple domains as conceptually comparable are, from our viewpoint, incomplete with respect to content, whether becoming so accidentally, pragmatically, or ideologically.

Another question to be asked is, "On what basis will we distinguish the multidomains of personality from those we judge as of a more narrow perspective?" Several criteria were used to select and develop the clinical domains described in the next section of this chapter: (a) that they be varied in the features they embody; they must not be limited to behaviors or cognitions but instead should encompass a full range of clinically relevant characteristics;

(b) that they parallel, if not correspond, to many of our profession's therapeutic modalities (e.g., self-oriented techniques for altering dysfunctional cognitions; group treatment procedures for modifying interpersonal conduct); and (c) that they not only be coordinated to the official *DSM* and *International Classification of Diseases* schemas of PD prototypes but also that each PD be represented by a distinctive characteristic within each clinical trait domain.

Our approach reflects historic models that are employed in the study of biology; that is, that they be systematically differentiated into structural and functional attributes. The science of anatomy investigates embedded and essentially permanent structures that serve, for example, as substrates for mood and memory. Its functional counterpart, physiology, is concerned with processes that regulate internal dynamics and external transactions. Together, structures and functions bind the organism together as a coherent entity. Dividing the characteristics of the psychological world into structural and functional realms is, of course, by no means a novel notion.

The term *trait domains* in personality study (see Millon, 1984, 2011) reflects descriptive attributes across several significant clinical realms (e.g., interpersonal conduct, cognitive style) within which evolutionary polarities are expressed and with which all PD categories may be further refined, distinguished, and compared. Trait domains were developed to formulate a schema that maximizes their clinical utility, notably to facilitate therapeutic choice and efficacy. This goal could help not only to identify which personality pathology pattern outlined in prior pages can best characterize a patient but also to specify which traits are prominent and therefore most suitable as therapeutic targets.

As noted, treatment-oriented trait domains should be composed of distinctive clinical features for each PD in each diagnostic domain (e.g., interpersonally unengaged for schizoids, interpersonally submissive for dependents, interpersonally exploitive for narcissists). The domains should parallel, if not correspond, to many of our profession's current therapeutic modalities (e.g., cognitive-behavioral techniques methods for altering dysfunctional cognitions; group therapy procedures for modifying interpersonal conduct).

Let us turn to the eight domains (Millon, 1984, 2011) that serve as trait content areas for the theory, dividing them into those we have termed *functional* and *structural*.

FUNCTIONAL DOMAINS

Functional characteristics represent dynamic processes that transpire within the intrapsychic world and between the individual's self and his or her psychosocial environment. Transactional processes take place through the medium of functional domains. For definitional purposes, we might say that functional domains represent expressive modes of regulatory action: behaviors, social conduct, cognitive processes, and unconscious mechanisms that manage, coordinate, and control the give-and-take of inner and outer life. Four functional domains relevant to the personality spectra are briefly described.

Emotional Expression

These inferred emotional attributes relate to the observables seen at the behavioral level of data, and are usually recorded by noting what and how the patient acts. Characteristics such as impassivity, fretfulness, impetuousness, impulsiveness, and resentfulness are among the varied forms of emotional expression worthy of note.

Interpersonal Conduct

A patient's style of relating to others also is noted essentially at the behavioral data level and may be captured in a number of ways, such as how the patient's actions impact on others, intended or otherwise; extrapolating from these observations, the clinician may construct an image of how the patient functions in relation to others, be it antagonistically, respectfully, aversively, secretively, and so on.

Cognitive Style

How the patient focuses and allocates attention, encodes and processes information, organizes thoughts, makes attributions, and communicates reactions and ideas to others represent data at the phenomenological level and are among the most useful indexes to the clinician of the patient's distinctive way of functioning. By synthesizing these signs and symptoms, it may be possible to identify indications of what may be termed an *impoverished style*, *distracted thinking*, or *cognitive flightiness*.

Intrapsychic Dynamics

Although the dynamics of self-protection, need gratification, and conflict resolution are consciously recognized at times, they represent data derived primarily at the intrapsychic level. Because these defense mechanisms are internal processes, they are more difficult to discern and describe than processes anchored closer to the observable world.

STRUCTURAL DOMAINS

In contrast to functional characteristics, structural attributes represent a deeply embedded and relatively enduring template of imprinted memories, attitudes, needs, fears, conflicts, and so on, that guide experience and transform the nature of ongoing life events. Psychic structures have an orienting and preemptive effect in that they alter the character of action and the impact of subsequent experiences in line with preformed inclinations and expectancies.

Self-Image

As the inner world of symbols is mastered through development, the swirl of events that buffets the young child gives way to a growing sense of order and continuity. One major configuration emerges to impose a measure of sameness on an otherwise fluid environment, the perception of self-as-object, a distinct, ever-present, and identifiable "I" or "me." Specific self-characteristics worthy of note would include a view of self as estranged, admirable, combative, discontented, and so on.

Intrapsychic Content

As noted previously, significant early experiences with others leave an inner imprint, a structural residue composed of memories, attitudes, and affects that serves as a substrate of dispositions for perceiving and reacting to life's ongoing events.

Intrapsychic Architecture

The overall architecture that serves as a framework for an individual's psychic interior may display weakness in its structural cohesion; exhibit deficient coordination among its components; and possess few mechanisms to maintain balance and harmony, regulate internal conflicts, or mediate external pressures. The concept also refers to the structural strength, interior congruity, and functional efficacy of the personality system.

Mood/Temperament

Few observables are clinically more relevant from the biophysical level of data analysis than the predominant character of an individual's affect and the intensity and frequency with which he or she expresses it. The meaning of behaviorally expressed momentary and transient extreme emotions is easy to decode. This is not so with the more subtle moods and feelings that insidiously and repetitively pervade the patient's ongoing relationships and experiences.

CHARACTERIZING EACH PERSONALITY WITH A FEW OF THE EIGHT TRAIT DOMAINS

Our model encourages an analysis of numerous trait domains, permitting primacy to emerge as they actually exist in the psychic makeup of the person. In contrast with the models of our esteemed integrative colleagues, no singular trait has primacy. In the following figures, readers can skim our view of the theory's 15 PDs and view the trait domains that correspond to three major monotaxic theoretical schools outlined in prior chapters—the interpersonal, the cognitive, and the intrapsychic—as presented by thinkers who espouse these views.

An initial Exhibit 15.1 is presented so that the reader can identify the 15 personalities and their corresponding trait features. For example, the letter C identifies in all later figures the trait noted as most characteristic of the Shy/ Reticent/Avoidant personality spectrum (from normal to abnormal).

Figure 15.1 portrays the Interpersonal Conduct trait domain for the 15 different personality pathologies. For example, the letter F indicates that the Sociable/Pleasuring/Histrionic Interpersonal trait is Attention-seeking.

Figure 15.2 portrays the Cognitive Style trait domain, and Figure 15.3 covers the traits noted as the Intrapsychic Content realm.

Interpersonal Conduct Domain

1st Best Fit	2nd Best Fit	3rd Best Fit	Characteristic Conduct
1	2	3	**A. Unengaged:** Is indifferent to the actions or feelings of others, possessing minimal "human" interests; ends up with few close relationships and a limited role in work and family settings (e.g., has few desires or interests).
1	2	3	**B. Secretive:** Strives for privacy, with limited personal attachments and obligations; drifts into increasingly remote and clandestine social activities (e.g., is enigmatic and withdrawn).
1	2	3	**C. Aversive:** Reports extensive history of social anxiety and isolation; seeks social acceptance, but maintains careful distance to avoid anticipated humiliation and derogation (e.g., is socially pananxious and fearfully guarded).
1	2	3	**D. Submissive:** Subordinates needs to a stronger and nurturing person, without whom will feel alone and anxiously helpless; is compliant, conciliatory, and self-sacrificing (e.g., generally docile, deferential, and placating).
1	2	3	**E. High-Spirited:** Is unremittingly full of life and socially buoyant; attempts to engage others in an animated, vivacious, and lively manner; often seen by others, however, as intrusive and needlessly insistent (e.g., is persistently overbearing).
1	2	3	**F. Attention-Seeking:** Is self-dramatizing, and actively solicits praise in a showy manner to gain desired attention and approval; manipulates others and is emotionally demanding (e.g., seductively flirtatious and exhibitionistic).
1	2	3	**G. Exploitive:** Acts entitled, self-centered, vain, and unempathic; expects special favors without assuming reciprocal responsibilities; shamelessly takes others for granted and uses them to enhance self and indulge desires (e.g., egocentric and socially inconsiderate).
1	2	3	**H. Provocative:** Displays a quarrelsome, fractious, and distrustful attitude; bears serious grudges and precipitates exasperation by a testing of loyalties and a searching preoccupation with hidden motives (e.g., unjustly questions fidelity of spouse/friend).

	1	2	3

I. Irresponsible: Is socially untrustworthy and unreliable, intentionally or carelessly failing to meet personal obligations of a marital, parental, employment, or financial nature; actively violates established civil codes through duplicitous or illegal behaviors (e.g., shows active disregard for rights of others).

J. Abrasive: Reveals satisfaction in competing with, dominating, and humiliating others; regularly expresses verbally abusive and derisive social commentary, as well as exhibiting harsh, if not physically brutal behavior (e.g., intimidates, coerces, and demeans others).

K. Defenseless: Feels and acts vulnerable and guilt-ridden; fears emotional abandonment and seeks public assurances of affection and devotion (e.g., needs supportive relationships to bolster hopeless outlook).

L. Deferential: Relates to others in a self-sacrificing, servile, and obsequious manner, allowing, if not encouraging others to exploit or take advantage; is self-abasing, accepting undeserved blame and unjust criticism (e.g., courts others to be exploitive and mistreating).

M. Contrary: Assumes conflicting roles in social relationships, shifting from dependent acquiescence to assertive independence; is obstructive toward others, behaving either negatively or erratically (e.g., sulky and argumentative in response to requests).

N. Paradoxical: Needing extreme attention and affection, but acts unpredictably and manipulatively and is volatile, frequently eliciting rejection rather than support; reacts to fears of separation and isolation in angry, mercurial, and often self-damaging ways (e.g., is emotionally needy, but interpersonally erratic).

O. Respectful: Exhibits unusual adherence to social conventions and proprieties; prefers polite, formal, and "correct" personal relationships (e.g., interpersonally proper and dutiful).

Figure 15.1. Interpersonal Conduct trait domain for the 15 different personality pathologies. A patient's style of relating to others may be captured in a number of ways, such as how his or her actions affect others, intended or otherwise; the attitudes that underlie, prompt, and give shape to these actions; the methods by which he or she engages others to meet his or her needs; and his or her way of coping with social tensions and conflicts. Extrapolating from these observations, the clinician may construct an image of how the patient functions in relation to others. From DICANDRIEN, Inc. Copyright 2006 by DICANDRIEN, Inc. Reprinted with permission.

Cognitive Style Domain

1st Best Fit	2nd Best Fit	3rd Best Fit	Characteristic Conduct
1	2	3	**A. Impoverished:** Seems deficient in human spheres of knowledge and evidences vague thought processes about everyday matters that are below intellectual level; social communications are easily derailed or conveyed via a circuitous logic (e.g., lacks awareness of human relations).
1	2	3	**B. Autistic:** Intrudes social communications with personal irrelevancies; there is notable circumstantial speech, ideas of reference, and metaphorical asides; is ruminative, appears self-absorbed and lost in occasional magical thinking; there is a marked blurring of fantasy and reality (e.g., exhibits peculiar ideas and superstitious beliefs).
1	2	3	**C. Distracted:** Is bothered by disruptive and often distressing inner thoughts; the upsurge from within of irrelevant and digressive ideation upsets thought continuity and interferes with social communications (e.g., withdraws into reveries to fulfill needs).
1	2	3	**D. Naive:** Is easily persuaded, unsuspicious, and gullible; reveals a Pollyanna attitude toward interpersonal difficulties, watering down objective problems and smoothing over troubling events (e.g., childlike thinking and reasoning).
1	2	3	**E. Scattered:** Thoughts are momentary and scrambled in an untidy disarray with minimal focus to them, resulting in a chaotic hodgepodge of miscellaneous and haphazard beliefs expressed randomly with no logic or purpose (e.g., intense and transient emotions disorganize thoughts).
1	2	3	**F. Flighty:** Avoids introspective thought and is overly attentive to trivial and fleeting external events; integrates experiences poorly, resulting in shallow learning and thoughtless judgments (e.g., faddish and responsive to superficialities).
1	2	3	**G. Expansive:** Has an undisciplined imagination and exhibits a preoccupation with illusory fantasies of success, beauty, or love; is minimally constrained by objective reality; takes liberties with facts and seeks to redeem boastful beliefs (e.g., indulges fantasies of repute/power).

1	2	3	**H. Mistrustful:** Is suspicious of the motives of others, construing innocuous events as signifying conspiratorial intent; magnifies tangential or minor social difficulties into proofs of duplicity, malice, and treachery (e.g., wary and distrustful).
1	2	3	**I. Deviant:** Construes ordinary events and personal relationships in accord with socially unorthodox beliefs and morals; is disdainful of traditional ideals and conventional rules (e.g., shows contempt for social ethics and morals).
1	2	3	**J. Dogmatic:** Is strongly opinionated, as well as unbending and obstinate in holding to his or her preconceptions; exhibits a broad social intolerance and prejudice (e.g., closed-minded and bigoted).
1	2	3	**K. Fatalistic:** Sees things in their blackest form and invariably expects the worst; gives the gloomiest interpretation of current events, believing that things will never improve (e.g., conceives life events in persistent pessimistic terms).
1	2	3	**L. Diffident:** Is hesitant to voice his or her views; often expresses attitudes contrary to inner beliefs; experiences contrasting and conflicting thoughts toward self and others (e.g., demeans own convictions and opinions).
1	2	3	**M. Cynical:** Skeptical and untrusting, approaching current events with disbelief and future possibilities with trepidation; has a misanthropic view of life, expressing disdain and caustic comments toward those who experience good fortune (e.g., envious or disdainful of those more fortunate).
1	2	3	**N. Vacillating:** Experiences rapidly changing, fluctuating, and antithetical perceptions or thoughts concerning passing events; contradictory reactions are evoked in others by virtue of his or her behaviors, creating, in turn, conflicting and confusing social feedback (e.g., erratic and contrite over own beliefs and attitudes).
1	2	3	**O. Constricted:** Constructs world in terms of rules, regulations, time schedules, and social hierarchies; is unimaginative, indecisive, and notably upset by unfamiliar or novel ideas and customs (e.g., preoccupied with lists, details, rules, etc.).

Figure 15.2. Cognitive Style trait domain. How the patient focuses and allocates attention, encodes and processes information, organizes thoughts, makes attributions, and communicates reactions and ideas to others represents key cognitive functions of clinical value. These characteristics are among the most useful indices of the patient's distinctive way of thinking. By synthesizing his or her beliefs and attitudes, it may be possible to identify indications of problematic cognitive functions and assumptions. From DICANDRIEN, Inc. Copyright 2006 by DICANDRIEN, Inc. Reprinted with permission.

Intrapsychic Content Domain

1st Best Fit	2nd Best Fit	3rd Best Fit	Characteristic Conduct
1	2	3	**A. Meager:** Inner representations are few in number and minimally articulated, largely devoid of the manifold percepts and memories, or the dynamic interplay among drives and conflicts that typify even well-adjusted persons.
1	2	3	**B. Chaotic:** Inner representations consist of a jumble of miscellaneous memories and percepts, random drives and impulses, and uncoordinated channels of regulation that are only fitfully competent for binding tensions, accommodating needs, and mediating conflicts.
1	2	3	**C. Vexatious:** Inner representations are composed of readily reactivated, intense, and anxiety-ridden memories, limited avenues of gratification, and few mechanisms to channel needs, bind impulses, resolve conflicts, or deflect external stressors.
1	2	3	**D. Immature:** Inner representations are composed of unsophisticated ideas and incomplete memories, rudimentary drives and childlike impulses, as well as minimal competencies to manage and resolve stressors.
1	2	3	**E. Piecemeal:** Inner representations are disorganized and dissipated, a jumble of diluted and muddled recollections that are recalled by fits and starts, serving only as momentary guideposts for dealing with everyday tensions and conflicts.
1	2	3	**F. Shallow:** Inner representations are composed largely of superficial yet emotionally intense affects, memories, and conflicts, as well as facile drives and insubstantial mechanisms.
1	2	3	**G. Contrived:** Inner representations are composed far more than usual of illusory ideas and memories, synthetic drives and conflicts, and pretentious, if not simulated, percepts and attitudes, all of which are readily refashioned as the need arises.
1	2	3	**H. Unalterable:** Inner representations are arranged in an unusual configuration of rigidly held attitudes, unyielding percepts, and implacable drives, which are aligned in a semidelusional hierarchy of tenacious memories, immutable cognitions, and irrevocable beliefs.

1	2	3	
1	2	3	*I. Debased:* Inner representations are a mix of revengeful attitudes and impulses oriented to subvert established cultural ideals and mores, as well as to debase personal sentiments and conventional societal attainments.
1	2	3	*J. Pernicious:* Inner representations are distinguished by the presence of aggressive energies and malicious attitudes, as well as by a contrasting paucity of sentimental memories, tender affects, internal conflicts, shame, or guilt feelings.
1	2	3	*K. Forsaken:* Inner representations have been depleted or devitalized, either drained of their richness and joyful elements or withdrawn from memory, leaving the person to feel abandoned, bereft, discarded.
1	2	3	*L. Discredited:* Inner representations are composed of disparaged past memories and discredited achievements, of positive feelings and erotic drives transposed onto their least attractive opposites, of internal conflicts intentionally aggravated, of mechanisms of anxiety reduction subverted by processes that intensify discomforts.
1	2	3	*M. Fluctuating:* Inner representations compose a complex of opposing inclinations and incompatible memories that are driven by impulses designed to nullify his or her own achievements and/or the pleasures and expectations of others.
1	2	3	*N. Incompatible:* Rudimentary and expediently devised, but repetitively aborted, inner representations have led to perplexing memories, enigmatic attitudes, contradictory needs, antithetical emotions, erratic impulses, and opposing strategies for conflict reduction.
1	2	3	*O. Concealed:* Only those inner affects, attitudes, and actions that are socially approved are allowed conscious awareness or behavioral expression, resulting in gratification being highly regulated, forbidden impulses sequestered and tightly bound, personal and social conflicts defensively denied, kept from awareness, all maintained under stringent control.

Figure 15.3. Intrapsychic Content trait domain. Significant experiences from the past leave an inner imprint, a structural residue composed of memories, attitudes, and affects that serve as a substrate of dispositions for perceiving and reacting to life's events. Analogous to the various organ systems in the body, both the character and the substance of these internalized representations of significant figures and relationships from the past can be differentiated and analyzed for clinical purposes. Variations in the nature and content of this inner world, or what are often called *object relations,* can be identified with one or another personality and lead us to employ the following descriptive terms to represent them. From DICANDRIEN, Inc., 2006. Copyright 2006 by DICANDRIEN, Inc. Reprinted with permission.

In concluding this extensive presentation, the authors wish to thank readers for bearing with them as they sought not only to portray the essential components of the evolutionary model but also to provide a rationale for why it can encompass other contemporary theoretical approaches.

REFERENCES

Bakan, D. (1966). *The duality of human existence: An essay on psychology and religion.* Chicago, IL: Rand McNally.

Bender, D. S. (2013). An ecumenical approach to conceptualizing and studying the core of personality psychopathology: A commentary on Hopwood et al. *Journal of Personality Disorders, 27,* 311–319. doi:10.1521/pedi.2013.27.3.311

Blatt, S. J. (2008). *Polarities of experience: Relatedness and self-definition in personality development, psychopathology, and the therapeutic process.* Washington, DC: American Psychological Association.

Bornstein, R. F. (2013). Combining interpersonal and intrapersonal perspectives on personality pathology: A commentary on Hopwood et al. *Journal of Personality Disorders, 27,* 296–302. doi:10.1521/pedi.2013.27.3.296

Bowers, K. S. (1977). There's more to Iago than meets the eye: A clinical account of personal consistency. In D. Magnusson & N. S. Endler (Eds.), *Personality at the crossroads* (pp. 65–81). Hillsdale, NJ: Erlbaum.

Clarkin, J. F. (2013). The search for critical dimensions of personality pathology to inform diagnostic assessment and treatment planning: A commentary on Hopwood et al. *Journal of Personality Disorders, 27,* 303–310. doi:10.1521/pedi.2013.27.3.303

Godel, K. (1931). *On formally undecidable propositions of* Principia Mathematica *and related systems.* Unpublished doctoral dissertation, University of Vienna.

Hempel, C. G. (1965). *Aspects of scientific explanation.* New York, NY: Free Press.

Hopwood, C. J., Wright, A. G. C., Ansell, E. B., & Pincus, A. L. (2013). The interpersonal core of personality pathology. *Journal of Personality Disorders, 27,* 270–295. doi:10.1521/pedi.2013.27.3.270

Horney, K. (1945). *Our inner conflicts.* New York, NY: Norton.

Lewontin, R. C. (1979). Sociobiology as an adaptationist program. *Behavioral Science, 24,* 5–14. doi:10.1002/bs.3830240103

Maslow, A. H. (1968). *Toward a psychology of being* (2nd ed.). New York, NY: Van Nostrand.

Millon, T. (1969). *Modern psychopathology: A biosocial approach to maladaptive learning and functioning.* Philadelphia, PA: Saunders.

Millon, T. (1981). *Disorders of personality: DSM–III, Axis II.* New York, NY: Wiley.

Millon, T. (1984). On the renaissance of personality assessment and personality theory. *Journal of Personality Assessment, 48*, 450–466. doi:10.1207/s15327752jpa4805_1

Millon, T. (1990). *Toward a new personology: An evolutionary model*. New York, NY: Wiley.

Millon, T. (1996). *Personality and psychopathology: Building a clinical science*. New York, NY: Wiley.

Millon, T. (2010). Using evolutionary principles for understanding psychopathology. In T. Millon, R. Krueger, & E. Simonsen (Eds.), *Contemporary directions in psychopathology: Scientific foundations of the* DSM–5 *and* ICD-11. New York, NY: Guilford Press.

Millon, T. (2011). *Disorders of personality: Introducing a* DSM/ICD *spectrum from normal to abnormal* (3rd ed.). Hoboken, NJ: Wiley.

Offer, D., & Sabshin, M. (Eds.). (1974). *Normality* (Rev. ed.). New York, NY: Basic Books.

Offer, D., & Sabshin, M. (Eds.). (1991). *The diversity of normal behavior*. New York, NY: Basic Books.

Prigogine, I. (1972). Thermodynamics of evolution. *Physics Today, 25*, 23–28, 38–44. doi:10.1063/1.3071090

Rushton, J. P. (1985). Differential K theory: The sociobiology of individual and group differences. *Personality and Individual Differences, 6*, 441–452. doi:10.1016/0191-8869(85)90137-0

Strack, S. (Ed.). (2006). *Differentiating normal and abnormal personality*. New York, NY: Springer.

Widiger, T. A. (2003). Personality disorder and Axis I psychopathology: The problematic boundary of Axis I and Axis II. *Journal of Personality Disorders, 17*, 90–108. doi:10.1521/pedi.17.2.90.23987

16

THE COGNITIVE–AFFECTIVE PROCESSING SYSTEM MODEL OF PERSONALITY PATHOLOGY: READY-MADE FOR THEORETICAL INTEGRATION

STEVEN K. HUPRICH AND SHARON M. NELSON

Regardless of which personality disorder (PD) theory one finds most interesting, virtually all value the role of cognition and cognitive processes in understanding the individual's personality. For instance, a patient with dependent PD believes she cannot function without the support of a loving, caring, and engaging partner. Such ideas and thoughts evoke distress, however, when her husband begins to work longer hours. Likewise, a young man with schizoid PD feels panic after learning that his family is moving and he will have to move out of the basement and adjust to a new home. He believes that his privacy is very important to him, that his parents do not have his best interest in mind, and that he does not want to move from a place in which he can be independent and by himself. His parents bring him into treatment because his anxious thoughts and affect are not something they can manage, particularly because he rarely shows any signs of emotional distress. In purely cognitive and cognitive-processing models of psychopathology, attention to

http://dx.doi.org/10.1037/14549-017
Personality Disorders: Toward Theoretical and Empirical Integration in Diagnosis and Assessment,
S. K. Huprich (Editor)

these thoughts and ideas is the explicit focal point, as well as the point of access by which the patient may be helped. Such models are based on the idea that one can logically infer from a person's self-reported thoughts, ideas, and/or behaviors (or lack thereof) what is happening internally that accounts for the way that person functions.

In this chapter, the focus is on a theory derived from observations of cognition, affect, and behavior. Though well-articulated cognitive theories of PDs have been offered by Aaron Beck and colleagues (Beck, Freeman, & Davis, 2004) and Jeffrey Young (1994), our focus here is on the cognitive–affective processing system (CAPS), a dynamic and expansive model of personality proposed by Walter Mischel and Yuishi Shoda (1995). On their own, Beck and Young's theories are formidable for what they offer toward an understanding of PDs (i.e., Huprich, 2004); however, we opt to focus on CAPS, not only because it incorporates many ideas from Beck and Young but most notably because of its potential to integrate the PD field with regard to assessment and diagnosis. In the sections to follow, we briefly review this model and its application for the assessment and conceptualization of PDs. This application of the model was first explained by Huprich and Bornstein (2007), who highlighted how it overcomes many of the shortcomings found in a number of existing assessment techniques and theories of PDs. We believe that such a model could effectively organize the disparate ideas and research on the PDs into one unified framework for understanding personality pathology without fundamentally losing the value or contributions that any one major theory or framework offers. Thus, CAPS seems to be ready made for theoretical integration.

THE COGNITIVE–AFFECTIVE PROCESSING SYSTEM

Overview

In response to what they saw as lacking in the extant models of personality, Mischel and Shoda (1995) introduced CAPS as a means of understanding personality organization. This model is an outgrowth of concerns expressed many years ago by Mischel (1968, 1973, 1984), who found trait models to be highly inadequate and inaccurate in describing and understanding personality. The CAPS model attempts to account for both trait and processing theories by considering the interaction of the individual and the situation, which is based upon internal cognitive and/or affective reactions of past experiences with similar features, and the patterns of variation that result.

In the CAPS, patterns of variability in affect and behavior are generally defined through the use of "if, then" statements. For example, rather than saying that someone has a problem with anger, a statement providing little room for variation in the understanding of the person's presentation, CAPS theory might articulate the problem this way: "If verbal criticism from a superior happens, then she or he becomes angry, but if criticism from a peer happens, then she or he remains pretty calm." Using an if, then statement in this case helps to provide a richer understanding of which contextual elements elicit the person's anger response and which do not. By breaking down the behavior or affect into these if, then contingencies, one begins to see specific consistencies in the pattern of an individual's personality. Outside observers likewise evaluate the responding behavior in light of the situation and subsequently provide a descriptive label to that person, such as "angry." Yet, as research has found, observers regularly identify these qualities within a contextual framework, thus maintaining some degree of situational specificity to the underlying label.

The CAPS model posits that an individual's personality is partially determined by the specific context an individual is in, while also acknowledging that the underlying personality system is stable (Mischel & Shoda, 2008). This personality system comprises the person's various mental representations, including encodings, expectancies and beliefs, affects, goals and values, and competency or self-regulatory plans (see Table 16.1). Mischel and Shoda referred to these various categories of mental representations as cognitive affective units, or CAUs. In any given situation, the CAUs interconnect in the mind to form a network that activates distinct patterns of cognitions, affects, and behavior. These interconnected networks of CAUs form the first of five levels of analysis in the CAPS model (see Figure 16.1).

The second level of analysis in the CAPS model is composed of the behavioral expressions that the individual exhibits as a result of the activation of the chain of CAUs. The subsequent behavior is perceived by an observer, which occurs at the third level of analysis. The fourth level of analysis comprises the situation or context—and its unique features—in which the individual finds

TABLE 16.1
Types of Cognitive–Affective Units

Encodings	Categories/constructs for the self, people, events, and situations
Expectations and beliefs	About the social world, about outcomes for behavior, and about one's self-efficacy
Affects	Feelings, emotions, and affective responses
Goals	Desirable outcomes and affective states, aversive outcomes and affective states, goals and life projects
Competencies and self-regulatory plans	Potential behaviors and scripts that one can do and plans and strategies for organizing action and for affecting outcomes and one's own behavior and internal states

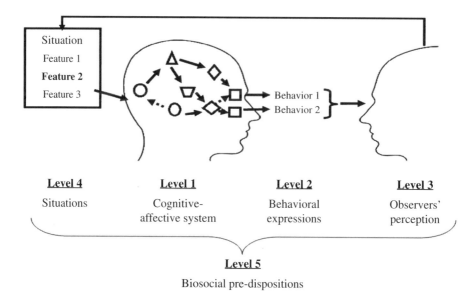

Figure 16.1. Five levels of analysis in the cognitive–affective processing system (CAPS) model. From "A Cognitive–Affective System Theory of Personality: Reconceptualizing Situations, Dispositions, Dynamics, and Invariance in Personality Structure," by W. Mischel & Y. Shoda, 1995, *Psychological Review, 102,* pp. 246–268. Copyright 1995 by American Psychological Association.

him- or herself. The fifth level consists of the individual's biogenetic predispositions, which can influence each of the other levels. There is a growing body of evidence to support the CAPS model at each level of analysis (Mischel & Shoda, 2008), as well as its usefulness for PD diagnosis (Rhadigan & Huprich, 2012; Roche, Pincus, Conroy, Hyde, & Ram, 2012). Furthermore, more recent studies of the biological influences on personality and its pathology are now being considered within each of these levels (see Chapter 7, this volume).

To demonstrate the effectiveness of the CAPS model in PD assessment, imagine the following scenario: An individual with a highly narcissistic personality is passed over for a promotion at work (Level 4/situation). This individual has CAUs that consist of *encodings* about the people around him not being as competent as he is, *beliefs* about his considerable ability, *expectations* of being recognized for his perceived superiority, *goals* of rising to the top of this company, *affects* involving a sense of shame over the apparent failure, and a direct attack to the individual's fragile self-esteem, as well as *self-regulatory plans* that do not provide for a stable, internal self-state. All of these different CAUs are connected in a network (Level 1/CAUs), and each is activated as a result of being in a situation in which the individual's self-esteem is wounded. These interconnected CAUs lead to the individual exhibiting what Kohut (1977) would call "narcissistic rage," or lashing out at the people with whom he works (Level 2/behavior), a behavior that coworkers then observe and characterize as extreme and unprofessional (Level 3/observer perceptions). The individual may then be further punished at work, or even fired, receiving an even greater injury to his self-esteem (Level 4/situation). This in turn activates a new series of CAU activations (Level 1), which may result in depression, further rage, and so on.

HOW CAPS ALLOWS FOR READY-MADE THEORETICAL INTEGRATION

In the sections below, we describe many ways in which CAPS is well suited to become a unifying framework for PD assessment and diagnosis. We describe how other major theories of PD may be dovetailed into a CAPS framework, we offer ideas for aligning other frameworks into a CAPS model, and we suggest specific research strategies.

CAPS Accounts for and Appreciates Cross-Situational Variation in Personality

CAPS has demonstrated that dispositional personality features, as manifested in certain behaviors and other observable outcomes, are highly consistent across situations, yet do not generalize across situations. This cross-situational variation is clearly relevant to assessing PDs, in which knowing the context in which a problem arises is critical. For instance, Huprich, Bornstein, and Schmitt (2011) noted that a patient who has a narcissistic personality may deny that people fail to appreciate his special accomplishments (a criterion of *DSM–IV* Narcissistic PD; American Psychiatric Association, 1994) provided that others frequently notice such things. However, if these things are not recognized, the patient may become angry or depressed and indeed acknowledge this problem. Indeed, mood state tends to evoke very specific changes in personality trait and PD symptom scores, thus leading to a specific way of presenting oneself in a depressed state that does not exist when one is not depressed (Bagby, Schuller, Marshall, & Ryder, 2004; Clark, Vittengl, Kraft, & Jarrett, 2003; Hirschfeld et al., 1983; Morey, 2010).

As another example, consider how a firm, loud voice is interpreted differently according to the context in which it is heard. For instance, if a person raises her voice and speaks loudly to make sure her ideas are heard in a meeting after she has already done most of the speaking during the meeting, this behavior may lead the clinician to suspect a more narcissistic personality. To test this idea, the clinician would look for other instances in which a need for attention is manifested across situations, such as speaking often and loudly or making a point of talking over others. Alternatively, if a person reports becoming loud and assertive because she dislikes another individual who recently disappointed her and characterizes the individual as "stupid" and "unrealistic," the therapist might be inclined to consider a borderline personality diagnosis. Regardless, in all situations, the clinician will search for confirming and disconfirming evidence by looking at behaviors in a given situation and making a judgment about the underlying motive. However, if the behavior or trait itself is simply left as a criterion by which to make a judgment, as is the case in the *Diagnostic and Statistical Manual of Mental Disorders* (DSM) system or within many trait models of personality pathology, important contextual information needed for an accurate assessment is lost. In fact, it could very well be the case that high levels of diagnostic overlap are seen in many samples partly because of a failure to provide important information about the context.

Another important contribution from the literature on context is found in studies of *priming*, in which the material or events that precede the assessment of individuals' personalities affect what the individuals subsequently report about themselves. That is, knowing what people were thinking about or exposed to immediately before an assessment affects what they tell the clinician about themself. Virtually all clinicians have experienced patients who report that they never do certain things (e.g., "I don't ever get angry at my sweet wife"), only later to tacitly admit that they actually do what they just denied (e.g., "My wife doesn't get our budget problems, and we can get into some pretty hot arguments about this"). In reviewing semistructured diagnostic interviews for PDs, Huprich et al. (2011) described how someone who has a narcissistic personality may endorse an item related to avoidant PD on a diagnostic interview after first saying no to the previous item, which actually assesses narcissistic PD. Thus, on the interview, the narcissistic patient actually meets criteria for avoidant PD instead of narcissistic PD. Bornstein (1998) demonstrated such assessment problems experimentally by noting that the type of instructions provided to someone with high levels of dependent features (assessed implicitly) evoked a higher occurrence of help-seeking responses.

We believe that most clinical judgment occurs from within an *interactionist* framework (see Chapter 9)—clinicians look for thoughts, feelings, behaviors, or actions that occur in a specific situation, and they make inferences about potential diagnosis exists on the basis of the context and nature of the patient's response. This is what Rhadigan and Huprich (2012) found in their pilot study of the CAPS model, in which clinicians were given greater detail and context about the DSM symptoms being expressed by patients versus being given just trait descriptions or a DSM description: Providing the context in which the symptoms occurred led to greater diagnostic accuracy. Although clinician judgment is frequently criticized for its many sources of error (e.g., Zimmerman, 2011), many clinicians do prefer a prototype-matching diagnostic system, which capitalizes on many of the ideas inherent in a CAPS model of assessment (Rhadigan & Huprich, 2012; Rottman, Ahn, Sanislow, & Kim, 2009; Spitzer, First, Shedler, Westen, & Skodol, 2008). Future research should study clinicians' internal consistency in making such judgments on the same patient in order to confirm whether the same processes are accurately used by different clinicians. Given past research on the CAPS model (see above), one could anticipate that clinicians will be highly consistent with each other when context is provided.

CAPS Actually Can Account for Cross-Situational Stability in Personality

Although context is important for accurate assessment, it is also important to see if similar behavior or response patterns occur across multiple situations. In fact, it could be that the more likely it is that a common response pattern is produced, the more likely it is that the pattern is a trait. As noted above, trait theories are regularly criticized for not giving attention to situational specificity for the expression of a given pattern normally described as a trait. However, there would be an easily quantifiable way to identify whether such a pattern is a trait, based upon the frequency in which the same pattern occurs over multiple situations. In fact, it is the premise of the five-factor model (FFM) that the regular expression (or lack of expression) of certain traits is pathological. Thus, it is the repeated use of a given set of CAUs with similar outcomes that defines a pathological aspect of personality. Such an idea was expressed by the *DSM–5* Personality and Personality Disorders Work Group, which suggested that assessing patients for pathological traits would improve upon PD assessment in the fifth edition of the *DSM* (Skodol et al., 2011).

That being said, CAPS is not a theory of traits. Mischel and Shoda (2008, p. 234) wrote,

> One of the most pernicious of these [previous assumptions about personality assessment] is the preemptive definition of personality psychology as a science of personality "traits," conceptualized as causal, genotypic entities that correspond to phenotypic behavioral dispositions. That automatically makes narrowly defined "traits" *the* target of investigation—as well as the bases for explanations. . . . These phenomena can be analyzed at each of the complementary levels . . . allowing an ultimately more comprehensive and cumulative science conception of personality and its diverse manifestations and antecedents.

Nevertheless, we believe that trait theory can be mapped into the CAPS framework. To do so effectively, the following research strategies may serve as a focal starting point:

- begin by assessing the behaviors or actions hypothesized to be associated with a given trait across a preset number of situations that a priori are believed to be ones in which a trait will and will not be expressed (this occurs at Level 2);
- determine how many times such behaviors occur in each situation and evaluate these relative to the a priori hypotheses; and
- determine if there is a situationally specific factor or set of factors that is associated with this behavior in the hypothesized situations.

Obviously, the more that the behavior is found to occur in a specific kind of situation or with a specific stimulus (which would be learned only after a careful examination of the situations), the more likely it is that the term *trait* may not be the best label (or, by contrast, it might be that the "trait" is present in a low level); however, if the behavior or action generalizes across situations that appear to share no common features or elements, the term *trait* would appear more appropriate. Nevertheless, it would be recognized that, for any given person, there are very likely situations or contexts in which such actions will not happen and that the collection of "traits" the individual possesses is therefore not a complete description or assessment of the individual.

This being the case, how do the personality trait domains (e.g., neuroticism, extraversion, agreeableness) fit into the CAPS model? We suggest that these domains are best understood as superordinate constructs that are individuals' self-attributed qualities (given that most of the extant research on trait domains is derived from a self-report methodology) and are found mainly—though not exclusively—within the CAUs (Level 1). These domains are broad ways in which CAUs are organized and how they translate into behaviors that individuals report doing (a self-report about what happens at Level 2). These CAUs are based in part upon biogenetic behavioral predispositions and also upon individuals' experiences, which makes them more accessible. In fact, it may be that the most empirically defined map we have of the organization of CAUs at the self-report level is found at the trait-domain level, though clearly this is only a small portion of what constitutes the CAUs. Moreover, according to Mischel and Shoda (2008), it is the idiographic pattern of CAUs that is most important to know when assessing consistency in a person's behavior.

As a final point, we would note that if repeated behaviors of the same kind (e.g., becoming angry and assertive) occur across multiple situations, it is likely that the person may have higher levels of impairment, in that she or he has not learned alternative routes toward resolving problems in ways that are socially acceptable and pleasing to others. The FFM and other trait models have assumed that very high or low levels of traits are associated with personality pathology. Yet, across trait-pathology studies, the findings are rather mixed as to which trait domains and facets are specifically associated with which PDs (Samuel & Widiger, 2008; Saulsman & Page, 2004). Efforts to expand FFM assessment are occurring in order to have self-attributed items that more accurately capture the magnitude by which the trait is high or low (see Widiger, Lynam, Miller, & Oltmanns, 2012). Yet, such efforts has produced very lengthy FFM scales for specific PDs, which include several subscales; it could be that the lack of specificity in the original FFM assessment tools is also associated with a failure to assess the context that drives the expression of a given "trait." In other words, overlooking context renders clinicians unable to adequately assess whether or not the trait applies to a client. From a research perspective, assessing these "traits" across situations could enhance considerably the mapping of trait models into a CAPS framework and potentially reduce the number of items necessary to assess maladaptive traits with self-report methods only. Doing this would require, however, a reworking of extant self-report instruments in order to identify those stimuli and situations that evoke certain traits to be expressed.

CAPS Accounts for Self–Other Discrepancies in Personality Perception

A pattern all too frequently found in the personality assessment literature, whether it is with individuals who have PDs or in nonclinical samples, is that self-reports do not converge well with the reports of others (Ganellen, 2007; Oltmanns & Turkheimer, 2006; see also Chapter 10, this volume). Put simply: People do not recognize or describe their own personalities the same way others do. This is very problematic when it comes to diagnosis and assessment, as any framework that puts most or all of its reliance on the self-report of the patient is setting itself up for an inherently one-sided view of the patient's functioning (Huprich et al., 2011; Westen, 1997; see Chapter 10). To be fair, it is impressive how much convergence occurs at the broad trait domain level when assessing self-reports of personality (Allik, 2005; McCrae & Costa, 2008). However, conflating the convergence of self-reported personality trait measures (e.g., their ecological validity) with a comprehensive, multimethod assessment of personality is an error in judgment (see Meyer et al., 2001, for a discussion of multimethod assessment). In fact, Mischel and Shoda (2008) noted that "in the studies in which . . . (situational-specificities of behavior) . . . are made available to lay perceivers, they seem to be linked to the social perceptions and inferences that are formed and suggest that perceivers may be intuitive interactionists" (p. 227).

Those who strongly support the use of self-report measures to organize the diagnostic system (e.g., Clark, 2007; Krueger et al., 2011; Widiger & Simonsen, 2005) often do not give enough attention to the self–other discrepancy problem and the important role that individual perception plays in understanding personality. It is well documented in the literature that patients with personality pathology will struggle in providing an accurate description of themselves. They have limited awareness of how their behaviors and actions affect others, may not have the requisite skills or capacities to act in more socially desirable ways, or may be motivated to appear healthier or unhealthier than they really are (depending upon the context; Ganellen, 2007; see also Chapter 10, this volume). Fortunately, CAPS provides a helpful framework in which the self–other discrepancy can be understood and discussed. This may be seen by the comparison of a Level 1 (cognitive–affective system) with a Level 3 (observer's perceptions) unit of analysis. More to the point, by its very nature, the CAPS model recognizes that personality exists within an observer-perceived framework. The view of both self and other must be appreciated to understand personality. Without both perspectives, only part of the model can be known, and it is left incomplete.

Thus, those interested in self–other agreement research should not only continue to assess self–other agreement but also look to what extent behavioral observations and expressions correspond most closely with which rater. This is something that has already been done, with a clear trend being that others' reports tend to correspond better with behaviors than do self-reports (John & Robins, 1994; Kolar, Funder, & Colvin, 1996). Further studies of the influence of context on person perception and self–other discrepancies would be helpful in further highlighting the convergence and divergence in multiple informant assessment, perhaps offering a more finely tuned description of certain types of personality pathology that would aid in the accuracy of detection (e.g., Besser & Zeigler-Hill, 2010).

CAPS Provides a Framework for Understanding Psychodynamic, Cognitive, and Interpersonal Theories of Personality and Psychopathology

Mischel and Shoda (2008) explicitly stated,

Consistent with the discovery initially within the psychodynamic-motivation tradition that much if not most of the mind operates at levels outside of awareness and plays out in automatic ways, CAPS is conceptualized as a network that operates rapidly and functions at multiple levels, often outside of conscious awareness. (p. 232)

CAPS provides a framework for understanding nonconscious processes that is jargon free (e.g., unconscious fantasies motivating a desire for power), but at the same time it allows one to test explicitly certain hypotheses about what happens at the nonconscious/unconscious level. Thus, priming studies and process-oriented assessment strategies (see Chapter 11) could readily be included within this model and their findings applied to how to structure the diagnostic system. Stated differently, this model is not just a cognitive theory of what happens in the mind and brain vis-à-vis cognitions, affects, expectancies, encodings, values, goals, and behavioral scripts. It is also a psychodynamic one that speaks to how such units interact in a dynamic and nonstatic way. Subsequently, it is not difficult to imagine how interpersonal relationships (i.e., interpersonal theory) could be studied within this framework, by looking not only at the CAUs associated with self- and other representations but also at corresponding behaviors, perceptions of others, and how individuals respond to each other. These types of frameworks are already being studied within interpersonal theory with more implicit methods (Roche, Pincus, Conroy, Hyde, & Ram, 2012; see also Chapter 14, this volume), and they could readily be discussed within the CAPS framework. Thus, given the powerful role of nonconscious processes in personality and its disorders (Kihlstrom, 2008; Robinson & Gordon, 2011; Schultheiss, 2008); a model that offers a place to study this level of analysis clearly has many advantages.

In using more typical cognitive terminology, CAPS specifically identifies that there are "hot," emotion-driven systems characteristic of a "reflexive affective personality system, just as much as it [CAUs] also contains a cool, more reflective, cognitive system" (Mischel & Shoda, 2008, p. 232). CAPS also notes that consequential behavior and actions involve both types of cognitive processes. Thus, PDs could be studied for the specific ways in which "hot" and "cold" CAUs are associated with behaviors relevant to PD and could be described for those processes that are governed by more rational or reflective thought and those that are governed by more affectively charged components.

CAPS Provides a Framework for Understanding Phenomenological Aspects of Personality

CAPS focuses on the unique construal of the situation by the individual and states that the person can best be understood by his or her unique phenomenology. For instance, George Kelly (1957/1969) and Carl Rogers (1961) each noted the powerful role that a person's unique construal of him- or herself and the situation plays when it comes to understanding the person.

They minimized the idea that most anything "objective" could be applied to understanding an individual's way of thinking, feeling, and behaving. Rogers (1961) especially was interested in the therapist's role in seeking to understand the person by striving to be as empathic as possible. Kohut (1977) as well noted the necessity of empathic immersion when understanding a patient, and more recent evidence-based treatments have identified the necessity of focusing upon internal, subjective representations of oneself and others when treating patients with PDs (e.g., Bateman & Fonagy, 2009; Clarkin, Levy, Lenzenweger, & Kernberg, 2007). Likewise, Westen (1997) captured some of this in his survey of clinicians, who valued most their subjective experience of the patient and the nature of the patient's interactions with others (i.e., how they perceived others and how others perceived them) when trying to assess and diagnose personality pathology. In short, phenomenological aspects of personality are part and parcel of understanding any person and formulating a way by which to help the person therapeutically.

Advocates of prototype assessment begin from the phenomenological framework (see Chapter 9). Such clinicians recognize that patients with a given personality style have a specific type of phenomenological experience that leads them to view themselves and interact with others in particular ways. Astute and experienced clinicians begin to recognize these patterns and thus form a generalized impression of the patient on the basis of this constellation of intrasubjective experience, which has historically led them to form an impression of what the patient is like. Within a CAPS framework, these generalized impressions can be studied empirically across levels: CAUs lead to particular behaviors, these behaviors lead to certain impressions, and these impressions are further developed as one gets to know the context in which patients' thoughts, feelings, and behaviors are expressed. Indeed, it is becoming well known that patients affect their therapists in regular or predictable ways (Colli, Tanzilli, Dimaggio, & Lingiardi, 2014). Such information can be empirically quantified, and CAPS offers the framework within which to understand these interactions.

CAPS Provides a Framework for Understanding Biogenetic Trait Aspects of Personality and Psychopathology

Trait models of personality and psychopathology recognize a biological or genetic predisposition toward the expression of the traits. Traits may be viewed as a repeated, consistent pattern of CAUs being activated across a number of situations. However, these traits and behavioral predispositions are now widely thought to be influenced by genes and their interaction with the environment (see Chapter 7) and are not viewed as just a unidimensional force that predetermines an individual's way of thinking, feeling, and acting. CAPS recognizes the profound influence of biogenetic factors by noting how their influence could be mapped in every level of analysis. Mischel and Shoda (2008) wrote, "These *pre*-dispositions interact with conditions throughout development and play out in ways that influence what the person thinks, feels, and does and the processing dynamics and behavioral signatures that come to characterize the individual" (p. 231). However, they added, "We emphasize the *pre* to underline that they are biological precursors that may manifest indirectly as well as directly, in diverse and complex form, at other levels of analysis" (pp. 230–231). Thus, CAPS does not suggest that personality organization be based upon biological foundations but rather upon the interaction of such material with the individual's cognitive–affective processing system and environment.

CAPS may arguably be one of the most optimal models upon which to frame biologically oriented studies of personality. As South notes in Chapter 7 of this volume, there is a long pathway from the identification of a biogenetic marker of personality to what it means about personality. For instance, some markers may be associated with a specific behavior, though a number of things are often unknown: how the marker is related to genetic expression, which kinds of biopsychosocial events evoke the genetic material, what mediates or moderates that expression, how a series of physiological processes become activated (and in which portions of the brain), how these areas interact, how brain activity evokes certain affective responses and cognitive patterns, how these patterns are consciously or nonconsciously experienced, what types of responses they evoke (and how detectable are such responses) and do others notice such responses, and—if so—what is the net effect of that person's responses on the social environment. At present, the field is far from mapping this level of specificity into how personality functions adaptively or maladaptively. LeDoux (1989, 1995), for instance, provided some important early discussion about the neurobiological terrain in which cognition, affect, and behavior occur, though ongoing research continues to develop such pathways with regard to psychopathology. In fact, this is what the Research Domain Criteria (RDoC) of the National Institute of Mental Health seeks to accomplish (http://www.nimh.nih.gov/research-priorities/rdoc/index.shtml). It is conceivable that findings from RDoC studies could be translated into the CAPS model and integrated with findings from other levels, such as cognitive, affective, behavioral, and interpersonal. Mischel and Shoda (2008) noted that biogenetic influences can be observed at every level of analysis, and over time these influences can be added into the CAPS model in order to better articulate greater specificity at which such influences act. To be consistent with the CAPS framework, however, RDoC systems would have to be understood by the context in which such systems are and are not activated and how the systems interact with each other within specific contexts to help determine behavior. Such ideas are already being examined in genetic modeling of personality and psychopathology (e.g., Chapter 7, this volume).

CLOSING THOUGHTS

CAPS offers a comprehensive, integrative framework within which many theories of personality and pathology can be understood. The field of PD assessment and diagnosis is in need of a unifying theory, and we believe that CAPS offers the best hope for meeting this need. CAPS is one of a few metatheories in which other extant theories may be placed. As a metatheory, CAPS has much to offer. In fact, as other authors have described so well in Chapters 3 and 12 through 15 herein, many efforts to integrate findings across theoretical models and research traditions are already under way.

In thinking about moving ahead, we offer the following general guidelines on how CAPS could be evaluated for becoming the preferred integrative theory by which PDs are assessed and diagnosed. First, we recommend that any diagnostic taxon—whether it be an existing category or type, a proposed category or type, a prototype, or a trait—be given equal consideration in the CAPS framework. Second, evidence must be provided for the support of the taxon across all five levels of the CAPS model. Third, for a taxon to be retained in future diagnostic manuals, a body of evidence must exist across all five levels of analysis, with special interest in showing how all five levels work together in concert. The greater the specificity and/or generalizability with which a taxon can be described, the more likely it should be that the taxon will be included in the *DSM*. Fourth, the clinical utility of proposed taxon must be evaluated: Do clinicians find the taxon useful, does it communicate useful information about a patient, and can other clinicians use the same taxon in a consistent way? Finally, it will be important to demonstrate that the taxon of interest is more useful and leads to greater diagnostic accuracy than do previous diagnostic labels. For instance, Rhadigan and Huprich (2012) found that a CAPS model built upon *DSM* descriptions of certain Axis II disorders led to greater accuracy than did decontextualized trait descriptions of the same disorders built upon the FFM.

We believe CAPS offers a model upon which most researchers and clinicians can agree. Clinical personality science is ready for integration, despite a cacophonous past. We hope that future architects of diagnostic manuals and treatment programs will be integrative in their thinking, such that a harmonious future can be actualized.

REFERENCES

Allik, J. (2005). Personality dimensions across cultures. *Journal of Personality Disorders, 19*, 212–232. doi:10.1521/pedi.2005.19.3.212

American Psychiatric Association. (1994). *Diagnostic and statistical manual of mental disorders* (4th ed.). Washington, DC: Author.

Bagby, R. M., Schuller, D. R., Marshall, M. B., & Ryder, A. G. (2004). Depressive personality disorder: Rates of comorbidity and personality disorders and relations to the five-factor model of personality. *Journal of Personality Disorders, 18*, 542–554. doi:10.1521/pedi.18.6.542.54796

Bateman, A., & Fonagy, P. (2009). Randomized controlled trial of outpatient mentalization-based treatment versus structured clinical management for borderline personality disorder. *The American Journal of Psychiatry, 166*, 1355–1364. doi:10.1176/appi.ajp.2009.09040539

Beck, A. T., Freeman, A. C., & Davis, D. D. (2004). *Cognitive therapy for personality disorders* (2nd ed.). New York, NY: Guilford Press.

Besser, A., & Zeigler-Hill, V. (2010). The influence of pathological narcissism on emotional and motivational responses to negative events: The roles of visibility and concern about humiliation. *Journal of Research in Personality, 44*, 520–534. doi:10.1016/j.jrp.2010.06.006

Bornstein, R. F. (1998). Implicit and self-attributed dependency strivings: Differential relationships to laboratory and field measures of help-seeking. *Journal of Personality and Social Psychology, 75*, 778–787. doi:10.1037/0022-3514.75.3.778

Clark, L. A. (2007). Assessment and diagnosis of personality disorder: Perennial issues and an emerging reconceptualization. *Annual Review of Psychology, 58*, 227–257. doi:10.1146/annurev.psych.57.102904.190200

Clark, L. A., Vittengl, J., Kraft, D., & Jarrett, R. B. (2003). Separate personality traits from states to predict depression. *Journal of Personality Disorders, 17*, 152–172. doi:10.1521/pedi.17.2.152.23990

Clarkin, J. F., Levy, K. N., Lenzenweger, M. F., & Kernberg, O. F. (2007). Evaluating three treatments for borderline personality disorder: A multiwave study. *The American Journal of Psychiatry, 164*, 922–928. doi:10.1176/appi.ajp.164.6.922

Colli, A., Tanzilli, A., Dimaggio, G., & Lingiardi, V. (2014). Patient personality and therapist response: An empirical investigation. *The American Journal of Psychiatry, 171*, 102–108. doi:10.1176/appi.ajp.2013.13020224

Ganellen, R. J. (2007). Assessing normal and abnormal personality functioning: Strengths and weaknesses of self-report, observer, and performance-based methods. *Journal of Personality Assessment, 89*, 30–40. doi:10.1080/00223890701356987

Hirschfeld, R. M. A., Klerman, G. L., Clayton, P. J., Keller, M. B., McDonald-Scott, P., & Larkin, B. H. (1983). Assessing personality: Effects of the depressive state on trait measurement. *American Journal of Psychiatry, 140*, 695–699.

Huprich, S. K. (2004). The evolution of cognitive therapy for personality disorders: Convergence in theories and therapies. [Review of the book *Cognitive therapy of personality disorders* (2nd ed.), by A. T. Beck, A. Freeman, & D. D. Davis]. *PsycCRITIQUES, 49*(Suppl. 2). doi:10.1037/040004

Huprich, S. K., & Bornstein, R. F. (2007). Categorical and dimensional assessment of personality disorders: A consideration of the issues. *Journal of Personality Assessment, 89*, 3–15. doi:10.1080/00223890701356904

Huprich, S. K., Bornstein, R. F., & Schmitt, T. A. (2011). Self-report methodology is insufficient for improving the assessment and classification of Axis II personality disorders. *Journal of Personality Disorders, 25*, 557–570.

John, O. P., & Robins, R. W. (1994). Accuracy and bias in self-perception: Individual differences in self-enhancement and the role of narcissism. *Journal of Personality and Social Psychology, 66*, 206–219. doi:10.1037/0022-3514.66.1.206

Kelly, G. A. (1969). Hostility [Presidential address, Clinical Division, American Psychological Association]. In B. Maher (Ed.), *Clinical psychology and personality: The selected papers of George Kelly* (pp. 267–280). New York, NY: Wiley. (Original work published 1957)

Kihlstrom, J. F. (2008). The psychological unconscious. In O. P. John, R. W. Robins, & L. A. Pervin (Eds.), *Handbook of personality* (3rd ed., pp. 583–602). New York, NY: Guilford Press.

Kohut, H. (1977). *The restoration of the self*. New York, NY: International Universities Press.

Kolar, D. W., Funder, D. C., & Colvin, C. R. (1996). Comparing the accuracy of personality judgments by the self and knowledgeable others. *Journal of Personality, 64*, 311–337. doi:10.1111/j.1467-6494.1996.tb00513.x

Krueger, R. F., Eaton, N. R., Clark, L. A., Watson, D., Markon, K. E., Derringer, J., . . . Livesley, W. J. (2011). Deriving an empirical structure of personality pathology for *DSM–5*. *Journal of Personality Disorders, 25*, 170–191. doi:10.1521/pedi.2011.25.2.170

LeDoux, J. E. (1989). Cognitive-emotional interactions in the brain. *Cognition and Emotion, 3*, 267–289. doi:10.1080/02699938908412709

LeDoux, J. E. (1995). Emotion: Clues from the brain. *Annual Review of Psychology, 46*, 209–235. doi:10.1146/annurev.ps.46.020195.001233

McCrae, R. R., & Costa, P. T., Jr. (2008). The five-factor theory of personality. In O. P. John, R. W. Robins, & L. A. Pervin (Eds.), *Handbook of personality* (3rd ed., pp. 159–181). New York, NY: Guilford Press.

Meyer, G. J., Finn, S. E., Eyde, L. D., Kay, G. G., Moreland, K. L., Dies, R. R., . . . Reed, G. M. (2001). Psychological testing and psychological assessment: A review of evidence and issues. *American Psychologist, 56*, 128–165. doi:10.1037/0003-066X.56.2.128

Mischel, W. (1968). *Personality and assessment*. New York, NY: Wiley.

Mischel, W. (1973). Toward a cognitive social learning reconceptualization of personality. *Psychological Review, 80*, 252–283. doi:10.1037/h0035002

Mischel, W. (1984). Convergences and challenges in the search for consistency. *American Psychologist, 39*, 351–364. doi:10.1037/0003-066X.39.4.351

Mischel, W., & Shoda, Y. (1995). A cognitive–affective system theory of personality: Reconceptualizing situations, dispositions, dynamics, and invariance in personality structure. *Psychological Review, 102*, 246–268. doi:10.1037/0033-295X.102.2.246

Mischel, W., & Shoda, Y. (2008). Toward a unified theory of personality: Integrating dispositions and processing dynamics within the cognitive–affective personality system. In O. P. John, R. W. Robins, & L. A. Pervin (Eds.), *Handbook of personality* (3rd ed., pp. 208–241). New York, NY: Guilford Press.

Morey, L. C. (2010). Personality disorders in childhood and adolescence: Conceptual challenges. *Journal of Psychopathology and Behavioral Assessment, 32*, 544–550. doi:10.1007/s10862-010-9200-y

Oltmanns, T. F., & Turkheimer, E. (2006). Perceptions of self and others regarding pathological personality traits. In R. F. Krueger & J. L. Tackett (Eds.), *Personality and psychopathology* (pp. 71–111). New York, NY: Guilford Press.

Rhadigan, C., & Huprich, S. K. (2012). The utility of the cognitive–affective processing system in the diagnosis of personality disorders: Some preliminary evidence. *Journal of Personality Disorders, 26*, 162–178. doi:10.1521/pedi.2012.26.2.162

Robinson, M. D., & Gordon, K. H. (2011). Personality dynamics: Insights from the personality social cognitive literature. *Journal of Personality Assessment, 93*, 161–176. doi:10.1080/00223891.2010.542534

Roche, M. J., Pincus, A. L., Conroy, D. E., Hyde, A. L., & Ram, N. (2012). Pathological narcissism and interpersonal behavior in daily life. *Personality Disorders: Theory, Research, and Treatment, 4*, 315–323. doi:10.1037/a0030798

Rogers, C. R. (1961). *On becoming a person*. Boston, MA: Houghton Mifflin.

Rottman, B. M., Ahn, W., Sanislow, C. A., & Kim, N. S. (2009). Can clinicians recognize *DSM–IV* personality disorders from five-factor model descriptions of patient cases? *The American Journal of Psychiatry, 166*, 427–433. doi:10.1176/appi.ajp.2008.08070972

Samuel, D. B., & Widiger, T. A. (2008). A meta-analytic review of the relationships between the five-factor model and *DSM–IV–TR* personality disorders: A facet level analysis. *Clinical Psychology Review, 28*, 1326–1342. doi:10.1016/j.cpr.2008.07.002

Saulsman, L. M., & Page, A. C. (2004). The five-factor model and personality disorder empirical literature: A meta-analytic review. *Clinical Psychology Review, 23*, 1055–1085. doi:10.1016/j.cpr.2002.09.001

Schultheiss, O. C. (2008). Implicit motives. In O. P. John, R. W. Robins, & L. A. Pervin (Eds.), *Handbook of personality* (3rd ed., pp. 603–633). New York, NY: Guilford Press.

Skodol, A. E., Bender, D. S., Morey, L. C., Clark, L. A., Oldham, J. M., Alarcon, R. D., . . . Siever, L. J. (2011). Personality disorder types proposed for *DSM–5*. *Journal of Personality Disorders, 25*, 136–169. doi:10.1521/pedi.2011.25.2.136

Spitzer, R. L., First, M. B., Shedler, J., Westen, D., & Skodol, A. (2008). Clinical utility of five dimensional systems for personality diagnosis. *Journal of Nervous and Mental Disease, 196*, 356–374. doi:10.1097/NMD.0b013e3181710950

Westen, D. (1997). Divergences between clinical and research methods for assessing personality disorders: Implications for research and the evolution of Axis II. *The American Journal of Psychiatry, 154*, 895–903.

Widiger, T. A., Lynam, D. R., Miller, J. D., & Oltmanns, T. F. (2012). Measures to assess maladaptive variants of the five-factor model. *Journal of Personality Assessment, 94*, 450–455. doi:10.1080/00223891.2012.677887

Widiger, T. A., & Simonsen, E. (2005). Alternative dimensional models of personality disorder: Finding common ground. *Journal of Personality Disorders, 19*, 110–130. doi:10.1521/pedi.19.2.110.62628

Young, J. E. (1994). *Cognitive therapy for personality disorders: A schema-focused approach* (Rev. ed.). Sarasota, FL: Professional Resource Press.

Zimmerman, M. (2011). A critique of the proposed prototype rating system for personality disorders in DSM–5. *Journal of Personality Disorders, 25*, 206–221. doi:10.1521/pedi.2011.25.2.206

17

THE LINK BETWEEN PERSONALITY THEORY AND PSYCHOLOGICAL TREATMENT: A SHIFTING TERRAIN

JOHN F. CLARKIN, NICOLE M. CAIN, AND W. JOHN LIVESLEY

Personality disorders are prevalent (10.56% median prevalence across studies; Lenzenweger, 2008) and debilitating, and they have a powerful impact on work functioning, interpersonal, and intimate relations. However, there are many impediments to the treatment of patients with a personality disorder, not the least of which are the controversies in defining personality disorder, the range of severity across the disorders, the difficulties in identifying the key dimensions of personality dysfunction, and the paucity of treatment research on the majority of the personality disorder types.

In this chapter, we briefly review the major theories of personality functioning and personality disorder that have been utilized in empirical efforts to treat patients with various personality disorders. Due to the major focus on borderline personality disorder (BPD) and the paucity of treatment research on the other personality disorders, we focus primarily on the treatments for BPD. We examine the limits of the use of personality disorder theory to date in informing manualized treatments and suggest future avenues of development.

http://dx.doi.org/10.1037/14549-018
Personality Disorders: Toward Theoretical and Empirical Integration in Diagnosis and Assessment,
S. K. Huprich (Editor)

With the background of the major theories reviewed in this volume, we examine the link between the major theories of personality disorder and how they inform the clinical tasks of client assessment and treatment articulation. The link between personality disorder theory and treatment is articulated in the treatment manuals that describe treatments for the personality disorders.

THEORY BEHIND THE DIAGNOSIS OF PERSONALITY DISORDER

Challenges for the Definition of Personality Disorder

The creation of a separate axis for the diagnosis of personality disorder in the third edition of the *Diagnostic and Statistical Manual of Mental Disorders* (*DSM–III*; American Psychiatric Association, 1980) was a boon to those interested in the personality disorders, and it provided a tremendous stimulus to the investigation of the pathology and treatment of these disorders. In the context of this chapter, it should be noted that the *DSM–III* heralded itself as being "atheoretical." In fact, the personality disorders in *DSM–III* were described with a mixture of attitudes, emotions, and behaviors, with the clear intent of staying close to phenomenology and striving for reliability of assessment. In retrospect, it seems clear that the architects of the *DSM–III* either were totally unaware of or ignored basic knowledge at the time of personality functioning and personality theory. They proceeded to describe personality dysfunction without a clear basis in a theory of personality functioning.

This phenomenological approach, admittedly very thin on theory, resulted in the often-noted problems and difficulties of *DSM–III* and the fourth edition of the *Diagnostic and Statistical Manual of Mental Disorders* (*DSM–IV*; American Psychiatric Association, 1994). The polythetic approach to the diagnosis of supposedly 10 distinct personality disorder categories has resulted in heterogeneity among patients in one diagnostic category (see Lenzenweger, Clarkin, Yeomans, Kernberg, & Levy, 2008) and rampant "comorbidity" of the personality disorders. These difficulties with the personality diagnostic system led to the intense discussions of the Personality and Personality Disorders Work Group (PPDWG) in preparation for the fifth edition of the *Diagnostic and Statistical Manual of Mental Disorders* (*DSM–5*; American Psychiatric Association, 2013).

One can perceive the use of personality theory behind two aspects of the *DSM–5* Section III approach to personality disorders: the revised definition of personality disorder and the use of traits to capture dysfunctional areas of functioning. The core of personality disorder is defined as disturbances in self- and interpersonal functioning. Self-functioning is described by the domains of identity and self-direction, and interpersonal functioning is described by the domains of empathy and intimacy. This definition, adapted by the PPDWG, is in line with a growing consensus in the field that self- and other function-ing is at the center of personality and personality disorder (Bender & Skodol, 2007; Gunderson & Lyons-Ruth, 2008; Hengartner, Müller, Rodgers, Rössler, & Ajdacic-Gross, 2013; Horowitz, 2004; Livesley, 2001; Meyer & Pilkonis, 2005; Pincus, 2005). This is a view that has long been espoused in object relations theory (Kernberg, 1984). These difficulties in identity and inter-personal functioning are intertwined, just as attention and memory contribute to conceptions of self and others and lead to the final common pathway of interpersonal behavior.

The revised and improved definition of personality disorder in DSM–5 Section III may lead to a more refined assessment of the core aspects of per-sonality disorder and, in turn, to advancements in the assessment of outcome of treatment for these individuals. To date, the treatments for personality disorder have concentrated on the reduction of symptom behaviors and feelings. Although various treatments have obtained significant changes in symptoms, the core issues of self-functioning and interpersonal functioning have received less attention. In the remainder of this chapter, we examine how the major theories of personality disorder conceptualize these central areas of self- and interpersonal functioning.

In the progression to DSM–5, there has been a perceptible shift in emphasis from categories of personality disorder (10 in DSM–IV to six in DSM–5, Section III) to dimensions of dysfunction. Both genes and neuro-cognitive dysfunction are not specific to a particular diagnostic category; rather, there are functions across diagnostic categories that are potential foci for therapeutic attention and change. It is now clear that molecular genetics will not provide a simple, gene-based classification of psychiatric illnesses. Rather, genetic findings will likely delineate specific biological pathways and domains of psychopathology (Craddock, 2013). In this regard, the National Institute of Mental Health declared an initiative to focus research not on categories of mental illness but on systems of neurocognitive functioning and dysfunction that extend across diagnostic categories (Sanislow et al., 2010). The changes to DSM–5 were based in the realization that the biological underpinnings of psychiatric disorders do not support current categories but rather suggest domains of dysfunction at various levels of severity (Hyman, 2011). To capture domains of dysfunction in addition to the core issues of self- and interpersonal functioning, the PPDWG introduced trait assessment.

Trait Theory and Assessment

With the introduction of traits into the diagnostic process of person-ality disorders in DSM–5 Section III, it is relevant to examine trait theory and the adequacy of trait assessment to planning treatment of individuals with personality pathology. Major dimensional models of personality and personality pathology based on traits converge on four higher-order traits: neuroticism/negative affectivity/emotional dysregulation, extraversion/positive affectivity, dissocial/antagonism, and constraint/compulsivity/conscientiousness (Trull, 2006). The *DSM–5* Section III has chosen to include five broad domains of personality trait variation: negative affectivity, detachment, antagonism, disinhibition, and psychoticism.

Traits describe individuals in terms of their stable patterns across environmental situations. This is basically a descriptive process, and, as such, trait theory fails to explain how or why the behaviors occur. It has been pointed out that only with the study of personality processes can one begin to understand how and why the personality traits have their impact (Hampson, 2012). With the combination of personality traits and personality processes (Caspi, Roberts, & Shiner, 2005; Cervone, 2005; Mischel & Shoda, 2008) one can achieve a fuller picture of personality functioning. This has implications for the clinical assessment of the individual with suspected personality pathology. The rating of salient traits and their severity is only the first step in treatment planning, and it must be followed with interview assessment of the situations in which the troublesome trait is manifested and details about the specific context.

THEORY OF PERSONALITY AS A BASIC FOUNDATION

It is commonly assumed that there is continuity between personality functioning and personality dysfunction. From this point of view, an empirically supported theory of personality functioning is a necessary foundation for progressing to a comprehensive understanding of personality dysfunction. Mischel and Shoda (2008) articulated a cognitive-affective processing model of personality functioning that is supported by years of empirical research in order to provide an overall framework in which the existing knowledge of personality functioning can be organized. This cognitive-affective processing system (CAPS) focuses on the processes by which individuals construe situations and themselves in adapting to the environment. Such a processing approach is most relevant to therapists who closely examine in the therapeutic context the cognitive-affective processing of the client with personality disorder. This metatheory emphasizes five levels of experience: (a) an organized pattern of activation of internal cognitive-affective units (e.g., conceptions of self and others, expectancies and beliefs, affects, goals and values, self-regulatory plans); (b) behavioral expressions of this internal processing system; (c) self- and other perception of these behaviors over time; (d) construction of one's typical environment; and (e) the predispositions at the biological and genetic levels of existence. This framework suggests that personality dysfunction can occur at multiple levels, and the assessment of these crucial areas could guide targets for intervention. Lacking a comprehensive theory of personality pathology, we suggest, the therapist should focus on the domains of dysfunction and how they are manifest in the client's particular environment.

CAPS theory has relevance beyond normal personality functioning. From this perspective, personality types are composed of individuals who have a common organization of relations among mediating units. For example, those individuals who share anxieties about interpersonal rejection and abandonment could be considered a type. These individuals scan the environment for cues about rejection. Anxiously expecting and primed to find such cues, they suffer from subsequent negative feelings of resentment and rage. It is not surprising that individuals with features of BPD were high on measures of rejection sensitivity (Ayduk et al., 2008). In addition and most relevant to interpersonal functioning, those with high rejection sensitivity combined with low executive control had increased borderline features, whereas those with high rejection sensitivity combined with high executive control had attenuated borderline features.

With the CAPS model of personality in mind, the therapist would attend both to observable behavior in the domains of dysfunction and to how the patient experiences his or her particular conceptualizations of self–other interactions, which guide behavior in specific environmental settings. With reference to these nodal points of interest from personality theory, we examine how major theories of personality dysfunction conceptualize and assess the cognitive-affective units or conceptions of self and other; in particular, how these are demonstrated in interpersonal behavior, perception of self over time, and the particular environments the individual seeks out.

In this chapter, the focus is on the use of personality disorder theory and how it informs psychological treatment. One can examine the link between personality disorder theory and psychological treatment by examining the treatment manuals that apply theory to intervention strategies. In our discussion of each theory and its use in treatment, we focus specifically on how the theory explicates self-functioning and interpersonal functioning (see Table 17.1).

PERSONALITY THEORY BEHIND COGNITIVE–BEHAVIORAL THERAPY

Theory

Cognitive and cognitive–behavioral theories of personality disorder emphasize the role of dysfunctional beliefs in the etiology and maintenance of personality pathology (Beck, Freeman, & Associates, 1990). Dysfunctional

TABLE 17.1
Self- and Interpersonal Functioning: Central Constructs and Related Treatment Strategies

Theory	Central construct	Related treatment strategy
Cognitive–affective processing system (CAPS)	Cognitive affective units	
Cognitive–behavioral	Schemas	Examination of dysfunctional schemas
Attachment	Internal working models	Focus on increasing mentalization
Object relations	Object relations dyad	Integration of the object relations dyads by clarification, confrontation, interpretation
Interpersonal	Interpersonal signatures	Examination of parataxic distortions

beliefs such as "I cannot tolerate unpleasant emotion," which often characterize individuals with BPD, reflect one or more conceptual themes that link a patient's developmental history, compensatory strategies, and dysfunctional reactions to current situations. If we incorporate the behavioral perspective, these dysfunctional reactions are often patterns of maladaptive learned behaviors that must be replaced through the learning of more adaptive responses to situations, often utilizing exposures and skills training. Principles of cognitive–behavioral therapy (CBT) have been extensively used to guide the development of dialectical behavior therapy (DBT; Linehan, 1993) and schema-focused psychotherapy (Young, 1990).

Relevance of Theory to Assessment and Treatment

Linehan (1993) described DBT as the application of a number of cognitive–behavioral intervention strategies to the problems of individuals with BPD. Thus, Linehan used the background of cognitive–behavioral theory and its related treatment strategies to an overall view of the coherence of the problems demonstrated by patients with BPD. Linehan conceptualized BPD as a dysfunction of the emotion regulation system resulting from biological irregularities combined with an invalidating environment. Given the nature of BPD, a number of aspects of DBT set it apart from traditional CBT, such as the focus on acceptance and validation of behavior as it is in the current moment, an emphasis on treating behaviors that interfere with therapy, an emphasis on developing a therapeutic alliance with the patient, and the use of dialectical processes to counter the patient's polarized thinking. The core strategies of DBT include behavior chain analysis to identify target problem behaviors and their antecedents and consequences, skills training and a discussion of alternative behavioral solutions, and dialectical strategies to elicit a commitment from the patient to engage in the recommended treatment procedures. DBT emphasizes that all of these strategies must be used in the context of a validating atmosphere created by the therapist.

ATTACHMENT THEORY AND TREATMENT OF PERSONALITY DISORDERS

Theory

Attachment theory has gained a great deal of enthusiasm in current approaches to understanding animal and human behavior. John Bowlby (1969/1982, 1973, 1980), the father of attachment theory, was a Darwin scholar who integrated ideas from the theory of evolution with object relations theory, control systems theory, evolutionary biology, ethology, and cognitive psychology (Simpson & Belsky, 2008).

Central to attachment theory is the concept of the attachment behavioral system with its inherent motivation for the child to seek the proximity of the caregiver, which in turn increases the likelihood of security and survival. This attachment system enables the child to respond with a range of behaviors with the goal of attaining proximity to the caregiver. Over time, the successes and failures in attaining proximity to the caregiver lead to individual differences in the quality of the attachment. Secure attachment involves the mental representation of the caregiver as available and responsive to one's needs. Secure attachment involves using the caregiver as a secure base that enables the child to explore the environment. In contrast, children with insecure attachment have internalized a nonresponsive caregiver, and the result is that these children experience anxiety and anger, especially in the face of threat from the environment. The mental representation constructed over time by the child through interactions with the caregiver was termed by Bowlby the *internal working model* (see Bretherton & Munholland, 2008, for further details). According to Bowlby (1969/1982), during the end of the first year and during the second and third years, the child constructs a working (i.e., imaginative, adaptive, and based on real-life experience) model of self and others in interaction.

Relevance of Theory to Assessment and Treatment

Bateman and Fonagy (2004) based mentalization-based therapy (MBT) on attachment theory combined with a comprehensive integration of developmental research. They posit that the disruption of early affectional bonds leads to maladaptive attachment bonds but also undermines a range of capabilities such as emotion regulation, attentional control, and the ability to make sense of the actions of oneself and others in terms of intentional mental states (i.e., mentalization). Often having a background of abuse and neglect, patients with BPD are prone to hyperactivating strategies (i.e., attempts to mentalize without an integration of cognition and affect) and deactivating strategies (i.e., minimizing and avoiding affectively charged content) in the face of environmental stress.

As the name of the treatment shows, the concept of mentalization is central to MBT, and this concept has become more differentiated by these authors. The central concept of mentalizing as the capacity to understand self and others in terms of mental states is seen as having four intersecting dimensions: implicit (reflexive, fast) versus explicit (focused awareness), internal (focus on own or others' internal states) versus external (focus on behavior), self (attention to self) and other (perceptive reading of others), and cognitive and affective mentalizing (Bateman & Fonagy, 2010). BPD is characterized by a bias toward implicit, automatic, nonconscious, intuitive, impressionist thinking about mental states that contributes to problematic interpersonal relations.

The aim of MBT is to develop a therapeutic process in which the mind of the patient is the central focus. The therapist establishes an enduring attachment relationship with the patient while stimulating the patient to mentalize. The objective is to assist patients in exploring more fully how they think and feel about themselves and others, how these thoughts and feelings influence their behavior, and how distortions in these thoughts and feelings lead to maladaptive actions. The therapeutic stance is one of curiosity and open-mindedness in exploring the patient's sense of self.

In a randomized clinical trial of MBT for self-harm in adolescents, MBT was more effective than treatment as usual in reducing self-harm and depression (Rossouw & Fonagy, 2012). Most important for the relationship between theory and clinical interventions, both attachment status and mentalization were independent mediators of the clinical outcomes. Rossouw and Fonagy (2012) concluded that these results were consistent with the hypothesis that positive change in mentalization and improvement in interpersonal functioning would be expected to bring about a change in self-harm.

OBJECT RELATIONS THEORY AND TREATMENT OF PERSONALITY DISORDERS

Theory

Object relations theory (Jacobson, 1964; Kernberg, 1980; Klein, 1957; Mahler, 1971) emphasizes that the drives of libido and aggression described by Freud are always experienced in relation to a specific other (i.e., an object). Internalized object relations are the building blocks of psychological structures and serve as the organizers of motivation and behavior. These building blocks are units composed of a representation of the self and a representation of the other, linked by an affect related to or representing a drive. These units of self, other, and the affect linking them are object relations dyads. It is not assumed that the "self" and the "object" in the dyad are accurate internal representations of the entirety of the self or the other; nor are they accurate representations of real interactions in the past. Rather, they are representations of the self and the other as these were experienced and internalized at specific, affectively charged moments in time in the course of early development and then processed by internal forces such as primary affects and fantasies.

Personality represents the integration of behavior patterns with their roots in temperament, cognitive capacities, character, and internalized value systems (Kernberg & Caligor, 2005). The individual with a healthy personality organization functions with an integrated and coherent concept of self and of significant others. The former includes both an internal, coherent sense of self and behaviors that reflect self-coherence. This coherent sense of self is basic to self-esteem, enjoyment, a capacity to derive pleasure from relationships with others and from commitments to work, and a sense of continuity through time. The individual with a normal personality organization has the capacity to experience a range of complex and well-modulated affects without the loss of impulse control. A coherent and integrated sense of self contributes to the realization of one's capacities, desires, and long-range goals. Likewise, a coherent and integrated conception of others contributes to a realistic evaluation of others, involving empathy and social tact and thus the ability to interact and relate successfully. The combination of an integrated sense of self and of others contributes to the capacity for mature interdependence with others, involving a capacity to make emotional commitments to others and simultaneously maintain self-coherence and autonomy.

Disruptions in the infant–caregiver interaction lead to deviations in this optimal developmental path that may lead to negative experiences taking on a more dominant role in the developing mind. Disruptions in the relationship between the child and caregivers and the presence of trauma have a profound effect upon the developing conception of self and others (Harter, 1999). Whereas early sexual abuse occurs in the history of some patients with BPD, the additional factors of caregiver neglect, indifference, and empathic failures have profound deleterious effects (Cicchetti, Beeghly, Carlson, & Toth, 1990; Westen, 1993). Children reared in these disturbed environments form insecure attachments with their primary caregivers (Cicchetti et al., 1990; Westen, 1993). Such attachments interfere with the development of capacities for effortful control and self-regulation, and the internalization of conceptions of self and other is compromised by intense negative affect and defensive operations that distort the information system in an attempt to avoid pain.

In the normally developing child, there is a gradual integration over the first few years of life of these extreme good and bad representations of self and other. The resulting internal representations of self and others are more complex and realistic, as they acknowledge the reality that all people are a mix of good and bad attributes and are capable of being satisfying at some times and frustrating at others. In future patients with BPD, this process of integration does not evolve, and a more permanent division between the idealized and persecutory sectors of peak affect experiences remains as a stable, pathological intrapsychic structure. This separation "protects" the idealized representations, which are imbued with warm, loving feelings toward the object perceived as satisfying, from the negative representations, which are associated with the affects of anxiety, rage, and hatred.

Relevance of Theory to Assessment and Treatment

In view of the centrality of disturbances in representations of self and other with related negative affects, the focus of transference-focused psychotherapy (TFP; Clarkin, Yeomans, & Kernberg, 2006) is the examination and eventual change in the self–other representations that the patient brings to the relationship with the therapist and that are reflected in his or her relationships with others in the present. The treatment begins with a carefully structured verbal contract that enables the patient and therapist to create a consistent setting in which the relationships with others and their internal representations can be examined for lack of reflection, polarized and affect-laden extremes, and gaps in understanding. TFP has been shown to significantly reduce symptoms (Clarkin, Levy, Lenzenweger, & Kernberg, 2007; Doering et al., 2010). Most important to the relationship between personality theory and its influence on the treatment, TFP has demonstrated a significant increase in mentalization (Levy et al., 2006), as hypothesized by the model.

CONTEMPORARY INTERPERSONAL THEORY AND TREATMENT OF PERSONALITY DISORDERS

Theory

Interpersonal behavior has often been viewed as a fundamental component of personality (Benjamin, 2003; Kiesler, 1996; Leary, 1957; Pincus & Ansell, 2012). The contemporary interpersonal theory of personality originated from Sullivan's (1953) relational model. Sullivan (1953) considered interpersonal relations and the self-concept to be central in the development of normal and abnormal personality and wrote, "Personality is the relatively enduring pattern of recurrent interpersonal situations which characterize a human life" (p. 111). Sullivan argued that the interpersonal situation underlies the development, maintenance, and flexibility of personality through the continuous adjustments that an individual makes in response to biological needs, security needs, and esteem needs.

Relevance of Theory to Assessment and Treatment

Contemporary interpersonal theory argues that the use of the Inventory of Interpersonal Problems (IIP; Alden, Wiggins, & Pincus, 1990) provides a useful way of conceptualizing the various types of interpersonal difficulties one sees in clinical practice across the range of personality disorders. The IIP provides a way to articulate the dynamic interpersonal processes that are both adaptive and maladaptive. It contains eight subscales that can be conceptually organized in a circular manner along the dimensions of dominance and affiliation. These dimensions provided the basis for Leary's (1957) interpersonal circumplex and are considered to be the basic elements of interpersonal behavior (Wiggins, 1991). Circumplex quadrants are often described as representing a mixture of the underlying dimensions (i.e., hostile dominance or friendly submissiveness), and they are useful summary descriptors of interpersonal behavior. The IIP also contains a general factor, which is equivalent to the mean level of interpersonal distress reported by the patient across his or her interpersonal interactions (Tracey, Rounds, & Gurtman, 1996). The maladaptive behaviors sampled by this measure can be considered extreme variants of the underlying interpersonal dispositions of the client.

Research using the IIP suggests that the core phenomenology of a subset of personality disorders may be substantially and uniquely described by relatively extreme and rigid interpersonal themes (Horowitz et al., 2006); in particular, the Paranoid (vindictive interpersonal problems), Schizoid (cold, avoidant interpersonal problems), Avoidant (avoidant, nonassertive interpersonal problems), Dependent (exploitable interpersonal problems), Histrionic (intrusive interpersonal problems), and Narcissistic (domineering, vindictive interpersonal problems) personality disorders (Wiggins & Pincus, 1989). Other personality disorders (e.g., Borderline) do not appear to consistently present with a single, prototypic interpersonal theme on the IIP (Wright et al., 2013). This finding is consistent with previous research (Lenzenweger et al., 2008) showing diverse clinical presentations associated with BPD.

Contemporary interpersonal theory argues that maladaptive interpersonal patterns are enacted both inside and outside of the therapy, thus giving the therapist the opportunity to understand and explore the etiology and maintenance of these disturbed interpersonal patterns with the client in the present moment. The therapist acts as a *participant observer* (Sullivan, 1953) in the therapeutic relationship. Pincus and colleagues (Cain & Pincus, in press; Pincus, 2005; Pincus & Hopwood, 2012) have articulated a treatment approach that integrates contemporary interpersonal theory with an object-relations-based understanding of personality structure (Clarkin et al., 2006). The underlying premise is that interpersonal situations occur not only between self and other but also in the mind via mental representations. Following Kernberg's (1975, 1984) object relations theory, these internalizations often consist of a self-representation, an other-representation, and a linking affect. Thus, treatment can proceed via an articulation of the internalizations of self and other in which a sequence of clarifications, confrontations, and well-timed interpretations of current interactions (Clarkin et al., 2006) is utilized to identify, challenge, and ultimately understand the etiology and maintenance of maladaptive interpersonal patterns. This process leads to increased interpersonal awareness and social learning.

HAS THE TIME ARRIVED FOR THEORETICAL INTEGRATION?

Is the field prepared to construct a comprehensive theory of personality dysfunction that could guide research pursuits and clinical interventions? A truly comprehensive theory of personality dysfunction would need to attend to a number of crucial issues including the following: relationship between normal and abnormal personality, relation of personality pathology and affect regulation, personality pathology in nonclinical samples as well as those from health-seeking samples, longitudinal course of personality pathology, the genetic and biological underpinnings of personality pathology, relationship of personality pathology to other domains of pathology, and the validity of the personality disorder constructs (Lenzenweger & Clarkin, 2005).

The review of personality theory in this chapter suggests that the field has multiple theories that can explain parts of personality functioning and dysfunction. Livesley (2001) suggested that our field is in a Kuhnian pretheoretical stage in which facts and more facts are articulated without a unifying theoretical understanding. Theoretical integration concerning the personality disorders will advance as the empirical research on the disorders progresses from the phenomenology of the overt disturbed behaviors to the mental representations of self and other, with an integration of social neurocognitive science that offers a window on how the brain functions under social circumstances.

Theoretical integration will take time, and the clinician cannot wait for the emergence of a comprehensive theory of the personality and personality disorders. Rather, the clinician needs a near-experience model of personality and personality dysfunction as a map to assessment and intervention. A framework for treatment integration must provide such a near-experience model.

The current review suggests that whereas the field is not prepared to generate a comprehensive theory of personality disorders to guide research and clinical practice, there are a limited number of general criteria for the treatment of individuals with personality disorder that can be articulated at the present time. Treatment must introduce structure, especially for the patients suffering from more severe personality disorders. In working with individuals who have deficits in self and interpersonal functioning, the therapist must attend constantly to the ongoing nature of the therapeutic alliance. The foci of intervention must begin with symptoms, especially dangerous ones such as suicidal behavior, followed by affect regulation, and only then can begin to concentrate on the central issues in personality disorder of the functioning of self and self in relationship to others. Initial assessment of patients can follow the guidelines of *DSM–5* Section III; that is, assessment of self- and other functioning, attention to categorical assignment, and assessment of key traits. The trait information must be enhanced by clinical interview assessment (see Clarkin & Livesley, in press) specifying in what environmental situations the troublesome traits are manifested.

The field of personality disorders is poised for a new round of treatment development studies, which is emerging in view of several conditions. First, the boundaries between the personality disorder categories in *DSM–5* are not clear. There is a growing awareness of shared domains of dysfunction across the personality disorder categories. These domains would include not only the essential components of self and interpersonal dysfunction but also the neurocognitive-psychological domains (and related traits) such as negative affect and affect dysregulation. Second, there is a need to approach a more comprehensive theory of personality disorder that integrates a conception of normal functioning, developmental pathways, and the neurobiological underpinnings for adjustment. Finally, treatment development for the personality disorders will focus on salient subgroups of patients with personality disorder, based less on heterogeneous categories (e.g., BPD) and more on identifiable domains of dysfunction matched to treatment modules.

ALTERNATIVES TO THEORETICAL
INTEGRATION AT THE PRESENT TIME

The field of psychotherapy has historically emphasized the schools of treatment with their related theories and groups of followers. This phenomenon has both helped clinicians to be immersed in a particular approach to treatment that fits their predilections and provides them with a support group. On the other hand, this emphasis can lead to competition and bias against other orientations (Larson, Broberg, & Kaldo, 2013), and it may result in the discarding of alternative approaches that might be quite helpful for our clients.

The field is currently shifting due to a number of current forces. We have noted movement away from the diagnosis of discrete personality disorders to a focus on the domains of dysfunction, conceptualized as dimensional in nature, whether seen as traits or as neurobiologically based domains of function. In this regard, one would not expect treatment development for the 10 (in *DSM–IV*) or six (in *DSM–5* Section III) personality disorders but rather treatment of dimensions of dysfunction across the disorders. Second, the empirically investigated treatments for BPD, the disorder that has attracted the lion's share of treatment development, have been shown to significantly reduce symptoms but with no discernible differences between the treatments.

In the face of these issues, the clinician has a limited number of choices. One can obtain special training in one of the empirically supported treatments and use that treatment for patients meeting the specific personality disorder diagnosis (e.g., BPD), and then use its general orientation for the other disorders with similar or related domains of dysfunction. Alternatively, one can look for general principles of treatment across the treatments and apply them with clinical judgment to patients with various combinations of personality disorder types.

With these issues in mind, we (Livesley, DiMaggio, & Clarkin, in press) are recommending an integrated treatment approach that is probably already the most popular approach by clinicians to the treatment of clients with personality disorders. Even though this is the situation, we think it remains important to articulate an integrated approach to the treatment of personality disorders in order to clarify the issues and refine the approach. An articulation of an integrated approach to treatment may also legitimize the wise integrative approaches of many clinicians who worry that in doing so they are violating the empirical treatment recommendations.

One way to tailor the treatment to the individual is to assess the individual for domains of dysfunction and match treatment modules to these domains. We (Livesley et al., in press) have termed this process *integrated modular treatment*. We describe modules of treatment as an interconnected series of therapist interventions (i.e., techniques) having a specific dysfunctional target. We have selected treatment modules from larger intervention packages that have been empirically investigated (e.g., Bateman & Fonagy, 2006; Clarkin et al., 2006; Linehan, 1993) or treatment modules devised by clinical researchers with experience intervening with specific target areas (e.g., Safran & Muran, 2000).

There are two overarching modules of treatment for those suffering from personality disorder: (a) general treatment modules that are used to structure the treatment, enhance motivation for change, and manage the relationship between patient and therapist; and (b) specific treatment modules for specific domains of dysfunction, such as affect dysregulation, interpersonal functioning, and domains of self-functioning (self-esteem and self-definition).

An integrated approach is an invitation to drop categorization of strategies and techniques related to therapy school (e.g., cognitive–behavioral, psychodynamic) and instead focus on patient domains of dysfunction and a variety of ways to approach them with effective treatment modules. Our attempt at an integrated treatment approach is a form of technical rather than theoretical integration, with a recognition that all theories of personality and its pathology have important points about selected aspects of personality functioning and that no comprehensive theory exists today.

SUMMARY AND CONCLUSIONS

There is an intense human need to understand the functioning of self and others. This function has survival value and, when successful, can lead to satisfying attempts to cooperate and compete with others. Architects of therapeutic interventions for the personality disorders forge links between personality theory and treatment interventions. As we have seen, the architects of treatments for severe personality disorder (several of which are empirically supported) have applied theories to central aspects of BPD pathology (i.e., self- and other functioning), with related constructs such as emotion dysregulation, an inability to mentalize or understand in depth the experience of self and others, and identity diffusion (see Table 17.1). A unifying element across the theories is the focus on the pathology of the individual with the particular personality disorder. The theories provide a somewhat different conceptualization of the problem domains but often lead to similar therapeutic interventions, such as attention to building a positive therapeutic alliance, providing structure, encouraging change, and closely examining how the patient relates to others. In this regard, the outcomes in the treatments and their positive change do not validate the individual theories but rather provide evidence that the common or overlapping strategies of intervention have been successful. Furthermore, whereas the treatment packages with multiple types of intervention have a significant effect on symptoms, few data are available on the mechanisms by which the treatments work or on the impact on self- and other functioning, the very heart of personality disorder.

Multiple personality disorder theories have guided the articulation of various treatments that have been empirically supported. We are in the interesting situation of having treatments informed by very different theories of personality disorder and functioning, all of which show significant improvement for patients' symptoms but without real differences in outcome between them (Levy, Ellison, Temes, & Khalsa, 2012). What is the meaning of this situation? Are the differences between the theories behind the treatments irrelevant? Could it be that the therapist needs a theory to guide his or her actions, but the particular theory is not that important? In this context, Bateman (2012) recently called for an increasingly coherent theory of personality disorder that could be translated into an understanding of mechanisms of change that, in turn, could inform a coherent treatment package. Such an effort will probably inform the next wave of treatment development for patients with personality disorders.

REFERENCES

Alden, L. E., Wiggins, J. S., & Pincus, A. L. (1990). Construction of circumplex scales for the Inventory of Interpersonal Problems. *Journal of Personality Assessment, 55,* 521–536. doi:10.1207/s15327752jpa5503&4_10

American Psychiatric Association. (1980). *Diagnostic and statistical manual of mental disorders* (3rd ed.). Washington, DC: Author.

American Psychiatric Association. (1994). *Diagnostic and statistical manual of mental disorders* (4th ed.). Washington, DC: Author.

American Psychiatric Association. (2013). *Diagnostic and statistical manual of mental disorders* (5th ed.). Arlington, VA: Author.

Ayduk, O., Zayas, V., Downey, G., Cole, A. B., Shoda, Y., & Michele, W. (2008). Rejection sensitivity and executive control: Joint predictors of borderline personality features. *Journal of Research in Personality, 42,* 151–168. doi:10.1016/j.jrp.2007.04.002

Bateman, A. W. (2012). Treating borderline personality disorder in clinical practice. *American Journal of Psychiatry, 169,* 560–563. doi:10.1176/appi.ajp.2012.12030341

Bateman, A. W., & Fonagy, P. (2004). *Psychotherapy for borderline personality disorder: Mentalization-based treatment.* Oxford, England: Oxford University Press.

Bateman, A., & Fonagy, P. (2006). *Mentalization-based treatment for borderline personality disorder: A practical guide.* Oxford, England: Oxford University Press.

Bateman, A., & Fonagy, P. (2010). Mentalization-based treatment and borderline personality disorder. In J. F. Clarkin, P. Fonagy, & G. O. Gabbard (Eds.), *Psychodynamic psychotherapy for personality disorders: A clinical handbook* (pp. 187–208). Washington, DC: American Psychiatric Publishing.

Beck, A. T., Freeman, A., & Associates. (1990). *Cognitive therapy of personality disorders*. New York, NY: Guilford Press.

Bender, D. S., & Skodol, A. E. (2007). Borderline personality as self–other representational disturbance. *Journal of Personality Disorders, 21,* 500–517. doi:10.1521/pedi.2007.21.5.500

Benjamin, L. S. (2003). *Interpersonal reconstructive therapy: Promoting change in nonresponders.* New York, NY: Guilford Press.

Bowlby, J. (1973). *Attachment and loss: Vol. 2. Separation: Anxiety and anger.* New York, NY: Basic Books.

Bowlby, J. (1980). *Attachment and loss: Vol. 3. Loss: Sadness and depression.* New York, NY: Basic Books.

Bowlby, J. (1982). *Attachment and loss: Vol. 1. Attachment* (2nd ed.). New York, NY: Basic Books. (Original work published 1969)

Bretherton, I., & Munholland, K. A. (2008). Internal working models in attachment relationships. In J. Cassidy & P. R. Shaver (Eds.), *Handbook of attachment: Theory, research, and clinical applications* (2nd ed., pp. 102–127). New York, NY: Guilford Press.

Cain, N. M., & Pincus, A. L. (in press). Treating maladaptive interpersonal signatures. In J. Livesley, G. DiMaggio, & J. F. Clarkin (Eds.), *An integrated modular approach to the treatment of the personality disorders.* New York, NY: Guilford Press.

Caspi, A., Roberts, B. W., & Shiner, R. (2005). Personality development. *Annual Review of Psychology, 56,* 453–484. doi:10.1146/annurev.psych.55.090902.141913

Cervone, D. (2005). Personality architecture: Within-person structures and processes. *Annual Review of Psychology, 56,* 423–452. doi:10.1146/annurev.psych.56.091103.070133

Cicchetti, D., Beeghly, M., Carlson, V., & Toth, S. (1990). The emergence of the self in atypical populations. In D. Cicchetti & M. Beeghly (Eds.), *The self in transition: Infancy to childhood* (pp. 309–344). Chicago, IL: University of Chicago Press.

Clarkin, J. F., Levy, K. N., Lenzenweger, M. F., & Kernberg, O. F. (2007). Evaluating three treatments for borderline personality disorder: A multiwave study. *American Journal of Psychiatry, 164,* 922–928. doi:10.1176/appi.ajp.164.6.922

Clarkin, J. F., & Livesley, W. J. (in press). Formulation and treatment planning. In W. J. Livesley, G. DiMaggio, & J. F. Clarkin (Eds.), *Integrated modular treatment for personality disorder.* New York, NY: Guilford Press.

Clarkin, J. F., Yeomans, F. E., & Kernberg, O. F. (2006). *Psychotherapy of borderline disorder: Focusing on object relations.* Washington, DC: American Psychiatric Publishing.

Craddock, N. (2013). Genome-wide association studies: What a psychiatrist needs to know. *Advances in Psychiatric Treatment, 19*, 82–88. doi:10.1192/apt.bp.110.007906

Doering, S., Horz, S., Rentrop, M., Fischer-Kern, M., Schuster, P., Benecke, C., . . . Buchheim, P. (2010). Transference-focused psychotherapy vs. treatment by community psychotherapists for borderline personality disorder: Randomized controlled trial. *British Journal of Psychiatry, 196*, 389–395. doi:10.1192/bjp.bp.109.070177

Gunderson, J. G., & Lyons-Ruth, K. (2008). BPD's interpersonal hypersensitivity phenotype: A gene-environment-developmental model. *Journal of Personality Disorders, 22*, 22–41. doi:10.1521/pedi.2008.22.1.22

Hampson, S. E. (2012). Personality processes: Mechanisms by which personality traits "get outside the skin." *Annual Review of Psychology, 63*, 315–339. doi:10.1146/annurev-psych-120710-100419

Harter, S. (1999). *The construction of the self: A developmental perspective.* New York, NY: Guilford Press.

Hengartner, M., Müller, M., Rodgers, S., Rössler, W., & Ajdacic-Gross, V. (2013). Interpersonal functioning deficits in association with *DSM–IV* personality disorder dimensions. *Social Psychiatry and Psychiatric Epidemiology, 49*, 317–325. doi:10.1007/s00127-013-0707-x

Horowitz, L. M. (2004). *Interpersonal foundations of psychopathology.* Washington, DC: American Psychological Association.

Horowitz, L. M., Wilson, K. R., Turan, B., Zolotsev, P., Constantino, M. J., & Henderson, L. (2006). How interpersonal motives clarify the meaning of interpersonal behavior: A revised circumplex model. *Personality and Social Psychology Review, 10*, 67–86. doi:10.1207/s15327957pspr1001_4

Hyman, S. E. (2011). Diagnosis of mental disorders in light of modern genetics. In D. Regier, W. Narrow, E. Kuhl, & D. Kupfer (Eds.), *The conceptual evolution of DSM–5* (pp. 3–18). Washington, DC: American Psychiatric Publishing.

Jacobson, E. (1964). *The self and the object world.* New York, NY: International Universities Press.

Kernberg, O. F. (1975). *Borderline conditions and pathological narcissism.* New York, NY: Aaronson.

Kernberg, O. F. (1980). *Internal world and external reality: Object relations theory applied.* New York, NY: Aronson.

Kernberg, O. F. (1984). *Severe personality disorders: Psychotherapeutic strategies.* New Haven, CT: Yale University Press.

Kernberg, O. F., & Caligor, E. (2005). A psychoanalytic theory of personality disorders. In M. Lenzenweger & J. F. Clarkin (Eds.), *Major theories of personality disorder* (2nd ed., pp. 114–156). New York, NY: Guilford Press.

Kiesler, D. J. (1996). *Contemporary interpersonal theory and research: Personality psychopathology, and psychotherapy.* Hoboken, NJ: Wiley.

Klein, M. (1957). *Envy and gratitude: A study of unconscious sources.* New York, NY: Basic Books.

Larson, B. P. M., Broberg, A. G., & Kaldo, V. (2013). Do psychotherapists with different theoretical orientations stereotype or prejudge each other? *Journal of Contemporary Psychotherapy, 43,* 169–178. doi:10.1007/s10879-013-9231-2

Leary, T. (1957). *Interpersonal diagnosis of personality.* New York, NY: Ronald Press.

Lenzenweger, M. F. (2008). Epidemiology of personality disorders. *Psychiatric Clinics of North America, 31,* 395–403. doi:10.1016/j.psc.2008.03.003

Lenzenweger, M. F., & Clarkin, J. F. (Eds.). (2005). *Major theories of personality disorder* (2nd ed.). New York, NY: Guilford Press.

Lenzenweger, M. F., Clarkin, J. F., Yeomans, F. E., Kernberg, O. F., & Levy, K. N. (2008). Refining the borderline personality disorder phenotype through finite mixture modeling: Implications for classification. *Journal of Personality Disorders, 22,* 313–331. doi:10.1521/pedi.2008.22.4.313

Levy, K. N., Ellison, W. D., Temes, C. M. & Khalsa, S. (2012, September). *The outcome of psychotherapy for borderline personality disorder: A meta-analysis.* Paper presented at the International Congress on Borderline Personality Disorder and Allied Disorders, Amsterdam, the Netherlands.

Levy, K. N., Meehan, K. B., Kelly, K. M., Reynoso, J. S., Weber, M., Clarkin, J. F., & Kernberg, O. F. (2006). Change in attachment patterns and reflective function in a randomized control trial of transference-focused psychotherapy for borderline personality disorder. *Journal of Consulting and Clinical Psychology, 74,* 1027–1040. doi:10.1037/0022-006X.74.6.1027

Linehan, M. M. (1993). *Cognitive-behavioral treatment of borderline personality disorder.* New York, NY: Guilford Press.

Livesley, W. J. (2001). Conceptual and taxonomic issues. In W. J. Livesley (Ed.), *Handbook of personality disorders: Theory, research, and treatment* (pp. 3–38). New York, NY: Guilford Press.

Livesley, W. J., DiMaggio, G., & Clarkin, J. F. (Eds.). (in press). *Integrated modular approach to the treatment of the personality disorder.* New York, NY: Guilford Press.

Mahler, M. S. (1971). A study of the separation–individuation process and its possible application to borderline phenomena in the psychoanalytic situation. *Psychoanalytic Study of the Child, 26,* 403–424.

Meyer, B., & Pilkonis, P. A. (2005). An attachment model of personality disorders. In M. F. Lenzenweger & J. F. Clarkin (Eds.), *Major theories of personality disorder* (2nd ed., pp. 231–281). New York, NY: Guilford Press.

Mischel, W., & Shoda, Y. (2008). Toward a unified theory of personality: Integrating dispositions and processing dynamics within the cognitive-affective processing system. In O. P. John, R. W. Robins, & L. A. Pervin (Eds.), *Handbook of personality: Theory and research* (3rd ed., pp. 208–241). New York, NY: Guilford Press.

Pincus, A. L. (2005). A contemporary integrative interpersonal theory of personality disorders. In M. F. Lenzenweger & J. F. Clarkin (Eds.), *Major theories of personality disorder* (2nd ed., pp. 282–331). New York, NY: Guilford Press.

Pincus, A. L., & Ansell, E. B. (2012). Interpersonal theory of personality. In J. Suls & H. Tennen (Eds.), *Handbook of psychology: Vol. 5. Personality and social psychology* (2nd ed., pp. 141–159). Hoboken, NJ: Wiley.

Pincus, A. L., & Hopwood, C. J. (2012). A contemporary interpersonal model of personality pathology and personality disorder. In T. A. Widiger (Ed.), *Oxford handbook of personality disorders* (pp. 372–398). New York, NY: Oxford University Press.

Rossouw, T. I., & Fonagy, P. (2012). Mentalization-based treatment for self-harm in adolescents: A randomized controlled trial. *Journal of the American Academy of Child & Adolescent Psychiatry, 51*, 1304–1313. doi:10.1016/j.jaac.2012.09.018

Safran, J. D., & Muran, J. C. (2000). *Negotiating the therapeutic alliance: A relational treatment guide*. New York, NY: Guilford Press.

Sanislow, C. A., Pine, D. S., Quinn, K. J., Kozak, M. J., Garvey, M. A., Heinssen, R. K., . . . Cuthbert, B. N. (2010). Developing constructs for psychopathology research: Research domain criteria. *Journal of Abnormal Psychology, 119*, 631–639. doi:10.1037/a0020909

Simpson, J. A., & Belsky, J. (2008). Attachment theory with a modern evolutionary framework. In J. Cassidy & P. R. Shaver (Eds.), *Handbook of attachment: Theory, research, and clinical applications* (2nd ed., pp. 131–157). New York, NY: Guilford Press.

Sullivan, H. S. (1953). *The interpersonal theory of psychiatry*. New York, NY: Norton.

Tracey, T. J., Rounds, J., & Gurtman, M. B. (1996). Examination of the general factor with the interpersonal circumplex structure: Application of the Inventory of Interpersonal Problems. *Multivariate Behavioral Research, 31*, 441–466. doi:10.1207/s15327906mbr3104_3

Trull, T. J. (2006). Dimensional models of personality disorder. In T. A. Widiger, E. Simonsen, P. J. Sirovatka, & D. Regier (Eds.), *Dimensional models of personality disorders: Refining the research agenda for DSM–V* (pp. 171–188). Washington, DC: American Psychiatric Publishing.

Westen, D. (1993). The impact of sexual abuse on self-structure. In D. Cicchetti & S. L. Toth (Eds.), *Rochester Symposium on Developmental Psychopathology: Vol. 5. Disorders and dysfunctions of the self* (pp. 223–250). Rochester, NY: University of Rochester Press.

Wiggins, J. S. (1991). Agency and communion as conceptual coordinates for the understanding and measurement of interpersonal behavior. In D. Cicchetti &

W. M. Grove (Eds.), *Thinking clearly about psychology: Essays in honor of Paul E. Meehl. Vol. 2: Personality and psychopathology* (pp. 89–113). Minneapolis: University of Minnesota Press.

Wiggins, J. S., & Pincus, A. L. (1989). Conceptions of personality disorders and dimensions of personality. *Psychological Assessment, 1,* 305–316. doi:10.1037/1040-3590.1.4.305

Wright, A. G. C., Hallquist, M. N., Morse, J. Q., Scott, L. N., Stepp, S. D., Nolf, K. A., & Pilkonis, P. A. (2013). Clarifying interpersonal heterogeneity in borderline personality disorder using latent mixture modeling. *Journal of Personality Disorders, 27,* 125–143. doi:10.1521/pedi.2013.27.2.125

Young, J. (1990). *Cognitive therapy for personality disorders: A schema-focused approach.* Sarasota, FL: Professional Resource Exchange.

INDEX

Ruscio, A. M., 71–72
Ruscio, J., 71–72
Russell, J. J., 351

Sadistic personality pattern, 379
Safran, J. D., 335, 359
Samstag, L. W., 335
Samuel, D. B., 53, 94
Sanislow, C. A., 94
Schedule for Nonadaptive and Adaptive Personality—2 (SNAP–2), 51, 263
Schema-focused psychotherapy, 418
Schema mode processing, 279–280
Schema Mode Questionnaire (SMQ), 280
Schichman, S., 299
Schizoid Personality Disorder
    attachment patterns associated with, 315, 321
    in statistical modeling, 119, 126
Schizoid personality pattern, 378
Schizophrenia, 177, 183, 280
Schizotypal Personality Disorder
    abnormal verbal associative patterns in, 280–281
    attachment patterns associated with, 321
    behavior genetics research on, 177
    in statistical modeling, 118, 122–124
Schizotypal personality pattern, 380
Schizotypy, 72
Schmitt, T. A., 89, 399
SCID–II. See Structured Clinical Interview for DSM–IV Axis II Personality Disorders
Science of personality disorders, 371–372. See also Evolutionary theory
SCORS (Social Cognitions and Object Relations Scale), 215–216, 219
Scree test, 117
Secure attachment, 297, 317, 319
Self-coherence, 421
Self-critical perfectionism, 295
Self-defeating personality pattern, 380
Self-definition
    in object relations theories, 206–207, 209–210
    in psychodynamic theory, 294–298

Self-determination theory, 296
Self-direction, 212
Self-functioning, 211–212, 414–415
Self-image, 384
Self–other differentiation, 210, 212–213, 219, 403–404
Self–Other Differentiation Scale, 219
Self-propagating strategy (evolutionary theory), 377
Self-report
    on Adult Attachment Interview, 319
    as explicit assessment tool, 256–260
    organizing diagnostic system based on, 404
    process-focused assessment with, 273–275
    unintended consequences of reliance on, 273–274
    value of, 90–91
Sensorimotor-autonomy phase (ontogenetic growth), 377
Sensory-attachment phase (ontogenetic growth), 376
Sequential activation, 281–282
Serotonin, 184
Sexual abuse, 421
Sexual seductiveness, 232–233
Shedler, J., 5, 89, 93, 94, 304
Shedler–Westen Assessment Procedure (SWAP–200)
    clinical case formulation with, 228–235
    method of, 264
    overview, 8
    therapist version of, 276
Shedler–Westen Assessment Procedure (SWAP–II), 240–247
Shoda, Y., 351, 396, 397, 401, 403–407, 416
Sieswerda, S., 280
Silk, K. R., 7
Simms, L. J., 46
Simonsen, Erik, 4
Single nucleotide polymorphisms (SNPs), 182–183
Skinner, B. F., 262
Skodol, A. E., 5, 6, 88, 94
Slade, A., 335
Smith, G. T., 48–49

ABOUT THE EDITOR

Steven K. Huprich, PhD, is a professor and director of clinical training at Wichita State University. He is the editor of the *Journal of Personality Assessment* and the 2013 recipient of the Theodore Millon Award in Personality Psychology. Dr. Huprich also serves as the secretary/treasurer for the International Society for the Study of Personality Disorders. He has authored nearly 100 peer-reviewed publications and chapters and over 200 presentations, as well as five other books. His work includes a book on the use of the Rorschach Inkblot Test to assess personality disorders, a general textbook on clinical psychology, an edited text on integrating personality assessment with the *DSM–5*, important concepts for new therapists in treating narcissistic personalities, and a text on the conceptual and empirical foundations of psychodynamic psychotherapy. Dr. Huprich has also published on the assessment of interpersonal dependency and relational influences on the assessment of borderline personality disorder. He has written about and presented on ways in which to integrate the manner by which personality disorders are conceptualized and assessed.

Dr. Huprich received his PhD from the University of North Carolina at Greensboro (1999) and completed his predoctoral internship at the State University of New York (SUNY) Upstate Medical University in Syracuse.

He held faculty appointments at Baylor University and Eastern Michigan University before moving to Wichita State University in 2014. Dr. Huprich's research interests have focused on the diagnosis, assessment, and validation of personality disorders, with particular attention to the *DSM–IV* proposal of depressive personality disorder. At the present time, he is exploring the validity of a self-representation construct known as malignant self-regard, which he believes helps account for the diagnostic comorbidity and clinical similarities in masochistic, self-defeating, depressive, and vulnerably narcissistic personalities.